Non-Alcoholic Fatty Liver Disease

Editor

PAUL J. GAGLIO

CLINICS IN LIVER DISEASE

www.liver.theclinics.com

Consulting Editor
NORMAN GITLIN

May 2016 • Volume 20 • Number 2

ELSEVIER

1600 John F. Kennedy Boulevard • Suite 1800 • Philadelphia, Pennsylvania, 19103-2899

http://www.theclinics.com

CLINICS IN LIVER DISEASE Volume 20, Number 2
May 2016 ISSN 1089-3261, ISBN-13: 978-0-323-41696-2

Editor: Kerry Holland
Developmental Editor: Meredith Clinton

Clinics in Liver Disease (ISSN 1089-3261) is published quarterly by Elsevier Inc., 360 Park Avenue South, New York, NY 10010-1710. Months of issue are February, May, August, and November. Business and Editorial Offices: 1600 John F. Kennedy Blvd., Ste. 1800, Philadelphia, PA 19103-2899. Customer Service Office: 3251 Riverport Lane, Maryland Heights, MO 63043. Periodicals postage paid at New York, NY and additional mailing offices. Subscription prices are $275.00 per year (U.S. individuals), $100.00 per year (U.S. student/resident), $453.00 per year (U.S. institutions), $395.00 per year (international individuals), $200.00 per year (international student/resident), $562.00 per year (international institutions), $340.00 per year (Canadian individuals), $200.00 per year (Canadian student/resident), and $562.00 per year (Canadian institutions). Foreign air speed delivery is included in all *Clinics* subscription prices. All prices are subject to change without notice. **POSTMASTER:** Send address changes to *Clinics in Liver Disease*, Elsevier Health Sciences Division, Subscription Customer Service, 3251 Riverport Lane, Maryland Heights, MO 63043. **Customer Service: Telephone: 1-800-654-2452 (U.S. and Canada); 314-447-8871 (outside U.S. and Canada). Fax: 314-447-8029. E-mail: journalscustomer service-usa@elsevier.com (for print support); journalsonlinesupport-usa@elsevier.com (for online support).**

Reprints. For copies of 100 or more of articles in this publication, please contact the Commercial Reprints Department, Elsevier Inc., 360 Park Avenue South, New York, NY 10010-1710. Tel.: 212-633-3874; Fax: 212-633-3820; E-mail: reprints@elsevier.com.

Clinics in Liver Disease is covered in *MEDLINE/PubMed (Index Medicus)*, Science Citation Index Expanded, Journal Citation Reports/Science Edition, and Current Contents/Clinical Medicine.

Contributors

CONSULTING EDITOR

NORMAN GITLIN, MD, FRCP (LONDON), FRCPE (EDINBURGH), FAASLD, FACP, FACG
Formerly, Professor of Medicine, Chief of Hepatology, Emory University; Currently, Consultant, Atlanta Gastroenterology Associates, Atlanta, Georgia

EDITOR

PAUL J. GAGLIO, MD, FACP, AGAF, FAASLD
Professor of Medicine at Columbia University Medical Center, Director, Hepatology Outreach, Columbia University College of Physicians and Surgeons, Center for Liver Disease and Transplantation, NY Presbyterian Hospital-Columbia University Medical Center, New York, New York

AUTHORS

PAUL D. BERK, MD, FACP
Professor of Medicine, Divisions of Digestive and Liver Diseases and Preventive Medicine, Department of Medicine, Columbia College of Physicians and Surgeons, Columbia University Medical Center, New York, New York

JEROME BOURSIER, MD, PhD
Hepato-Gastroenterology Department, University Hospital, Angers, France; HIFIH Laboratory, UPRES 3859, SFR 4208, LUNAM University, Angers, France

ELISABETTA BUGIANESI, MD, PhD
Professor, Division of Gastroenterology and Hepatology, Department of Medical Sciences, A.O. Città della Salute e della Scienza di Torino, University of Turin, Turin, Italy

KRISTINA R. CHACKO, MD
Assistant Professor, Department of Medicine, Albert Einstein College of Medicine, Bronx, New York

MICHAEL R. CHARLTON, MD, FRCP
Professor of Medicine, Chief of Hepatology and Medical Director of Liver Transplantation, Intermountain Transplant Center, Intermountain Medical Center, Murray, Utah

TRAVIS B. DICK, PharmD, MBA, BCPS
Department of Pharmacy, Intermountain Medical Center, Murray, Utah

ANNA MAE DIEHL, MD
Division of Gastroenterology, Department of Medicine, Duke University Medical Center, Durham, North Carolina

PAUL J. GAGLIO, MD, FACP, AGAF, FAASLD
Professor of Medicine at Columbia University Medical Center, Director, Hepatology
Outreach, Columbia University College of Physicians and Surgeons, Center for Liver
Disease and Transplantation, NY Presbyterian Hospital-Columbia University Medical
Center, New York, New York

SWAYTHA GANESH, MD
Division of Gastroenterology, Hepatology and Nutrition, University of Pittsburgh Medical
Center, Pittsburgh, Pennsylvania

NIDHI P. GOYAL, MD, MPH
Division of Gastroenterology, Hepatology, and Nutrition, Department of Pediatrics,
University of California, San Diego, San Diego, California; Department of
Gastroenterology, Rady Children's Hospital, San Diego, California

BILAL HAMEED, MD
Assistant Professor of Medicine; Program Director, Transplant Hepatology,
Division of Gastroenterology, University of California San Francisco, San Francisco,
California

WILLIAM N. HANNAH Jr, MD
Associate Dean of SAUSHEC, Department of Medicine, San Antonio Military Medical
Center, Joint Base San Antonio; Assistant Professor, Uniformed Services University, Fort
Sam Houston, San Antonio, Texas

STEPHEN A. HARRISON, MD
Chief of Hepatology, Division of Gastroenterology, Department of Medicine, San Antonio
Military Medical Center, Joint Base San Antonio; Professor, Uniformed Services
University, Fort Sam Houston, San Antonio, Texas

LINDA HENRY, PhD
Betty and Guy Beatty Center for Integrated Research, Inova Fairfax Hospital, Falls
Church, Virginia

RAMY IBRAHIM KAMAL JOUNESS, MD
Division of Gastroenterology and Hepatology, Department of Medical Sciences, A.O.
Città della Salute e della Scienza di Torino, University of Turin, Turin, Italy

HARMIT S. KALIA, DO
Department of Medicine, Montefiore Einstein Liver Center, Montefiore Medical Center,
Albert Einstein College of Medicine, Bronx, New York

PUSHPJEET KANWAR, MD
Department of Gastroenterology and Hepatology, New York Methodist Hospital,
Brooklyn, New York

DAVID E. KLEINER, MD, PhD
Chief, Post-mortem Section Director, Laboratory Information System, Laboratory of
Pathology, Center for Cancer Research, National Cancer Institute, Bethesda, Maryland

AARON KOENIG, MS
Betty and Guy Beatty Center for Integrated Research, Inova Fairfax Hospital, Falls
Church, Virginia

KRIS V. KOWDLEY, MD
Department of Transplant Hepatology, Swedish Medical Center, Seattle, Washington

HALA R. MAKHLOUF, MD, PhD
Program Director, Cancer Diagnosis Program, Pathology Investigation and Resources Branch, Division of Cancer Treatment and Diagnosis, National Cancer Institute, Bethesda, Maryland; Professor, Department of Pathology, Ain Shams University, Faculty of Medicine, Cairo, Greater Cairo, Egypt

ANDREA MARENGO, MD
Division of Gastroenterology and Hepatology, Department of Medical Sciences, A.O. Città della Salute e della Scienza di Torino, University of Turin, Turin, Italy

VAISHALI PATEL, MBBS
Fellow in Transplant Hepatology, Section of Hepatology, Department of Gastroenterology, Hepatology and Nutrition, Virginia Commonwealth University, Richmond, Virginia

TUAN PHAM, MD
Division of Gastroenterology and Hepatology, University of Utah, Salt Lake City, Utah

JOHN REINUS, MD
Professor of Clinical Medicine, Department of Medicine, Albert Einstein College of Medicine, Bronx, New York

VINOD K. RUSTGI, MD, MBA
Medical Director, Liver Transplantation, Professor of Medicine and Surgery, The Thomas Starzl Transplant Institute, University of Pittsburgh Medical Center Montefiore, Pittsburgh, Pennsylvania

ARUN J. SANYAL, MBBS, MD
Charles Caravati Professor of Medicine, Chair of Center of Clinical and Translational Research and Former Division Chair, Section of Hepatology, Department of Gastroenterology, Hepatology and Nutrition, Virginia Commonwealth University, Richmond, Virginia

MEHMET SAYINER, MD
Betty and Guy Beatty Center for Integrated Research, Inova Fairfax Hospital, Falls Church, Virginia

JEFFREY B. SCHWIMMER, MD
Division of Gastroenterology, Hepatology, and Nutrition, Department of Pediatrics, University of California, San Diego, San Diego, California; Department of Gastroenterology, Rady Children's Hospital, San Diego, California

RICHARD STERLING, MD, MSc
Professor of Medicine, Chief of Hepatology and Program Director of Transplant Hepatology Fellowship, Section of Hepatology, Department of Gastroenterology, Hepatology and Nutrition, Virginia Commonwealth University, Richmond, Virginia

NORAH TERRAULT, MD, MPH
Professor of Medicine and Surgery; Director, Viral Hepatitis Center, Division of Gastroenterology, University of California San Francisco, San Francisco, California

ELIZABETH C. VERNA, MD, MS
Division of Digestive and Liver Diseases, Department of Medicine, Columbia College of Physicians and Surgeons, Columbia University Medical Center, New York, New York

ZOBAIR M. YOUNOSSI, MD, MPH
Betty and Guy Beatty Center for Integrated Research; Department of Medicine, Center for Liver Diseases, Inova Fairfax Hospital, Falls Church, Virginia

Contents

Nonalcoholic fatty liver disease (NAFLD) is a common cause of chronic liver disease with increasing prevalence, which can progress to cirrhosis and liver failure. Because of the obesity epidemic and increasing prevalence of metabolic syndrome, NAFLD and its progressive form, nonalcoholic steatohepatitis, are seen more commonly in different parts of the world. This article reviews the worldwide epidemiology of NAFLD and nonalcoholic steatohepatitis. The PubMed database was used to identify studies related to epidemiology of NAFLD in the adult population. It is estimated that the epidemic of obesity will continue to fuel the burden of NAFLD and its long-term complications.

Nonalcoholic fatty liver disease (NAFLD) is emerging as the most common cause of liver disease in the United States. The prevalence varies dramatically when comparing individuals of different races and ethnicities. Rates are highest in Hispanic patient populations compared with non-Hispanic whites and African Americans, despite similar rates of the metabolic syndrome and risk factors. This observation remains poorly characterized; variations in genes that effect lipid metabolism may play a role. This article describes the prevalence of NAFLD in patients of different races or ethnicities, and discusses pathophysiologic mechanisms that may explain why these differences exist.

Nonalcoholic steatohepatitis (NASH) and the metabolic syndrome (MetS) are highly prevalent in the Western population. Their pathogenesis is closely linked to insulin resistance, which serves as a therapeutic target for the management of these conditions. This article reviews the research supporting the influence of MetS on NASH and includes studies supporting their similar epidemiology, pathogenesis, and treatment.

Obesity and its major comorbidities, including type 2 diabetes mellitus, nonalcoholic fatty liver disease (NAFLD), obesity cardiomyopathy, and certain cancers, have caused life expectancy in the United States to decline in recent years. Obesity is the increased accumulation of triglycerides (TG), which are synthesized from glycerol and long-chain fatty acids (LCFA) throughout the body. LCFA enter adipocytes, hepatocytes, and cardiomyocytes via specific, facilitated transport processes. Metabolism of increased cellular TG content in obesity may lead to comorbidities such as NAFLD and cardiomyopathy. Better understanding of LCFA transport processes may lead to successful treatment of obesity and NAFLD.

Recent progress has allowed a more comprehensive study of the gut microbiota. Gut microbiota helps in health maintenance and gut dysbiosis associates with chronic metabolic diseases. Modulation of short-chain fatty acids and choline bioavailability, lipoprotein lipase induction, alteration of bile acid profile, endogenous alcohol production, or liver inflammation secondary to endotoxemia result from gut dysbiosis. Modulation of the gut microbiota by pre/probiotics gives promising results in animals, but needs to be evaluated in humans before use in clinical practice. Gut microbiota adds complexity to the pathophysiology of nonalcoholic fatty liver disease but represents an opportunity to discover new therapeutic targets.

Nonalcoholic fatty liver disease (NAFLD) is a diagnosis of exclusion. Most patients are asymptomatic, and diagnosed incidentally. Most patients remain undiagnosed. A high index of suspicion and serologic work-up to rule out alternative causes of liver disease is required. In NALFD, fibrosis correlates with outcomes, including mortality. To diagnose, assess severity, and monitor fibrosis, two noninvasive methods can be used; however, noninvasive tests are more helpful at extremes of fibrosis: excluding it or diagnosing advanced fibrosis. Liver biopsy is usually reserved for cases whereby noninvasive tests fail to accurately determine the degree of fibrosis or the diagnosis is unclear.

Nonalcoholic fatty liver disease (NAFLD) is the liver disease associated with obesity, diabetes, and the metabolic syndrome. Although steatosis is a key histologic feature, liver biopsies of patients with NAFLD can show a wide range of findings. Nonalcoholic steatohepatitis (NASH) is a progressive subtype of NAFLD first defined by analogy to alcoholic hepatitis. Young children may have an alternate pattern of progressive NAFLD characterized by a zone 1 distribution of steatosis, inflammation, and fibrosis. Several grading and staging systems exist, but all require adequate biopsies. Although NASH generally shows fibrosis progression over time, some patients show regression of disease.

Liver-related mortality is the third cause of death in patients with nonalcoholic fatty liver disease, but the long-term prognosis basically depends on the presence and severity of liver damage. Thus, life expectancy in patients with simple steatosis is not different from the general population, but liver-related mortality is significantly higher in patients with nonalcoholic steatohepatitis (NASH), particularly in those with advanced fibrosis. Progression of liver disease is observed in up to one-third of patients with NASH. The long-term hepatic prognosis mostly depends on the histologic stage at initial liver biopsy, but multiple risk factors may concur.

Nonalcoholic fatty liver disease (NAFLD) is the most common cause of chronic liver disease in the United States. Childhood NAFLD is associated with hepatic and nonhepatic morbidity and mortality. Nonhepatic associations include cardiovascular, metabolic, pulmonary, and psychological disorders. Cardiovascular conditions observed in childhood include left ventricular dysfunction. Furthermore, childhood obesity is associated with greater odds of having hepatocellular carcinoma as an adult. Evidence suggests that NAFLD may begin in utero in children of diabetic mothers. Thus rigorous efforts for structured diagnosis and follow-up are a priority to better develop the understanding of outcomes in pediatric NAFLD.

Nonalcoholic fatty liver disease (NAFLD) is the hepatic manifestation of the metabolic syndrome. NAFLD is the most common liver disease in developed countries. Weight reduction of 3% to 5% is associated with improved steatosis; reductions of 5% to 7% are necessary for decreased inflammation; with 7% to 10%, individuals may experience NAFLD/NASH remission and regression of fibrosis. No specific dietary intervention has proven beneficial beyond calorie restriction. Physical activity without weight loss seems to decrease hepatic steatosis. Bariatric surgery is associated with decreased cardiovascular risk and improved overall mortality in addition to reduction in hepatic steatosis, inflammation, and fibrosis.

Weight loss, regular exercise, and diet composition modification seem to improve biochemical and histologic abnormalities. Other therapies directed at insulin resistance, oxidative stress, cytoprotection, and fibrosis may also offer benefits. Insulin sensitizers and vitamin E seem to be the most promising; however, they cause side effects. A multifaceted approach of lifestyle modifications, weight loss, and pharmacotherapy can be used in combination, but no single treatment approach has proved universally applicable to the general population with nonalcoholic steato-hepatitis (NASH). Continuous clinical and preclinical studies on existing and potential drugs are needed to improve treatment of nonalcoholic fatty liver disease/NASH.

Nonalcoholic fatty liver disease is the most common cause of liver disease in the United States. There are no drug therapies approved for the treatment of nonalcoholic steatohepatitis (NASH). Multiple different pathways are involved in the pathogenesis and each can be the target of the therapy. It is possible that more than 1 target is involved in disease development and progression. Multiple clinical trials with promising agents are underway. Because NASH is a slowly progressive disease and treatment likely to be of prolonged duration, acceptance and approval of any agent will require information on long-term clinical benefits and safety.

Nonalcoholic fatty liver disease (NAFLD) is an important cause of liver disease that is often associated with the metabolic syndrome. There is a growing awareness that extrahepatic complications occur in individuals with NAFLD, especially an increased risk of cardiovascular disease. Development of diabetes mellitus, chronic kidney disease, colorectal cancer, and endocrinopathies has been linked to NAFLD. This article reviews the extrahepatic complications affecting individuals with NAFLD and the pathogenesis underlying their development.

Nonalcoholic fatty liver disease (NAFLD) is prevalent in the general population and a growing indication for liver transplant. Longer wait times and challenges with pretransplant survivorship are expected, underscoring the need for improved management of attendant comorbidities. Recognition with potential modification of obesity, sarcopenia, chronic kidney disease, and cardiovascular disease in patients with NAFLD may have important implications in the pretransplant and posttransplant periods. Although patients with NAFLD have generally favorable postoperative outcomes, they are at risk for developing recurrent disease in their allograft, driving the need for pharmacotherapies and dietary innovations appropriate for use in the posttransplant period.

CLINICS IN LIVER DISEASE

THE CLINICS ARE AVAILABLE ONLINE!
Access your subscription at:
www.theclinics.com

Preface

Nonalcoholic Fatty Liver Disease

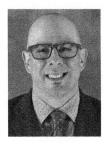

Paul J. Gaglio, MD, FACP, AGAF, FAASLD
Editor

Due to the current obesity epidemic, nonalcoholic fatty liver disease (NAFLD) affects a significant portion of the US patient population, and it represents one of the most common causes of liver disease in the Western world. Over the last several years, significant progress has been made related to understanding the natural history, pathobiology, and treatment of this condition. It is recognized that NAFLD encompasses a spectrum of liver histology ranging from isolated fatty liver to steatohepatitis with cirrhosis. NAFLD may be present in both adults and children and can progress to end-stage liver disease with resultant cirrhosis, portal hypertension, and hepatocellular carcinoma. In addition, several extrahepatic conditions may be linked to NAFLD, including cardiovascular disease, insulin-requiring and type 2 diabetes mellitus, obstructive sleep apnea, colonic adenomas, and polycystic ovarian syndrome. In this issue of *Clinics in Liver Disease*, a group of distinguished experts in the field provide an update related to various aspects of NAFLD.

The epidemiology of NAFLD in the United States and the rest of the world is introduced by Drs M Sayiner, A Koenig, L Henry, and Z Younossi, and a discussion of racial and ethnic differences in NAFLD is provided by Drs H Kalia and P Gaglio. Next, the pathobiology of NAFLD related to the metabolic syndrome is reviewed by Drs P. Kanwar and K Kowdley, followed by a discussion of the effect of lipids and insulin resistance on this condition by Drs P Berk and E Verna. Emerging data related to the influence of the gut microbiome on NAFLD are presented by Drs J Boursier and AM Diehl. The next group of articles covers clinical aspects and natural history of NAFLD; Drs V Patel, A Sanyal, and R Sterling describe the clinical presentation and evaluation of patients with NAFLD, and the histology of NAFLD and NASH in adults and children is discussed by Drs D Kleiner and H Makhlouf. This is followed by a review of the progression and natural history of NAFLD in adults by Drs A Marengo, RI Jouness, and E Bugianesi, and in children, by Drs N Goyal and J Schwimmer.

Our understanding of optimal therapy for NAFLD is evolving rapidly; Drs W Hannah and S Harrison illustrate the effect of weight loss, diet, exercise, and bariatric surgery,

Clin Liver Dis 20 (2016) xiii–xiv
http://dx.doi.org/10.1016/j.cld.2016.02.001
1089-3261/16/$ – see front matter © 2016 Published by Elsevier Inc.

liver.theclinics.com

and current pharmacologic therapies are reviewed by Drs S Ganesh and V Rustgi. NAFLD therapies on the horizon are introduced by Drs B Hameed and N Terrault. Several additional aspects of NAFLD are covered by Drs K Chacko and J Reinus, who present information on extrahepatic manifestations of NAFLD, including a discussion of a "mimic" of NAFLD, specifically, lysosomal acid lipase deficiency. Drs T Pham, T Dick, and M Charlton conclude this issue with an article on the present and future role of liver transplantation in managing patients with NAFLD.

It is hoped that this issue of *Clinics in Liver Disease* will provide health care providers and other interested individuals a convenient reference for understanding multiple aspects of NAFLD and provide a framework to facilitate patient diagnosis, and ultimately, treatment for this condition. Further advances in understanding the pathobiology, natural history, and optimal therapy for NAFLD are eagerly anticipated.

Paul J. Gaglio, MD, FACP, AGAF, FAASLD
Professor of Medicine
Columbia University Medical Center
Columbia University College
of Physicians and Surgeons
Center for Liver Disease and Transplantation
NY Presbyterian Hospital-Columbia
University Medical Center
622 West 168th Street, PH 14, Room 202 F
New York, NY 10032, USA

E-mail address: pg2011@cumc.columbia.edu
Websites: https://www.linkedin.com/in/pauljgagliomd
http://www.columbiadoctors.org/prof/pjgaglio

Epidemiology of Nonalcoholic Fatty Liver Disease and Nonalcoholic Steatohepatitis in the United States and the Rest of the World

Mehmet Sayiner, MD[a], Aaron Koenig, MS[a], Linda Henry, PhD[a], Zobair M. Younossi, MD, MPH[a,b,*]

KEYWORDS

• Epidemiology • NAFLD • NASH • Prevalence

KEY POINTS

• Nonalcoholic fatty liver disease (NAFLD) and its progressive form, nonalcoholic steatohepatitis (NASH), are common causes of chronic liver disease with an increasing worldwide prevalence.
• Because of the differences in diagnostic modalities, prevalence estimates of NAFLD/NASH differ widely across populations.
• Although histologic evaluation with liver biopsy is the gold standard for diagnosing NASH, emerging noninvasive modalities, such as transient elastography, are increasingly used for evaluation of fibrosis in patients with NASH.
• The population studied and their associated risk factors are potential reasons for the variances in prevalence rates.
• As the rate of obesity, diabetes, and metabolic syndrome continue to increase, NAFLD and NASH will bring a tremendous impact on health care in the upcoming years.

BACKGROUND

Nonalcoholic fatty liver disease (NAFLD) is one of the most common causes of chronic liver disease in adults.[1] NAFLD is a spectrum of liver disease ranging from simple steatosis to steatohepatitis, fibrosis, and cirrhosis.[2] Although not all patients with NAFLD

Dr Z.M. Younossi is a consultant to BMS, Gilead, Abbvie, Intercept and GSK. Drs M. Sayiner, A. Koenig, and L. Henry have nothing to disclose.
[a] Betty and Guy Beatty Center for Integrated Research, Inova Fairfax Hospital, Claude Moore Health Education and Research Building, 3300 Gallows Road, Falls Church, VA 22042, USA;
[b] Department of Medicine, Center for Liver Diseases, Inova Fairfax Hospital, 300 Gallows Road, Falls Church, VA 22042, USA
* Corresponding author. Betty and Guy Beatty Center for Integrated Research, Claude Moore Health Education and Research Building, 3300 Gallows Road, Falls Church, VA 22042.
E-mail address: zobair.younossi@inova.org

Clin Liver Dis 20 (2016) 205–214
http://dx.doi.org/10.1016/j.cld.2015.10.001
1089-3261/16/$ – see front matter
liver.theclinics.com

develop liver-related complications, patients with nonalcoholic steatohepatitis (NASH) are at an increased risk of developing fibrosis, cirrhosis, or hepatocellular carcinoma.[3] NASH is currently the second indication for liver transplantation and will become the leading indication for liver transplantation in the next two decades.[4] Known risk factors for NAFLD and NASH include metabolic conditions, such as diabetes and obesity, and age, gender, and race/ethnicity.[5] Although the prevalence of NAFLD is well described in the Western World, the global epidemiology of NAFLD is less well described.

In this study, we reviewed the literature (2000-2015) to assess epidemiology of NAFLD in adults. Incidence, prevalence and risk factors were summarized.

NONALCOHOLIC FATTY LIVER DISEASE/NONALCOHOLIC STEATOHEPATITIS DIAGNOSIS

There are several diagnostic modalities used in the diagnosis of NAFLD and NASH. The accuracy of of these modalities can vary, which can impact the assessment of epidemiology of NAFLD. For more information on this topic please see Kleiner DE and Makhlouf HR: Histology of Nonalcoholic Fatty Liver Disease and Nonalcoholic Steatohepatitis in Adults and Children, in this issue.

NONALCOHOLIC FATTY LIVER DISEASE/NONALCOHOLIC STEATOHEPATITIS INCIDENCE

There is a paucity of data regarding the incidence of NAFLD. In the literature, the numbers differ widely, and the incidence rates are most likely underreported. In a Japanese study, Sung and colleagues[6] followed up nearly 11,500 patients for 5 years to determine if a change in fatty liver status had an effect on incident hypertension. Fatty liver status was assessed at baseline and in the follow-up period by using ultrasound. In this study, 10% of participants developed fatty liver in 5 years and in 5% of the cohort, fatty liver at baseline resolved during follow-up. In another study from Israel, Zelber-Sagi and coworkers[7] in a 7-year prospective study evaluated the incidence and remission of NAFLD. Their incidence rate was found to be 19%, almost double compared with the study by Sung and colleagues.[6]

In another Japanese study with a longer follow-up period, data from atomic bomb survivors were used. In this study, 1635 patients without NAFLD were followed for 11.6 years. The incidence of NAFLD was found to be 19.9 per 1000 person-years.[8] In a recent study of Wong and colleagues[9] 565 patients were followed. The development of fatty liver was assessed by using MRI and transient elastography. The population incidence of NAFLD at 3 to 5 years was 13.5% (34 per 1000 person-years). The obvious variations in these incidence rates suggest that further studies, using consistent diagnostic modalities, are needed to provide a more accurate assessment of the incidence of NAFLD worldwide.

NONALCOHOLIC FATTY LIVER DISEASE/NONALCOHOLIC STEATOHEPATITIS WORLDWIDE PREVALENCE BY CONTINENT
North America

Despite the limitation of the diagnostic modalities, it is clear that NAFLD and NASH have reached epidemic proportions in the United States and North America. In one recent study the US population prevalence of NAFLD was estimated using data from the National Health and Nutrition Examination Survey (NHANES) III database (**Fig. 1**). Patients were diagnosed with NAFLD if moderate to severe hepatic steatosis was found on the ultrasound in the absence of other causes of liver disease. Furthermore, NAFLD patients with elevated liver enzymes in the presence of diabetes mellitus

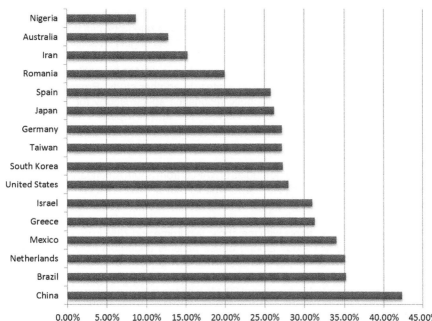

Fig. 1. Global prevalence of NAFLD (Nigeria,[28] Australia,[32] Iran,[56] Romania,[57] Spain,[22] Japan,[33] Germany,[58] Taiwan,[37] South Korea,[36] United States,[10] Israel,[7] Greece,[25] Mexico,[3] Netherlands,[26] Brazil,[18] and China[45]).

(DM) or insulin resistance were presumed to have NASH. From these data, the prevalence of NAFLD in the United States was determined to be 18.8% and NASH was 2.6%, whereas the prevalence of NAFLD among overweight people was 28%.[10] In another study also using NHANES III data, the prevalence of NAFLD according to ultrasonography was approximately the same at 19%. Additionally, in a study using the same database but establishing NAFLD with liver enzymes, the prevalence of NAFLD was reported to be 24%.[11,12]

In general, it is not easy to establish the prevalence of NASH in the general population because of the need of histologic evaluation. Therefore, the prevalence of NASH has been usually reported from selected patient populations. A recent study that enrolled military personnel and their dependents revealed the prevalence of NAFLD as 46% with the highest rate in Hispanics (58.3%) followed by whites (44.4%) and African Americans (35.1%). In addition, all patients with a positive ultrasound that suggested hepatic steatosis were offered a liver biopsy. NASH prevalence was found to be 12.2% among the entire cohort and 29.9% among patients with a positive ultrasound.[13] It is important to place these data in the context of rates reported from the autopsy series in which steatohepatitis was reported in 18.5% of the markedly obese patients and 2.7% of lean patients.[14] In another study, the prevalence of NASH in the living donor liver transplantation donor population was found to be approximately 1.1%.[15] Although both populations of study were highly selected, it seems reasonable to suggest that the prevalence of NASH in the US general population is between 1% and 3%.

One important demographic factor that may impact the prevalence of NAFLD is ethnicity. In a recent study by Fleischman and colleagues[3] prevalence rates of NAFLD were assessed in 6814 patients according to their ethnic background. In this study, NAFLD was determined via computed tomography scans. Although the prevalence of NAFLD in the entire cohort was 29%, the subgroup analysis showed that Hispanics of Mexican origin had a significantly higher prevalence rate (33%) as compared with Hispanics of Dominican (16%) and Puerto Rican (18%) origins. A similar prevalence rate was reported by Foster and colleagues[16] in which the prevalence of NAFLD among Hispanics was 28%. However, the prevalence of NAFLD in African Americans was only 11%, whereas it was 15% in whites. In another study, Browning and colleagues[17] used proton nuclear magnetic resonance spectroscopy for NAFLD diagnosis and reported an overall prevalence of 31%. Again, Hispanics had the highest prevalence rate of 45% followed by whites (33%) and African Americans (24%).

South America

There are only a few epidemiologic studies of NAFLD from South America. In a study from Brazil, Karnikowski and colleagues[18] reported that prevalence of NAFLD may be 35.2% among middle-aged patients. In another study, where asymptomatic men and women were evaluated with hepatic ultrasound, the prevalence of NAFLD was 36% in the total cohort but was 74% in patients with metabolic syndrome and 73% in obese patients.[19] Finally, in a more recent study among obese patients undergoing bariatric surgery, NAFLD was found in 95% of patients and histologic diagnosis of NASH was 66.7%.[20] In addition to the studies from Brazil, the prevalence of ultrasound-documented NAFLD in Chile has been reported to be around 23.4% with the rate increasing with age.[21]

Europe

The prevalence of NAFLD also varies greatly among European countries. In a multicenter, cross-sectional population study from Spain, ultrasound-documented NAFLD was reported to be 33.4% in men and 20.3% in women (overall prevalence of 25.8%).[22] In another study conducted in Spain, investigators evaluated the presence of NAFLD in patients with gallstones. After clinical examination, abdominal ultrasound, and applying exclusion criteria, liver biopsies from eligible patients were taken during laparoscopic cholecystectomy operation. These investigators reported that 51.6% of patients with gallstones had histologic evidence of NAFLD and 10.2% of the total cohort had NASH. It is noteworthy that 36.7% of the cohort was obese and 25.6% met the criteria for metabolic syndrome.[23]

In Italy, the prevalence of NAFLD was present in 78.8% of patients with metabolic syndrome.[24] These high rates are similar to other countries where prevalence of NAFLD has been reported to be very high in a high-risk population.

In a Greek study, Zois and colleagues[25] evaluated liver biopsies of 498 autopsies. They reported that hepatic steatosis was present in 31.3% of patients and steatohepatitis was present in 39.8% of cases.

In northern Europe, the prevalence of NAFLD among the elderly population was reported to be approximately 35.1%.[26] Finally, in a large population-based study in the United Kingdom, Alazawi and colleagues[27] evaluated the presence of NAFLD in patients with abnormal liver function test results. Although they stated that NAFLD affected 10% to 30% of United Kingdom population, it was found that, among the recorded liver-related diagnoses, NAFLD was the number one diagnosis with a prevalence of 42.9%. Furthermore, it was stated that not all patients with liver-related diagnosis had abnormal liver enzymes. In fact, 55.7% of NAFLD patients had normal liver enzyme tests.

Africa

There are even fewer publications about the prevalence of NAFLD in Africa. Nevertheless, the reported prevalence of NAFLD in African countries seems to be lower than those reported from other parts of the world. In a study in Nigeria, the prevalence of

NAFLD was found to be 8.7%. In the same study, NAFLD was more common in people with diabetes but this difference was not statistically significant (9.5% vs 4.5%).[28] It was stated that the reason for this lower prevalence may be attributed to lower intraperitoneal fat content.[29] However, in contrast, another study conducted in the same geographic area reported the prevalence of fatty liver in 13.3% of human immunodeficiency virus–infected individuals. Obviously, this high prevalence is most likely related to other causes of fatty liver, such as highly active antiretroviral therapy in the region.[30]

In a South African study, Kruger and colleagues[31] investigated the prevalence of NAFLD and NASH in obese patients. The rate of fatty infiltration on ultrasound was 87%. Among the NAFLD cohort who agreed to undergo liver biopsy, NASH prevalence was 36%. These rates are similar to those reported from the obese population undergoing weight reduction surgery in the other regions of the world.[5,6]

Australia

Again, there is a paucity of data about the epidemiology of NAFLD in NASH from Australia. In one study of 1170 participant, the prevalence of NAFLD was estimated to be 12.8%. NAFLD was significantly more prevalent in females and none of the participants had a diagnosis of diabetes.[32]

Asia

The prevalence of NAFLD/NASH was measured in different parts of Asia by community surveys using radiologic modalities. In Japan, the prevalence of NAFLD has shown an increasing trend over the last two decades, which has been attributed to changing lifestyle of the population. The rate increased from 13% before 1990 to 26.2% (32% in men, 17% in women) in 2008.[33]

In China, the prevalence of NAFLD has been estimated to be between 12% and 15% for the general adult population. Furthermore, in some parts of China where obesity is more common, NAFLD prevalence is 51%.[34]

In a recent study (2012) conducted in Hong Kong, Wong and colleagues[35] assessed hepatic fat accumulation through proton magnetic resonance spectroscopy. Furthermore, all patients underwent a liver stiffness measurement by transient elastography. The authors reported the prevalence of NAFLD to be 27.3% with the prevalence rates higher in men (36.8%) compared with women (22.7%). Using elastography, 3.7% of NAFLD patients and 1% of non-NAFLD participants had advanced fibrosis.

In South Korea, the prevalence of NAFLD was reported to be 27.3% in a large population survey. Again, the prevalence was significantly higher in men than women (34.4% vs 12.2%).[36] Interestingly, a study from Taiwan among healthy elderly people reported a similar prevalence rate for NAFLD (27.2%).[37] Finally, studies from India, Sri Lanka, Malaysia, Singapore, and Indonesia showed that the prevalence of NAFLD ranges from 9% to 45%. In these studies, the lowest estimates came from the rural areas where people were poorer and more physically active.[33]

RISK FACTORS FOR NONALCOHOLIC FATTY LIVER DISEASE/NONALCOHOLIC STEATOHEPATITIS

Age

The prevalence of NAFLD and associated fibrosis increases with age (**Fig. 2**).[5] In a recent study, Shima and colleagues[38] studied the influence of age and lifestyle on the development and progression of NAFLD. In this study, multivariate analysis revealed that age was significantly associated with NASH in NAFLD patients.

In another study, Brea and Puzo[39] reported that the prevalence of NAFLD increased with age, from less than 20% in people younger than age 20 to more than 40% in

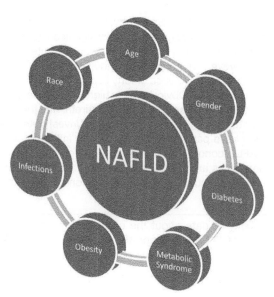

Fig. 2. Risk factors for NAFLD.

patients older than 60 years of age. In a retrospective study by Frith and colleagues[40] among elderly patients, participants were categorized according to their age. An association between increasing age and the degree of fibrosis was described. NASH and cirrhosis were more common in patients greater than 50 years of age compared with younger group. Older age is not only a risk factor for hepatic steatosis, but also individuals with older age have a greater likelihood of mortality and disease progression to fibrosis and hepatocellular carcinoma.[41] It is possible that the relationship between age and fibrosis progression may be attributable to the longer duration of disease in the elderly patients with NAFLD.

Gender

There are conflicting data about the association of gender with the prevalence of NAFLD. Although some studies suggest a higher prevalence in males, others suggest that NAFLD is more common among females.[42] In a study of Stepanova and colleagues,[43] although there was no significant difference of age or race among study population, NASH was significantly higher in females. In another study among younger-aged individuals, NAFLD was also more prevalent in females.[32] In contrast, other studies suggest that male gender is a risk factor for NAFLD.[5,41,44] In a study from Hong Kong among nearly 2500 patients, male gender was found to be associated with NAFLD. In this study, males constituted 53% of patients in NAFLD, whereas only 40% of control subjects without NAFLD were male.[45] Furthermore, another study by Williams and colleagues[13] reported that NAFLD patients were more likely to be male.[46] Although the exact reason for these discrepancies is not known, the study definition and diagnostic modalities may explain some of the differences.

Race

Race is another risk factor for NAFLD/NASH and is discussed in Kalia HS and Gaglio PJ: The Prevalence and Pathobiology of Nonalcoholic Fatty Liver Disease in Patients of Different Races or Ethnicities, in this issue.

Metabolic Disorders

DM is a worldwide health problem, affecting nearly 350 million people.[1–10] It is a metabolic disease caused by abnormalities either in insulin secretion, action, or both. DM and NAFLD are particularly closely related.[47,48] NAFLD prevalence has been found to be increased in patients with type 2 DM with increasing evidence that those with DM are at increased risk for NASH development.[46,49] It was previously shown in a NHANES study that type 2 DM is an independent predictor of NAFLD.[50] Actually, there is evidence that the reverse scenario is also true. In persons with no diabetes, NAFLD can be a predictor of incident diabetes.[51]

The relationship of obesity and steatosis has been known for a long time. The rising epidemic of obesity has become associated with an increase in metabolic syndrome and NAFLD. Results from a study using NHANES data found that both obesity and NAFLD are increasing in the United States population.[52] In a recent study, NAFLD was found in 65.7% and NASH in 33.6% of patients undergoing bariatric surgery, whereas a study by Lazo and Clark[53] found an even higher prevalence of NAFLD and NASH in obese patients undergoing bariatric surgery (91% and 37%, respectively).

A study in Japan found that individuals who met the criteria for metabolic syndrome were more likely to develop NAFLD in the follow-up period.[54] The association between NAFLD and metabolic syndrome can be the consequence of insulin resistance. It has been speculated that insulin resistance induces increased fatty acid transport from adipose tissue to liver, causing steatosis.[55]

The risk of NAFLD has been found to be increased in patients with polycystic ovarian syndrome, where more than 40% of patients with polycystic ovarian syndrome have NAFLD. The reason for this is thought to also be related to insulin resistance.[46]

SUMMARY

It is increasingly clear that NAFLD and NASH are highly prevalent in the United States and the around the world. However, the prevalence of NAFLD and NASH differs significantly according to the diagnostic method used and the population studied. With the impact of different risk factors, the range for NAFLD prevalence varied from 4.5% in patients with no diabetes in Africa to 99% in patients undergoing bariatric surgery.

Studies within the last 10 to 20 years have led clinicians to understand this common problem. Yet, it is obvious that the prevalence of NAFLD and NASH is still increasing despite the known risk factors. As the rate of obesity, diabetes, and metabolic syndrome continue to increase, NAFLD and NASH may significantly impact health care use in the upcoming years and with the development of long-term complications, such as cirrhosis and hepatocellular carcinoma. Although there are numerous questions to be solved in this topic, ongoing studies will help clinicians to understand how to cope with the emerging effects of NAFLD in the near future.

REFERENCES

1. Angulo P. Nonalcoholic fatty liver disease. N Engl J Med 2002;346:1221–31.
2. Brunt EM. Nonalcoholic steatohepatitis. Semin Liver Dis 2004;24:3–20.
3. Fleischman MW, Budoff M, Zeb I, et al. NAFLD prevalence differs among Hispanic subgroups: the Multi-Ethnic Study of Atherosclerosis. World J Gastroenterol 2014;20:4987–93.

4. Charlton MR, Burns JM, Pedersen RA, et al. Frequency and outcomes of liver transplantation for nonalcoholic steatohepatitis in the United States. Gastroenterology 2011;141:1249–53.

5. Vernon G, Baranova A, Younossi ZM. Systematic Frequency and outcomes of liver transplantation for nonalcoholic steatohepatitis in the United States review: the epidemiology and natural history of non-alcoholic fatty liver disease and non-alcoholic steatohepatitis in adults. Aliment Pharmacol Ther 2011;34: 274–85.

6. Sung KC, Wild SH, Byrne CD. Development of new fatty liver, or resolution of existing fatty liver, over five years of follow-up, and risk of incident hypertension. J Hepatol 2014;60:1040–5.

7. Zelber-Sagi S, Lotan R, Shlomai A, et al. Predictors for incidence and remission of NAFLD in the general population during a seven-year prospective follow-up. J Hepatol 2012;56:1145–51.

8. Tsuneto A, Hida A, Sera N, et al. Fatty liver incidence and predictive variables. Hypertens Res 2010;33:638–43.

9. Wong VW, Wong GL, Yeung DK, et al. Incidence of non-alcoholic fatty liver disease in Hong Kong: a population study with paired proton-magnetic resonance spectroscopy. J Hepatol 2015;62:182–9.

10. Younossi ZM, Stepanova M, Negro F, et al. Nonalcoholic fatty liver disease in lean individuals in the United States. Medicine (Baltimore) 2012;91:319–27.

11. Clark JM. The epidemiology of nonalcoholic fatty liver disease in adults. J Clin Gastroenterol 2006;40(Suppl 1):S5–10.

12. Clark JM, Brancati FL, Diehl AM. Nonalcoholic fatty liver disease. Gastroenterology 2002;122:1649–57.

13. Williams CD, Stengel J, Asike MI, et al. Prevalence of nonalcoholic fatty liver disease and nonalcoholic steatohepatitis among a largely middle-aged population utilizing ultrasound and liver biopsy: a prospective study. Gastroenterology 2011;140:124–31.

14. Wanless IR, Lentz JS. Fatty liver hepatitis (steatohepatitis) and obesity: an autopsy study with analysis of risk factors. Hepatology 1990;12:1106–10.

15. Yamamoto K, Takada Y, Fujimoto Y, et al. Nonalcoholic steatohepatitis in donors for living donor liver transplantation. Transplantation 2007;83:257–62.

16. Foster T, Anania FA, Li D, et al. The prevalence and clinical correlates of nonalcoholic fatty liver disease (NAFLD) in African Americans: the multiethnic study of atherosclerosis (MESA). Dig Dis Sci 2013;58:2392–8.

17. Browning JD, Szczepaniak LS, Dobbins R, et al. Prevalence of hepatic steatosis in an urban population in the United States: impact of ethnicity. Hepatology 2004; 40:1387–95.

18. Karnikowski M, Cordova C, Oliveira RJ, et al. Non-alcoholic fatty liver disease and metabolic syndrome in Brazilian middle-aged and older adults. Sao Paulo Med J 2007;125:333–7.

19. Oni ET, Kalathiya R, Aneni EC, et al. Relation of physical activity to prevalence of nonalcoholic Fatty liver disease independent of cardiometabolic risk. Am J Cardiol 2015;115:34–9.

20. Feijo SG, Lima JM, Oliveira MA, et al. The spectrum of non alcoholic fatty liver disease in morbidly obese patients: prevalence and associate risk factors. Acta Cir Bras 2013;28:788–93.

21. Riquelme A, Arrese M, Soza A, et al. Non-alcoholic fatty liver disease and its association with obesity, insulin resistance and increased serum levels of C-reactive protein in Hispanics. Liver Int 2009;29:82–8.

22. Caballeria L, Pera G, Auladell MA, et al. Prevalence and factors associated with the presence of nonalcoholic fatty liver disease in an adult population in Spain. Eur J Gastroenterol Hepatol 2010;22:24–32.
23. Garcia-Monzon C, Vargas-Castrillon J, Porrero JL, et al. Prevalence and risk factors for biopsy-proven non-alcoholic fatty liver disease and non-alcoholic steatohepatitis in a prospective cohort of adult patients with gallstones. Liver Int 2015; 35(8):1983–91.
24. Soresi M, Noto D, Cefalu AB, et al. Nonalcoholic fatty liver and metabolic syndrome in Italy: results from a multicentric study of the Italian Arteriosclerosis society. Acta Diabetol 2013;50:241–9.
25. Zois CD, Baltayiannis GH, Bekiari A, et al. Steatosis and steatohepatitis in postmortem material from Northwestern Greece. World J Gastroenterol 2010;16: 3944–9.
26. Koehler EM, Schouten JN, Hansen BE, et al. Prevalence and risk factors of nonalcoholic fatty liver disease in the elderly: results from the Rotterdam study. J Hepatol 2012;57:1305–11.
27. Alazawi W, Mathur R, Abeysekera K, et al. Ethnicity and the diagnosis gap in liver disease: a population-based study. Br J Gen Pract 2014;64:e694–702.
28. Onyekwere CA, Ogbera AO, Balogun BO. Non-alcoholic fatty liver disease and the metabolic syndrome in an urban hospital serving an African community. Ann Hepatol 2011;10:119–24.
29. Guerrero R, Vega GL, Grundy SM, et al. Ethnic differences in hepatic steatosis: an insulin resistance paradox? Hepatology 2009;49:791–801.
30. Lesi OA, Soyebi KS, Eboh CN. Fatty liver and hyperlipidemia in a cohort of HIV-positive Africans on highly active antiretroviral therapy. J Natl Med Assoc 2009; 101:151–5.
31. Kruger FC, Daniels C, Kidd M, et al. Non-alcoholic fatty liver disease (NAFLD) in the Western Cape: a descriptive analysis. S Afr Med J 2010;100:168–71.
32. Ayonrinde OT, Olynyk JK, Beilin LJ, et al. Gender-specific differences in adipose distribution and adipocytokines influence adolescent nonalcoholic fatty liver disease. Hepatology 2011;53:800–9.
33. Farrell GC, Wong VW, Chitturi S. NAFLD in Asia–as common and important as in the West. Nat Rev Gastroenterol Hepatol 2013;10:307–18.
34. Fan JG, Farrell GC. Epidemiology of non-alcoholic fatty liver disease in China. J Hepatol 2009;50:204–10.
35. Wong VW, Chu WC, Wong GL, et al. Prevalence of non-alcoholic fatty liver disease and advanced fibrosis in Hong Kong Chinese: a population study using proton-magnetic resonance spectroscopy and transient elastography. Gut 2012;61:409–15.
36. Jeong EH, Jun DW, Cho YK, et al. Regional prevalence of non-alcoholic fatty liver disease in Seoul and Gyeonggi-do, Korea. Clin Mol Hepatol 2013;19:266–72.
37. Shen HC, Zhao ZH, Hu YC, et al. Relationship between obesity, metabolic syndrome, and nonalcoholic fatty liver disease in the elderly agricultural and fishing population of Taiwan. Clin Interv Aging 2014;9:501–8.
38. Shima T, Seki K, Umemura A, et al. Influence of lifestyle-related diseases and age on the development and progression of non-alcoholic fatty liver disease. Hepatol Res 2015;45:548–59.
39. Brea A, Puzo J. Non-alcoholic fatty liver disease and cardiovascular risk. Int J Cardiol 2013;167:1109–17.
40. Frith J, Day CP, Henderson E, et al. Non-alcoholic fatty liver disease in older people. Gerontology 2009;55:607–13.

41. Attar BM, Van Thiel DH. Current concepts and management approaches in nonalcoholic fatty liver disease. ScientificWorldJournal 2013;2013:481893.

42. Hashimoto E, Yatsuji S, Kaneda H, et al. The characteristics and natural history of Japanese patients with nonalcoholic fatty liver disease. Hepatol Res 2005;33:72–6.

43. Stepanova M, Rafiq N, Makhlouf H, et al. Predictors of all-cause mortality and liver-related mortality in patients with non-alcoholic fatty liver disease (NAFLD). Dig Dis Sci 2013;58:3017–23.

44. Than NN, Newsome PN. A concise review of non-alcoholic fatty liver disease. Atherosclerosis 2015;239:192–202.

45. Fung J, Lee CK, Chan M, et al. High prevalence of non-alcoholic fatty liver disease in the Chinese: results from the Hong Kong liver health census. Liver Int 2015;35:542–9.

46. Mishra A, Younossi ZM. Epidemiology and natural history of non-alcoholic fatty liver disease. J Clin Exp Hepatol 2012;2:135–44.

47. Firneisz G. Non-alcoholic fatty liver disease and type 2 diabetes mellitus: the liver disease of our age? World J Gastroenterol 2014;20:9072–89.

48. Leite NC, Villela-Nogueira CA, Cardoso CR, et al. Non-alcoholic fatty liver disease and diabetes: from physiopathological interplay to diagnosis and treatment. World J Gastroenterol 2014;20:8377–92.

49. Leite NC, Villela-Nogueira CA, Pannain VL, et al. Histopathological stages of nonalcoholic fatty liver disease in type 2 diabetes: prevalences and correlated factors. Liver Int 2011;31:700–6.

50. Younossi ZM, Stepanova M, Afendy M, et al. Changes in the prevalence of the most common causes of chronic liver diseases in the United States from 1988 to 2008. Clin Gastroenterol Hepatol 2011;9:524–30.e1 [quiz: e60].

51. Verderese JP, Younossi Z. Interaction of type 2 diabetes and nonalcoholic fatty liver disease. Expert Rev Gastroenterol Hepatol 2013;7:405–7.

52. Flegal KM, Carroll MD, Kit BK, et al. Prevalence of obesity and trends in the distribution of body mass index among US adults, 1999-2010. JAMA 2012;307:491–7.

53. Lazo M, Clark JM. The epidemiology of nonalcoholic fatty liver disease: a global perspective. Semin Liver Dis 2008;28:339–50.

54. Hamaguchi M, Kojima T, Takeda N, et al. The metabolic syndrome as a predictor of nonalcoholic fatty liver disease. Ann Intern Med 2005;143:722–8.

55. Younossi ZM, McCullough AJ. Metabolic syndrome, non-alcoholic fatty liver disease and hepatitis C virus: impact on disease progression and treatment response. Liver Int 2009;29(Suppl 2):3–12.

56. Eshraghian A, Dabbaghmanesh MH, Eshraghian H, et al. Nonalcoholic fatty liver disease in a cluster of Iranian population: thyroid status and metabolic risk factors. Arch Iran Med 2013;16:584–9.

57. Radu C, Grigorescu M, Crisan D, et al. Prevalence and associated risk factors of non-alcoholic fatty liver disease in hospitalized patients. J Gastrointestin Liver Dis 2008;17:255–60.

58. Volzke H, Robinson DM, Kleine V, et al. Hepatic steatosis is associated with an increased risk of carotid atherosclerosis. World J Gastroenterol 2005;11:1848–53.

The Prevalence and Pathobiology of Nonalcoholic Fatty Liver Disease in Patients of Different Races or Ethnicities

Harmit S. Kalia, DO[a], Paul J. Gaglio, MD[b],*

KEYWORDS

• NAFLD • Race • Ethnicity • PNPLA

KEY POINTS

- The prevalence of nonalcoholic fatty liver disease (NAFLD) is higher in Hispanics compared with non-Hispanic whites and African Americans.
- Several components of the metabolic syndrome exist at higher rates when comparing Hispanic with non-Hispanic white patients.
- The increase prevalence of NAFLD in Hispanics is not explained by differences in rates of the metabolic syndrome.
- Genetic polymorphisms in genes that influence lipid metabolism, such as patatin-like phospholipase domain-containing protein-3, may play a role in effecting both the amount of hepatic triglyceride content and injury, and may influence the prevalence of NAFLD in different patient populations.

INTRODUCTION

During the last several decades, nonalcoholic fatty liver disease (NAFLD) has emerged as an important cause of liver dysfunction. It is currently one of the most common causes of liver disease in the United States and is rapidly increasing as an indication for liver transplantation. At present, most data related to NAFLD, including histology, risk factors, and natural history, have been garnered from studies in white subjects. However, it is becoming increasingly apparent that multiple aspects of NAFLD differ

The authors have nothing to disclose.
[a] Department of Medicine, Montefiore Einstein Liver Center, Montefiore Medical Center, Albert Einstein College of Medicine, 111 East 210th Street, Rosenthal 2 Red Zone, Bronx, NY 10467, USA; [b] Center for Liver Disease and Transplantation, Columbia University Medical Center, PH-14, 622 West 168th Street, New York, NY 10032, USA
* Corresponding author.
E-mail address: pg2011@cumc.columbia.edu

Clin Liver Dis 20 (2016) 215–224
http://dx.doi.org/10.1016/j.cld.2015.10.005
1089-3261/16/$ – see front matter © 2016 Elsevier Inc. All rights reserved.

liver.theclinics.com

when analyzing subjects of different races or ethnicities. Several recently published manuscripts demonstrate a nonuniform distribution of NAFLD in different subject populations. This article discusses the prevalence of NAFLD in patients of different races or ethnicities, and examines the pathophysiologic mechanisms that may explain why these differences exist.

DIFFERENCES IN THE METABOLIC SYNDROME BASED ON RACE OR ETHNICITY

It is clear that the metabolic syndrome, which includes insulin resistance (IR), obesity, dyslipidemia, and hypertension, has been identified as a significant risk factor for the development of NAFLD. When analyzing the presence of various components of the metabolic syndrome, it is apparent that its prevalence exists at a higher rate in African American and Hispanic patients. Multiple publications have documented a greater frequency of obesity and diabetes in US African American and Hispanic patient populations.[1–3] A recent publication comparing non-Hispanic blacks with Mexican Americans identified overweight and obesity rates of 70% and 73%, respectively, compared with 62% in whites.[4] An analysis of self-reported rates of obesity in the United States revealed an overall rate of 26.7%; however, 36.8% of non-Hispanic blacks and 30.7% of Hispanics identified themselves as obese.[5] In addition to obesity, diabetes has been reported to be more prevalent in African Americans and Hispanics compared with non-Hispanic whites.[6,7] Finally, multiple additional components of the metabolic syndrome, including dyslipidemia, have also been reported to be more prevalent in US minority populations,[8] with initial presentation when these patients enter adolescence.[9]

Based on the increased rates of the various components of the metabolic syndrome in African American and Hispanic patients, it could be assumed that the prevalence of NAFLD in these patient populations is increased compared with non-Hispanic whites. However, despite increased rates of obesity, diabetes, and other components of the metabolic syndrome in African Americans, data suggest that the incidence of NAFLD is lower than expected in this patient population compared with other patient demographics, specifically non-Hispanic white and Hispanic patients (**Fig. 1**).

Demographics of Nonalcoholic Fatty Liver Disease in Non-Hispanic White, African American, and Hispanic Patients

Published data assessing NAFLD vary significantly based on how NAFLD is defined. As an example, some studies use either laboratory, radiologic, or histologic criteria,

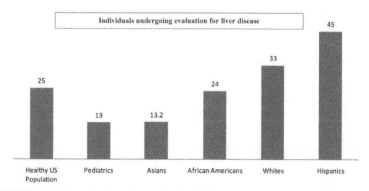

Fig. 1. NAFLD prevalence in the US population (%).

or different combinations of these parameters, to demonstrate the prevalence of NAFLD.

Laboratory assessment of nonalcoholic fatty liver disease

A recently published study in 181 children attending a pediatric obesity clinic (147 non-Hispanic black and 33 non-Hispanic white) revealed that non-Hispanic white children were significantly more likely to have an abnormal alanine aminotransferase (ALT), a surrogate marker for NAFLD compared with black children.[10] Several additional studies of note, including more than 100 children and 832 adults, revealed abnormal ALT and concern for the presence of NAFLD in up to 23% of Hispanic subjects compared with less than 10% of the general population.[11,12] Another study performed with 333 US subjects revealed significant differences in ALT when comparing patients of different races or ethnicities with a mean ALT of 60, 53, and 39 IU/L, and a corresponding diagnosis of "definite or probable NAFLD," in 28%, 18%, and 3% of Hispanic, non-Hispanic white, and African American subjects, respectively.[13]

Radiologic assessment of nonalcoholic fatty liver disease

Radiologic studies have also revealed differences when comparing rates of NAFLD in subjects of various races or ethnicities. Radiologic techniques used to diagnose NAFLD in these studies include ultrasonography, computed tomography (CT), or MRI scanning including MR spectroscopy. The distribution of hepatic triglyceride content using proton MR spectroscopy was assessed in 2287 subjects from a multiethnic patient population. The frequency of hepatic steatosis varied significantly based on ethnicity. The highest rates were found in Hispanics (45%), followed by non-Hispanic white (33%) and African American patients (24%).[14] A recent study by Wagenknecht and colleagues[15] evaluated 1142 adults of Hispanic and African American descent in the Insulin Resistant Atherosclerosis (IRAS) Family Study. CT scans of the abdomen were used to evaluate liver-spleen density ratio and abdominal fat distribution. The prevalence of NAFLD in Hispanics was 24% compared with 10% in African Americans. A recently published study that performed ultrasonography as a modality to assess abnormal liver tests in 442 subjects revealed that 52% of Mexican Americans in the study population met radiologic criteria for NAFLD.[16]

Liver biopsy assessment of nonalcoholic fatty liver disease in patients of different races or ethnicities

Despite limitations related to sampling error and morbidity associated with the procedure, liver biopsy remains the gold standard for diagnosing NAFLD. In addition, liver biopsy can differentiate more benign forms of NAFLD (isolated fatty liver disease) from more advanced forms of NAFLD, including nonalcoholic steatohepatitis (NASH) and NASH with fibrosis. Solga and colleagues[17] prospectively studied 189 subjects who had liver biopsies performed during bariatric surgery. African Americans assessed in this study were younger (mean age 37 vs 44) and had a higher body mass index (BMI), 61.5 versus 54.4 kg/m^2, compared with non-Hispanic whites. However, liver biopsy results revealed that African American had lower rates of moderate or severe steatosis, inflammation, and fibrosis compared with non-Hispanic whites.[17] In a retrospective analysis of liver biopsy data in 238 adults with NAFLD, Mohanty and colleagues[18] evaluated the influence of ethnicity related to the presence of liver histology in subjects with NAFLD. In this study, African Americans had lower grades of steatosis compared with non-Hispanic whites, and a trend toward lower grades of inflammation and lower stages of fibrosis. A study by Kallwitz and colleagues[19] revealed that African-American subjects who underwent liver biopsy at the time of bariatric surgery displayed a decreased amount of steatosis and fibrosis compared with non-Hispanic white and Hispanic subjects, whereas there were no differences in the rates and histologic characteristics of NAFLD when comparing non-Hispanic white with Hispanic patients. However, several recently published studies analyzing histology data indicate a higher rate of advanced NAFLD in Hispanics. Bambha and colleagues[20] analyzed more than 1000 liver biopsies in individuals of different races or ethnicities on behalf of the NASH Clinical Research Network. In this study, the frequency of NASH was 63% in Hispanic, 62% in non-Hispanic whites, and 52% in non-Hispanic blacks. In addition, when comparing Hispanic with non-Hispanic subjects, advanced fibrosis was less frequently identified. However, more pronounced lobular inflammation (NASH) was evident in the Hispanic subjects. The decreased prevalence of advanced fibrosis was hypothesized to be due to the younger age of the Hispanic subjects in the study. Weston and colleagues[13] performed an analysis of a racially diverse patient population in Alameda County, California, assessing serum transaminases, ultrasound, or CT scans with confirmatory liver biopsy and found that of the 159 subjects with "definite or probable NAFLD," 28% were Hispanic compared with 18% Asians and 3% African Americans. Other studies assessing liver biopsies in Hispanics noted a higher rate of Mallory bodies compared with white and black subjects,[18] potentially indicating greater rates of advanced histologic injury in Hispanic patients with NAFLD.

Is the prevalence of nonalcoholic fatty liver disease similarly elevated in all Hispanic or Latino groups?

Given the disproportionate burden of NAFLD in Hispanics, it is important to note that not all Hispanic subgroups are equally affected. Kallwitz and colleagues[21] studied a large cohort of over 12,000 individuals who participated in the Hispanic Community Health Study/Study of Latinos. Hispanic adults, including individuals of Mexican, Dominican, Puerto Rican, Cuban, Central American, and South American descent, were analyzed. Data on subjects with abnormal aminotransferases in the absence of other causes for chronic liver disease were collected. Multivariate analysis revealed that the overall prevalence of NAFLD was 19% in this population and was highest in patients of Central American, South American, or Mexican heritage, whereas subjects with Cuban, Puerto Rican, and Dominican backgrounds had lower rates of NAFLD (**Fig. 2**). These observations were not explained by differences in rates of the metabolic syndrome, physical activity, obesity, or diet when comparing individuals from different countries.

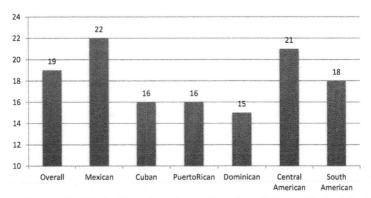

Fig. 2. Prevalence of NAFLD in Hispanic patients. (*Data from* Kallwitz ER, Daviglus ML, Allison MA, et al. Prevalence of suspected nonalcoholic fatty liver disease in Hispanic/Latino individuals differs by heritage. Clin Gastroenterol Hepatol 2015;13(3):569–76.)

Clinical Features and Histology of Nonalcoholic Fatty Liver Disease in Asians

Several interesting differences have been identified when comparing NAFLD in Asian with non-Asian subjects. Weston and colleagues[13] reported that Asians with NAFLD had a significantly lower BMI than other racial groups (compared with Hispanics, African Americans, and Caucasians). A similar observation was noted in a prospective study by Chang and colleagues[22] who assessed 15,347 Korean men. Interestingly, the group with a normal BMI ranging from 18.5 to 22.9 who demonstrated weight gain of greater than 2.3 kg had a significantly increased risk of manifesting NAFLD on ultrasound. This study should raise suspicion that NAFLD may be present when assessing the cause of abnormal liver tests in Asians because NAFLD may exist despite normal BMI compared with the more common phenomenon of elevated BMI and the presence of NAFLD in Western patients.

In a study from Iran, Bahrami and colleagues[23] identified a cohort of 53 subjects with biopsy-proven NASH. Subjects in this study had a mean BMI of 29.3. Although the rate of diabetes was only 5.7%, 54.7% of these patients had IR when assessed by more sensitive techniques, and dyslipidemia was noted in 75.5%. Of note, 13.2% of the subjects did not have any of the standard risk factors for NASH but still demonstrated NASH on liver biopsy. Interestingly, the presence of IR did not correlate with histologic grade or stage of liver injury. Similarly, Mohanty and colleagues[18] have recently published that, despite having a lower BMI than other groups, Asian subjects had more significant histologic injury with increased lobular inflammation and higher grades of ballooning compared with other ethnicities. A potential explanation for this observation was described in a cohort of Chinese subjects with NAFLD who demonstrated low adiponectin and high tumor necrosis factor (TNF)-alpha levels,[24] both of which have been shown to contribute to the development of NAFLD and NASH.

In a cross-sectional study from an ethnically diverse area in the United Kingdom, data were collected for more than 600,000 adults. Demographics, liver diagnoses, and other clinical information were analyzed. This revealed that the highest incidence of abnormal liver tests was present in Bangladeshi (18.4%), Pakistani (17.6%), and Indian (14.8%) individuals compared with non-Hispanic white (13.5%), African (11.8%), and Caribbean (10.2%) subjects.[25] It is thus important for clinicians to recognize that NAFLD may exist in Asian patients and may not correlate with elevated BMI.

Pathobiology of Nonalcoholic Fatty Liver Disease in Patients of Different Races or Ethnicities

The seemingly incongruous disconnect between the prevalence of the metabolic syndrome and incidence of NAFLD when comparing patients of different races or ethnicities deserves further mention. Several investigators have noted that, despite similar or increased rates of the metabolic syndrome, including intraperitoneal adipose content, IR, and obesity, African Americans seemed to be more resistant to the development of hepatic steatosis.[14,15,20] Furthermore, the lower frequency of hepatic steatosis observed in African Americans was not explained by differences in BMI, IR, ethanol ingestion, or medication use compared with Hispanics.[26] Adding to the complexity of this issue is the observation that individuals of African descent have decreased rates of visceral fat compared with patients of other races or ethnicities.[27,28] Several investigators have hypothesized that increased visceral fat exacerbates NAFLD by worsening IR and liberating proinflammatory cytokines that accelerate the progression from simple steatosis to more advanced forms of NAFLD.[29] It can therefore be hypothesized that genetic factors may play a role in how components of the metabolic syndrome influence the emergence of NAFLD in patients of different races or ethnicities.

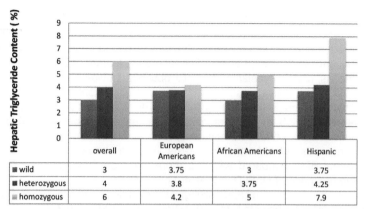

Fig. 3. Hepatic triglyceride content related to PNPLA I148M genetic polymorphism. (*Data from* Romeo S, Kozlitina J, Xing C, et al. Genetic variation in PNPLA3 confers susceptibility to nonalcoholic fatty liver disease. Nat Genet 2008;40(12):1461–5.)

Role of Genetic Polymorphisms in Patatin-like Phospholipase Domain-Containing Protein-3

The pathophysiologic and genetic determinants of NAFLD may be different when comparing different races or ethnicities. Several investigators have performed genome wide association analyses that identified a higher rate of genetic mutations of the patatin-like phospholipase domain-containing protein (PNPLA) 3 rs738409 gene in Hispanic populations.[30,31] This genetic polymorphism has been identified as a risk for more advanced forms of NAFLD. The PNPLA family of genes affects lipid metabolism. Patients with specific genetic polymorphisms in this gene have been found to have significant elevation in hepatic fat, triglyceride content and inflammation. This mutation or allele was twice as common in Hispanic Americans as in African Americans (40% vs 19%), and correlated with a greater prevalence of NAFLD in

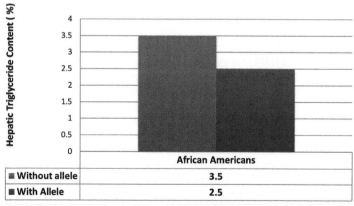

Fig. 4. Hepatic triglyceride content in African Americans with and without PNPLA3 S453I genetic polymorphism. (*Data from* Romeo S, Kozlitina J, Xing C, et al. Genetic variation in PNPLA3 confers susceptibility to nonalcoholic fatty liver disease. Nat Genet 2008;40(12):1461–5.)

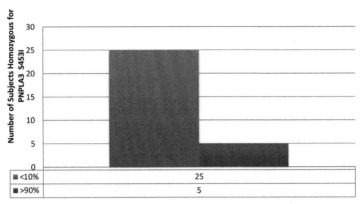

Fig. 5. Hepatic triglyceride content in patients homozygous for PNPLA3 S453I allele. (*Data from* Romeo S, Kozlitina J, Xing C, et al. Genetic variation in PNPLA3 confers susceptibility to nonalcoholic fatty liver disease. Nat Genet 2008;40(12):1461–5.)

Hispanic Americans compared with African Americans (24 vs 9%). An additional genetic mutation of the PNPLA3 rs738409 gene-encoding I148M has consistently been identified as a risk for more severe histologic features of NAFLD.[31] This single nucleotide mutation is strongly associated with increased hepatic fat levels with a more than twofold greater incidence in homozygotes compared with nonaffected individuals. In addition, the observation of significant elevation in serum levels of ALT was strongly associated with this genetic mutation and was limited to Hispanic subjects.[30,31] The highest frequency of this allele was found in Hispanic subjects (49%) with lower frequencies found in European Americans (23%) and African Americans (17%)[31] (**Fig. 3**). A similar strong association with NAFLD has also been identified in pediatric populations expressing this mutation, with increased hepatic fat content as well as more severe hepatocyte ballooning, lobular inflammation, and perivenular fibrosis.[32,33] This genetic variant has also been identified in Asian Indians with NAFLD.[34] Of note, no associations were observed between this PNPLA3 variant related to BMI, IR, homeostatic model assessment (HOMA)-IR, plasma levels of triglyceride, or total cholesterol.[30,31]

The influence of additional genetic variations in PNPLA has recently been identified. The PNPLA3 variant at position S453I is associated with diminished hepatic triglyceride content. This allele has been found in higher frequencies in African Americans, with diminished rates in European Americans and Hispanics (**Figs. 4** and **5**). These results suggest that certain inherited variations in lipid metabolism may influence the development and progression of NAFLD. Genetic variations at PNPLA3 confer either a markedly increased or decreased risk of severe histologic features of NAFLD, and influence the effect of components of the metabolic syndrome related to the development and progression of NAFLD, and may explain the observed differences in rates of NAFLD in patients of different races or ethnicities.

SUMMARY

NAFLD is rapidly emerging as the most common cause of liver injury in the United States. The prevalence of NAFLD varies dramatically when comparing individuals of different races and ethnicities. Rates of NAFLD are highest in Hispanic patient populations compared with non-Hispanic whites and African Americans, despite similar or higher rates of the metabolic syndrome. In addition, NAFLD in Asian patients is being increasingly recognized and may be present in patients with a normal BMI. An adequate explanation for the disconnect between rates of the metabolic syndrome and prevalence of NAFLD in patients of different races or ethnicities remains elusive, although variations in genes that effect lipid metabolism, such as PNPLA, may play a role. It is likely that future therapies for NAFLD will incorporate strategies to recognize and diagnose the disease and take advantage of differences in lipid metabolism and/ or genetic differences in patients of different races or ethnicities to achieve optimal management.

REFERENCES

1. Brancati FL, Kao WH, Folsom AR, et al. Incident type 2 diabetes mellitus in African American and white adults: the Atherosclerosis Risk in Communities Study. JAMA 2000;283:2253–9.
2. Hedley AA, Ogden CL, Johnson CL, et al. Prevalence of overweight and obesity among US children, adolescents, and adults, 1999-2002. JAMA 2004;291: 2847–50.
3. Crespo CJ, Loria CM, Burt VL. Hypertension and other cardiovascular disease risk factors among Mexican Americans, Cuban Americans, and Puerto Ricans from the Hispanic Health and Nutrition Examination Survey. Public Health Rep 1996;111(Suppl 2):7–10.
4. Flegal KM, Carroll MD, Ogden CL, et al. Prevalence and trends in obesity among US adults, 1999-2008. JAMA 2010;303:235–41.
5. Centers for Disease Control and Prevention (CDC). Vital signs: state-specific obesity prevalence among adults United States, 2009. MMWR Morb Mortal Wkly Rep 2010;59(30):951–5.
6. Hausmann LR, Ren D, Sevick MA. Racial differences in diabetes-related psychosocial factors and glycemic control in patients with type 2 diabetes. Patient Prefer Adherence 2010;4:291–9.
7. Kirk JK, D'Agostino RB Jr, Bell RA, et al. Disparities in HbA1c levels between African-American and non-Hispanic white adults with diabetes: a meta-analysis. Diabetes Care 2006;29(9):2130–6.
8. Karlamangla AS, Merkin SS, Crimmins EM, et al. Socioeconomic and ethnic disparities in cardiovascular risk in the United States, 2001-2006. Ann Epidemiol 2010;20(8):617–28.
9. Walker SE, Gurka MJ, Oliver MN, et al. Racial/ethnic discrepancies in the metabolic syndrome begin in childhood and persist after adjustment for environmental factors. Nutr Metab Cardiovasc Dis 2012;22:141–8.
10. Louthan MV, Theriot JA, Zimmerman E, et al. Decreased prevalence of nonalcoholic fatty liver disease in black obese children. J Pediatr Gastroenterol Nutr 2005;41:426–9.
11. Quiros-Tejeira RE, Rivera CA, Ziba TT, et al. Risk for nonalcoholic fatty liver disease in Hispanic youth with BMI > or =95th percentile. J Pediatr Gastroenterol Nutr 2007;44:228–36.
12. Riquelme A, Arrese M, Soza A, et al. Non-alcoholic fatty liver disease and its association with obesity, insulin resistance and increased serum levels of C-reactive protein in Hispanics. Liver Int 2009;29:82–8.
13. Weston SR, Leyden W, Murphy R, et al. Racial and ethnic distribution of nonalcoholic fatty liver in persons with newly diagnosed chronic liver disease. Hepatology 2005;41(2):372–9.

14. Browning JD, Szczepaniak LS, Dobbins R, et al. Prevalence of hepatic steatosis in an urban population in the United States: impact of ethnicity. Hepatology 2004; 40:1387–95.
15. Wagenknecht LE, Scherzinger AL, Stamm ER, et al. Correlates and heritability of nonalcoholic fatty liver disease in a minority cohort. Obesity 2009;17: 1240–6.
16. Pan JJ, Fisher-Hoch SP, Chen C, et al. Burden of nonalcoholic fatty liver disease and advanced fibrosis in a Texas Hispanic community cohort. World J Hepatol 2015;18:1586–94.
17. Solga SF, Clark JM, Alkhuraishi AR, et al. Race and comorbid factors predict nonalcoholic fatty liver disease histopathology in severely obese patients. Surg Obes Relat Dis 2005;1(1):6–11.
18. Mohanty SR, Troy TN, Huo D, et al. Influence of ethnicity on histological differences in non-alcoholic fatty liver disease. J Hepatol 2009;50:797–804.
19. Kallwitz ER, Guzman G, TenCate V, et al. The histologic spectrum of liver disease in African-American, non-Hispanic white, and Hispanic obesity surgery patients. Am J Gastroenterol 2009;104:64–9.
20. Bambha K, Belt P, Abraham M, et al. Ethnicity and nonalcoholic fatty liver disease. Hepatology 2012;55:769–80.
21. Kallwitz ER, Daviglus ML, Allison MA, et al. Prevalence of suspected nonalcoholic fatty liver disease in Hispanic/Latino individuals differs by heritage. Clin Gastroenterol Hepatol 2015;13(3):569–76.
22. Chang Y, Ryu S, Sung E, et al. Weight gain within the normal weight range predicts ultrasonographically detected fatty liver in healthy Korean men. Gut 2009; 58(10):1419–25.
23. Bahrami H, Daryani NE, Mirmomen S, et al. Clinical and histological features of nonalcoholic steatohepatitis in Iranian patients. BMC Gastroenterol 2003;3: 27–33.
24. Wong VW, Hui AY, Tsang SW, et al. Metabolic and adipokine profile of Chinese patients with nonalcoholic fatty liver disease. Clin Gastroenterol Hepatol 2006; 4(9):1154–61.
25. Alazawi W, Mathur R, Abeysekera K, et al. Ethnicity and the diagnosis gap in liver disease: a population-based study. Br J Gen Pract 2014;64:694–702.
26. Guerrero R, Vega GL, Grundy SM, et al. Ethnic differences in hepatic steatosis: an insulin resistance paradox? Hepatology 2009;49(3):791–801.
27. Sumner AE, Micklesfield LK, Ricks M, et al. Waist circumference, BMI, and visceral adipose tissue in white women and women of African descent. Obesity 2010;19:671–4.
28. Carroll JF, Chiapa AL, Rodriquez M, et al. Visceral fat, waist circumference, and BMI: impact of race/ethnicity. Obesity 2008;16(3):600–7.
29. Qureshi K, Abrams GA. Metabolic liver disease of obesity and role of adipose tissue in the pathogenesis of nonalcoholic fatty liver disease. World J Gastroenterol 2007;13(26):3540–53.
30. Wagenknecht LE, Palmer ND, Bowden DW, et al. Association of PNPLA3 with non-alcoholic fatty liver disease in a minority cohort: the Insulin Resistance Atherosclerosis Family Study. Liver Int 2011;31(3):412–6.
31. Romeo S, Kozlitina J, Xing C, et al. Genetic variation in PNPLA3 confers susceptibility to nonalcoholic fatty liver disease. Nat Genet 2008;40(12):1461–5.
32. Valenti L, Alisi A, Galmozzi E, et al. I148M patatin-like phospholipase domain-containing 3 gene variant and severity of pediatric nonalcoholic fatty liver disease. Hepatology 2010;52(4):1274–80.

33. Sookoian S, Pirola CJ. Meta-analysis of the influence of I148M variant of patatin-like phospholipase domain containing 3 gene (PNPLA3) on the susceptibility and histological severity of nonalcoholic fatty liver disease. Hepatology 2011;53(6): 1883–94.

34. Bhatt SP, Nigam P, Misra A, et al. Genetic variation in the patatin-like phospholipase domain-containing protein-3 (PNPLA-3) gene in Asian Indians with nonalcoholic fatty liver disease. Metab Syndr Relat Disord 2013;11:329.

The Metabolic Syndrome and Its Influence on Nonalcoholic Steatohepatitis

Pushpjeet Kanwar, MD[a], Kris V. Kowdley, MD[b],*

KEYWORDS

- Metabolic syndrome • Risk factors • Nonalcoholic steatohepatitis • NAFLD
- Hepatocellular carcinoma

KEY POINTS

- Nonalcoholic fatty liver disease (NAFLD) is the most common liver disorder in the Western world; its subtype, nonalcoholic steatohepatitis (NASH), can progress to cirrhosis and hepatocellular carcinoma.
- The metabolic syndrome (MetS) is associated with NASH; insulin resistance (IR) is central in their pathogenesis and is the potential linking mechanism.
- The treatment of NASH is based on its pathogenesis and therefore primarily involves reduction in IR and modification of MetS risk factors.
- Individuals with NAFLD and MetS have a significantly higher overall, cardiovascular, and liver-related mortality versus those without MetS; NAFLD patients without MetS have a similar prognosis as those without liver disease.

INTRODUCTION

The metabolic syndrome (MetS) is a constellation of cardiovascular risk factors that identify patients at increased risk of diabetes type 2 and cardiovascular disease.[1] These factors include obesity, hyperglycemia, hypertension, dyslipidemia, and insulin resistance (IR). It was first described by Reaven as Syndrome X in 1988.[2] Since then, its definition has undergone multiple changes, but the fundamental criteria have remained the same. However, experts generally agree that presence of IR is a key ingredient in understanding the pathogenesis and making a diagnosis of MetS.[3]

Nonalcoholic fatty liver disease (NAFLD) is considered the most common liver disorder worldwide[4] and is an umbrella term used for patients with hepatic steatosis

The authors have nothing to disclose.
[a] Department of Gastroenterology and Hepatology, New York Methodist Hospital, 506, 6th Street, Brooklyn, NY 11215, USA; [b] Department of Transplant Hepatology, Swedish Medical Center, 1101, Madison Street, Suite 200, Seattle, WA 98104, USA
* Corresponding author.
E-mail address: kris.kowdley@swedish.org

Clin Liver Dis 20 (2016) 225–243
http://dx.doi.org/10.1016/j.cld.2015.10.002
1089-3261/16/$ – see front matter © 2016 Elsevier Inc. All rights reserved.

when alcohol, medication, and genetic disorder as a possible etiology have been ruled out.[5] Its increase in the Western countries has accompanied the obesity epidemic.[6] Patients with simple steatosis involving greater than 5% of the liver without any hepatocyte injury (ballooning) are considered to have nonalcoholic fatty liver (NAFL).[7] Nonalcoholic steatohepatitis (NASH) is a pathologic entity involving necroinflammation and hepatocyte injury in a steatotic liver.[8] NAFL disease (NAFLD) has been described as a hepatic manifestation of MetS owing to its close association with MetS and its "cardiometabolic" risk factors.[9]

DEFINITIONS OF THE METABOLIC SYNDROME AND NONALCOHOLIC STEATOHEPATITIS

The current definition of MetS is also called the "harmonization definition" and it is based on a joint statement by various organizations and professional medical societies.[10] Based on this definition, a diagnosis of MetS is based on presence of 3 of 5 factors, which include triglycerides (TG) 150 mg/dL or greater, high-density lipoprotein-cholesterol (HDL-C) of less than 40 mg/dL in men and less than 50 mg/dL in women, hypertension defined as systolic blood pressure 130 mm Hg or greater or diastolic blood pressure 85 mm Hg or greater, hyperglycemia defined as fasting glucose 100 g/dL or greater, and increased waist circumference, defined by country- and population-specific criteria.[10] Patients on treatment for hypertension, high TGs, low HDL-C and hyperglycemia were also included in this definition.[10]

The diagnosis of NASH involves the presence of steatosis, inflammation, and ballooning (**Table 1**).[8] A histologic scoring system called NAFLD activity score (NAS) was developed for NAFLD patients to evaluate improvement in liver biopsy in therapeutic trials.[11] A score of 0 to 3 is given depending on the amount of steatosis with 0 for less than 5%, 1 for 5% to 33%, 2 for 33% to 66%, and 3 for greater than 66%. Similarly, a score of 0 to 3 is given for lobular inflammation depending on the number of foci of inflammatory foci. Ballooning injury is important and a score of 0, 1, or 2 is assigned if there are no, few, or many ballooned hepatocytes, respectively.[8] Moreover, this scoring system also used specific histologic criteria that focused on the severity and zonal pattern of parenchymal remodeling to "stage" the fibrosis from 0 to 4 in NAFLD patients (Kleiner DE, Brunt EM 2005). Although a threshold NAS of 5 or greater has been used by certain investigators to differentiate between a diagnosis of steatohepatitis and those without steatohepatitis, a recent study clarified that this NAS cutoff of 5 is not accurate in making this distinction.[11]

Table 1
Definition and criteria for MetS and NASH

MetS	NASH
Obesity: increased waist circumference[a]	Steatosis: >5% of liver parenchyma
HTN: systolic ≥130 mm Hg or diastolic ≥85 mm Hg	Inflammation: lobular
Hyperglycemia: Fasting glucose >100 g/dL	Hepatocyte ballooning
TG ≥150 mg/dL	Absence of alcohol abuse
HDL-C <40 mg/dL in men and <50 mg/dL in women	Absence of medication side effect

Abbreviations: HLD-C, high-density lipoprotein cholesterol; HTN, hypertension; MetS, the metabolic syndrome; NASH, nonalcoholic steatohepatitis; TG, Triglycerides.
[a] Based on population- and ethnicity-specific criteria.

EPIDEMIOLOGY OF THE METABOLIC SYNDROME AND NONALCOHOLIC STEATOHEPATITIS

Although the prevalence of MetS in the United States has slightly decreased in the last decade from 26% to 23% based on the National Health and Nutrition Examination Survey (NHANES) data from 1999 to 2010, the prevalence of some of its constituents such as abdominal obesity has increased from 45% to 56%.[12] Another study used the "harmonization definition" and showed a higher prevalence of MetS in adult population at 34%.[13] One study used older NHANES data and showed that 8% of patients had both NAFLD and MetS.[14] Significantly greater abnormal values of MetS risk factors were noted in patients with both NAFLD and MetS compared with those with only MetS or NAFLD. The prevalence of NAFLD was 30% and it increased with the number of MetS criteria met in those patients. Patient without any MetS risk factors had a NAFLD prevalence of 17%, whereas those with all 5 MetS criteria had a prevalence of 91%.[14] Although MetS is considered a syndrome found mainly in the Western population, because European studies have also shown a high prevalence at 10% to 26%, recent data from many Asian countries including India, Turkey, and Iran have shown similar results.[15] Therefore, MetS is emerging as a global health problem.

Although 20% to 30% of the US population seems to be afflicted with this seemingly benign disease,[16] approximately one-third of NAFLD patients may have NASH, which is the more aggressive form of NAFL.[17] Although other estimates predict that 10% to 15% of NAFLD patients have NASH,[7] the prevalence of NASH in the general population in the United States is about 3% to 5%.[16] About 20% of NASH patients may progress to cirrhosis[7] and death in 30% to 40% of those with cirrhosis will be related to end-stage liver disease[18] (**Fig. 1**). Although NAFLD is considered a disease of the Western world, many of the Asian countries are not far behind with prevalence similar to the United States and Europe noted in countries such as India, Korea, and Japan.[19–21] Not surprisingly, this increase in the prevalence of NAFLD in Asia has

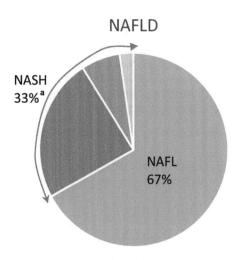

■ NAFL   ■ NASH   ▪ Cirrhosis   ▪ Death due to ESLD

Fig. 1. Approximately 20% of nonalcoholic steatohepatitis (NASH) patients develop cirrhosis and about 30% to 40% of those with cirrhosis die owing to end-stage liver disease (ESLD). [a] The estimates for prevalence of NASH in nonalcoholic fatty liver disease (NAFLD) patients varies from 10% to 33% based on various definitions.

been accompanied by an increase in obesity, hypertension, MetS, and type 2 diabetes.[22]

PATHOGENESIS OF THE METABOLIC SYNDROME AND NONALCOHOLIC STEATOHEPATITIS

Although genetics and lifestyle factors play an important role, IR is the major driving force for MetS and its risk factors.[23] Because visceral adiposity is a marker of IR,[24] it is not surprising that the mechanism of development of MetS starts in the adipose tissue where adipokines and free fatty acids (FFA) play a central role in the pathogenesis of MetS.[25]

Similarly, FFA accumulation with subsequent TG accumulation leads to hepatic steatosis in IR individuals.[26] However, recent literature suggests that TG might have a protective affect because its inhibition leads to decreased steatosis but increased hepatocyte injury.[27] In contrast, hepatic accumulation of FFA and cholesterol leads to hepatocyte damage, which is mediated by oxidative stress and direct lipotoxicity causing mitochondrial dysfunction.[28,29]

ROLE OF DIET

Multiple animal studies have shown that high fructose corn syrup in the diet and use of trans-fatty acids is responsible of development of NASH.[30–32] Furthermore, when these trans-fats were removed from their diet, there was improvement in NASH.[33] Use of a high cholesterol and saturated fat diet in mice led to development of features of MetS, NASH, and fibrosis.[34] Studies in humans have suggested that NASH patients have a higher saturated fat intake and low polyunsaturated fat intake.[35] The saturated fat intake also correlated with MetS and IR.[35]

ROLE OF GENETIC FACTORS

Asian Indian men can develop NASH despite lack of MetS features. These patients have a certain genetic predisposition, such as apolipoprotein C3 gene polymorphisms, that increases their risk of hepatic IR and NAFLD.[36] A genome-wide association analysis of a multiethnic population showed that Hispanics have the highest prevalence of a missense mutation in the *PNPLA3* gene that makes them at increased risk of NAFLD and hepatic IR.[37] Another polymorphism in the same gene is more common in African Americans and is associated with decreased liver steatosis.[37]

Insulin Resistance: The Bridge Connecting the Metabolic Syndrome and Nonalcoholic Steatohepatitis

Although the pathogenesis of MetS and NASH includes a number of common mechanisms and factors, IR plays a role in almost every pathway that leads to these 2 disease processes.

Role of Free Fatty Acids

In MetS, studies have suggested that IR is the cause and result of increase in plasma FFA.[38] This increase in plasma FFA occurs owing to decrease in the inhibitory action of insulin on lipolysis because there is peripheral IR in individuals with visceral adiposity.[39] Subsequently, FFA metabolites such as diacylglycerol and ceramides accumulate in skeletal muscle and liver and cause phosphorylation of insulin receptor substrate-1 by activating protein kinase C.[25] This phosphorylation inhibits insulin-dependent activation of phosphatidylinositol 3-kinase,[40] which leads to hepatic IR, thereby causing increased hepatic gluconeogenesis owing to loss of inhibitory action of insulin. Subsequently, glucose is shunted toward the lipogenesis pathway, leading to hepatic steatosis.[41] Although most of the hepatic lipid accumulation occurs owing to hepatic inflow of FFA, de novo lipogenesis can also contribute to liver steatosis in individuals on high carbohydrate diet.[7,42]

Role of Toll-like Receptors

Toll-like receptors (TLRs) are receptors of the innate immune system that are expressed in multiple tissues, including spleen and peripheral leukocytes.[43] They sense pathogens and produce inflammatory signals. FFAs interact with TLRs such as TLR-2 and TLR-4 on monocytes leading to proinflammatory gene expression.[44] This leads to phosphorylation of insulin receptor substrate-1 by activation of IkB kinase and c-Jun N-terminal kinase,[45] thereby leading to hepatic IR as described. TLR-4 knockout mice are protected from the development of saturated fat-induced IR and diet-induced obesity.[46] Similarly, murine models have also suggested a role of TLRs in NASH. In 1 study, TLR-9 was shown to signal production of IL-1β and thereby lead to steatohepatitis[47] (**Table 2**). Furthermore, several studies have suggested a role of TLR-4 in the progression of NAFLD and TLR-4 knockout mice have a lesser risk of steatohepatitis, even when fed on diets responsible for NAFLD.[48] A recent study also suggested an association between NAS and liver messenger RNA levels of TLR-2, -4, and -9.[49]

Table 2
The common pathogenesis: various mechanisms involved in pathogenesis of IR and NASH

	Mechanism of Action	Role in IR and NASH
FFA	FFA metabolites cause IRS-1 phosphorylation	FFA leads to hepatic IR and subsequent hepatic steatosis
TLR	TLR interact with FFA to cause IRS-1 phosphorylation by activating JNK and IKK TLR-9 can signal production of IL-β	Leads to hepatic IR and subsequent hepatic steatosis IL-β leads to NASH Various TLR have been associated with NASH and TLR-4 knockout mice have lower risk of NASH
Adipokines	Adiponectin depletion is seen in IR, MetS, and NASH A concept of leptin resistance is suggested in these patients because it counteracts the action of insulin	Adiponectin may have a therapeutic potential owing to its antioxidant and antiinflammatory activity Leptin levels are high in IR and NAFLD patients.
Inflammatory signals	Macrophages release TNF-α, IL-β, and IL-6 that activate JNK and IKK	Leads to hepatic IR and subsequent hepatic steatosis TNF-α antibodies can improve NAFLD
Mitochondrial dysfunction	Increased FFA uptake and their incomplete oxidation causes IR Oxidative stress leads to production of ROS, which causes necrosis	NASH is associated with decreased expression of genes involved in production of mitochondria

Abbreviations: FFA, Free fatty acids; IKK, IkB kinase; IL, interleukin; IR, insulin resistance; IRS-1, insulin receptor substrate-1; JNK, c-Jun N- terminal kinase; NAFLD, nonalcoholic fatty liver disease; NASH, nonalcoholic steatohepatitis; ROS, reactive oxygen species; TLR, Toll-like receptors; TNF, tumor necrosis factor.

ROLE OF ADIPOKINES
Leptin

Leptin is an adipokine that opposes the action of insulin by counteracting its lipogenic effect and decreasing TG synthesis without increasing plasma FFA levels.[50,51] In obese and IR individuals, there is blunting of the hypothalamic response to leptin.[52] Furthermore, obese patients have high leptin levels, suggesting a concept of leptin resistance.[53] This leads to development of IR as leptin resistance leads to accumulation of TGs in adipose, pancreas, muscle, and liver.[54] Similarly, NAFLD patients have high leptin levels and they correlate with steatosis, suggesting a role of leptin resistance in NAFLD as well.[55]

Adiponectin

Adiponectin is an adipokine that has an inverse relationship with IR and can therapeutically reverse it.[56] Moreover, low levels of adiponectin have been shown to be associated with type 2 diabetes mellitus, obesity, and MetS.[54,57] Adiponectin inhibits gluconeogenesis, causes FFA oxidation, and has antiinflammatory properties.[26] Many of these benefits may be deficient in NASH patients; studies have suggested that low adiponectin levels and reduced expression of adiponectin and its receptor correlate with the severity of NASH.[58–61] A recent study evaluated the role of adipokines in NAFL and NASH, and showed that NASH patients have lower adiponectin levels, higher hepatic IR, and a greater adipose IR index as compared with NAFL patients. Moreover, NASH patients had impaired pancreatic β-cell function, which was not seen in NAFL patients.[62]

Other Inflammatory Signals

Macrophages infiltrate adipose tissue in obese individuals and inflammatory factors such as tumor necrosis factor-α, interleukin-6 and interleukin-1β are released, which activate c-Jun N-terminal kinase and Iκβ kinase leading to IR.[63] These cytokines also play an important role in pathogenesis of NASH.[63] Antibodies to tumor necrosis factor-α have also been shown to improve NAFLD in mouse models.[64]

Mitochondrial Dysfunction

Individuals with IR have mitochondrial dysfunction owing to increased FFA uptake and their incomplete oxidation.[65] This leads to oxidative stress and production of reactive oxygen species owing to energy depletion, respiratory chain deficiency, and subsequent necrosis or apoptosis.[29,66] Furthermore, mitochondrial dysfunction causes IR, thus propagating this vicious cycle.[4]

All these mechanisms are not independent of each other and work together in this complex pathogenesis.[67] In 1 study, leptin-deficient mice, when fed a diet high in unsaturated fat, developed NASH, which was associated with depleted adiponectin levels and reduced expression of genes associated with production of mitochondria. Moreover, recombinant adiponectin infusion led to increased expression of mitochondrial genes in certain hepatocytes.[61]

Relationship Between Insulin Resistance and the Metabolic Syndrome Risk Factors

All the risk factors for MetS are associated with IR. Studies have shown that β-cell "burnout" occurs owing to chronic hyperglycemia in IR patients. This leads to high basal insulin levels but a lower response rate to hyperglycemia.[68] Moreover, high FFA levels inhibit release of insulin from β-cells in response to glucose, leading to further hyperglycemia and β-cell dysfunction.[69]

IR individuals lose the vasodilator effect of insulin,[70] but retain the sodium reabsorption effect in the kidneys,[71] thus leading to overall vasoconstriction and causing hypertension. This higher sodium reabsorption rate has also been shown to occur in MetS patients.[72] Furthermore, the renin–angiotensin system (RAS) may also play a role as seen in mice models where angiotensin derived from adipocytes leads to increased fat mass by causing adipocyte cell growth and differentiation.[73] Subsequently, it is secreted into the blood stream, leading to high levels of angiotensin, thereby causing vasoconstriction and thus hypertension.[74]

High plasma FFA load to the liver in IR individuals leads to elevated TG synthesis in the liver as very low-density lipoprotein,[75,76] which subsequently leads to higher plasma TG levels.[77] Furthermore, transfer of cholesterol esters from HDL-C to very low-density lipoprotein and high renal clearance of HDL-C leads to low HDL-C levels as seen in MetS.[41,78]

Recent Developments in the Pathogenesis of Nonalcoholic Steatohepatitis

As described, the pathogenesis of NASH involves hepatic TG accumulation triggered by IR and subsequent oxidative stress and lipid peroxidation through various mechanisms leading to hepatocyte injury. This 2-hit pathogenesis has been discarded in favor of a multiple-hit hypothesis where signals from adipose tissue and gut promote hepatic inflammation.[79] The role of microbiota in the development of NASH has been evaluated recently. Human and animal studies have suggested that obese participants have different prevalences of certain commensal bacteria as compared with their leaner counterparts.[80,81] In 1 study, the authors showed an improvement in insulin sensitivity when feces from lean donors was infused into male recipients with MetS.[82] This study also showed that butyrate-producing bacteria were increased in the feces of the recipients. Furthermore, another study showed that oral butyrate when given to fat-fed rats protected them from developing NAFLD and reduced IR in these rodents.[83]

In summary, the hypothesis of peripheral IR leading to the hepatic steatosis that causes hepatic IR and subsequent oxidative stress leading to NASH is oversimplified and this pathway is likely bidirectional (**Fig. 2**). Furthermore, the pathogenesis of MetS and NASH is more complex and, although IR plays a pivotal role, other mechanisms are also at play and further research into those pathways are necessary for better understanding of these disease processes, which may guide us in evaluating superior treatment options.

CORRELATION BETWEEN THE METABOLIC SYNDROME AND NONALCOHOLIC STEATOHEPATITIS

Although the pathogenesis of MetS and NASH have a similar pathway, studies to correlate these 2 conditions are essential to prove their association clinically. Although multiple studies showed that ultrasonographically diagnosed NAFLD is associated with MetS and its features,[84–87] studies involving histologic analysis were lacking. In 2003, Marchesini and colleagues[9] were able to show that NAFLD patients with MetS had a higher risk of developing NASH after correcting for age, sex, and body

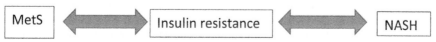

Fig. 2. The relationship between the metabolic syndrome (MetS), insulin resistance and nonalcoholic steatohepatitis (NASH) is bidirectional.

mass index (BMI). The prevalence of MetS in NASH patients was 88% compared with 53% in NAFL patients. Similar results were seen in a recent Korean study where patients with NASH had a significantly higher association with MetS compared with healthy controls.[88] Moreover, NASH patients with MetS when compared with those without MetS had a significantly higher IR based on their homeostasis model assessment of IR, suggesting a possible additive effect of NASH and MetS on IR.

Studies in children have revealed comparable results with 1 study from the United States showing that both MetS and IR have a significant association with NASH. Moreover, children with NASH and MetS had a high risk of developing advanced fibrosis.[89] Another pediatric study from Europe had comparable findings and suggested that MetS and the biochemical variables associated with it had a high correlation with the histologic features of NASH.[90] Conversely, a smaller study from Turkey involving 81 adult NAFLD patients did not show an increased prevalence of MetS in NASH patients compared with those with simple steatosis.[91]

Despite these few studies that evaluated data without any specific BMI criteria, most of the histologic data in MetS patients has been obtained in morbidly obese patients undergoing bariatric surgeries. These studies involving severely obese adults showed that there is a high correlation between MetS or its features with NASH.[92–94] One study involving morbidly obese patients evaluated a scoring system for NASH and reported that 82% of NASH patients had MetS compared with only 48% in those without NASH.

Despite the overwhelming data suggesting correlation of MetS with NAFLD and NASH, most of these studies were cross-sectional and association does not prove causality. However, a recent Chinese study followed patients over an average of 4.8 years and showed that 82 of 255 MetS patients developed NAFLD.[95] Although this study was limited by a lack of histologic analysis, it does suggest a high risk of developing NAFLD. A prospective study involving liver biopsies and multiethnic population is needed to determine the risk of developing NASH in MetS patients.

Role of the Metabolic Syndrome Risk Factors as Predictors for Nonalcoholic Steatohepatitis

Studies from all parts of the world and involving various ethnicities have evaluated the association of MetS risk factors and NASH and have shown high correlation with most of the risk factors. The landmark study by Marchesini and colleagues[9] showed that NASH patients had significantly higher prevalence of hypertension, hyperglycemia, and low HDL-C as compared with patients with NAFL. Moreover, the NASH patients had a higher BMI and waist circumference. These findings have been corroborated in studies comparing individual components and NASH. A study from Spain showed that almost 70% of obese patients have NASH and 41% of them develop significant fibrosis.[96] Another study from Australia involving severely obese patients showed that IR, elevated alanine aminotransferase levels and hypertension independently predict NASH.[97] Similarly, a Chinese study evaluated 95 NAFLD patients and compared the NASH and non-NASH patients and found that diagnosis of NASH significantly correlated with higher TG, BMI, and waist-to-hip ratio, among other variables.[98] A study from Europe showed that a diagnosis of NASH corresponded to high TG, low HDL-C, and high ferritin.[99] Similarly, a study involving bariatric surgery patients from the United States showed that 58% of NASH patients had high TG compared with only 32% in individuals with simple steatosis.[100] Another American study involving morbidly obese patients analyzed predictors of NASH and showed that the prevalence of hypertension and hyperlipidemia was significantly higher in NASH patients as compared with those with NAFL.[101]

Role of Glucose Intolerance

Multiple studies have evaluated the role of hyperglycemia in NASH. A study from Taiwan showed that high fasting glucose, hypertension, and MetS were associated with increased risk of NASH.[92] Similarly, a Scandinavian study showed that abnormal glucose tolerance was an independent risk factor for NASH.[102] MetS can itself increase the risk of developing impaired glucose tolerance as shown by Love-Osborne and colleagues[103] in a study involving adolescents. A study from Israel followed 141 patients with NAFLD over 7 years and showed that NAFLD has a high prediction rate for developing prediabetes and is a stronger risk factor than MetS.[104] Another prospective study from Sri Lanka followed NAFLD patients from 2007 to 2010. About 20% of NAFLD patients developed type 2 diabetes mellitus at the end of the study, which further emphasizes the bidirectional nature of the pathogenesis of NAFLD.[105]

TREATMENT

Several treatment options for NASH have been examined and based on the likely pathophysiologic mechanisms. Therefore, various management strategies use ways to decrease IR and improve risk factors for MetS or possibly protect the liver from oxidative stress that might lead to NASH.[106]

Decrease in Insulin Resistance

Lifestyle changes
Presently, weight loss through diet and exercise is considered the definitive treatment for NASH[4] (**Table 3**). Studies have shown that dietary changes involving calorie

Table 3
Treatment of NASH based on its pathophysiology, which depends on IR and MetS

Pathophysiology	Treatment	Comments
Decrease in insulin resistance through weight loss	Diet and exercise Bariatric surgery	Treatment of choice Bariatric surgery is useful in reversing NASH in morbidly obese patients
Insulin sensitizing agents	TZDs Metformin	TZDs can be useful until discontinued, concern for side effects Metformin lacks significant response in NASH
Reduction in oxidative stress	Vitamin E	May help to improve NASH but no effect on fibrosis
Modification of MetS risk factors: hyperlipidemia	Antihyperlipidemic drugs: statins, fibrates, and ezetimibe	Large RCTs are lacking but smaller studies have also not shown any benefit Ezetimibe may be useful but there is concern for side effects
Modification of MetS risk factors: hypertension, RAS pathway inhibition leads to reversal of fibrogenesis	RAS blockers such as telmisartan and valsartan	May have use in improving NASH and fibrosis Further large RCTs are needed

Abbreviations: IR, insulin resistance; MetS, metabolic syndrome; NASH, nonalcoholic steatohepatitis; RAS, renin angiotensin system; RCT, randomized controlled trials; TZDs, thiazolidinediones.

restriction by following a low carbohydrate, low fat diet along with physical activity can lead to improvement in liver histology.[107] A recent Chinese study involving more than 1000 patients showed that lifestyle changes involving change in dietary habits, physical activity, and behavioral therapy lead to significant improvement in BMI, waist circumference, IR, NAFLD, and MetS rate after 1 year compared with control group.[108] Weight loss of 7% or greater through change in diet, exercise, and behavioral therapy can lead to reversal of NASH.[109]

Pharmaceutical insulin sensitization

Pharmacologic therapy should be used if lifestyle changes fail to cause improvement or patients are unable to follow the dietary and exercise recommendations.[7] It may also be beneficial in patients at high risk for the development of advanced fibrosis.[106] Pharmacologic agents useful in NASH include medications that cause decrease in IR or oxidative stress.

Thiazolidinediones such as pioglitazone and rosiglitazone are insulin-sensitizing agents that have shown promising results. In the PIVENS (Pioglitazone, Vitamin E, or Placebo for Nonalcoholic Steatohepatitis) trial, pioglitazone showed improvement in histology in nondiabetic NASH patients although the improvement in NAS of 2 or greater did not attain significance.[110] Smaller studies did show significant improvement in histology and insulin sensitivity with pioglitazone.[111,112] Similar smaller studies with rosiglitazone have shown comparable results, although some of the beneficial effects of these drugs can be lost on discontinuation of the drug.[113,114] Overall, thiazolidinediones cause improvement in liver histology in NASH patients, although there is some concern for ankle edema and weight gain as potential side effects.[115] Metformin is another insulin-sensitizing agent, but studies have not shown any significant biochemical or histologic response in NASH patients.[116]

Bariatric surgery

Multiple studies have shown that bariatric surgery in morbidly obese patients can cause significant improvement in histology after weight loss associated with these surgeries. One study followed 18 NASH patients over 2 years after bariatric surgery and showed that about 60% weight loss can cause resolution of steatosis in 84%, disappearance of fibrosis in three-quarters of patients and of ballooning in one-half of the subjects.[117] Another prospective study followed 381 morbidly obese patients after bariatric surgery and showed that after 1 and 5 years there was significant improvement in every histologic feature of NASH, except for slight worsening of fibrosis in about 20% patients at 5 years.[118] Furthermore, improvement in IR corresponded with the improvement in liver histology at 1 year and was maintained at the 5-year follow-up. These findings have been confirmed by metaanalyses that showed that bariatric surgery leads to improvement in steatosis, necroinflammation, and fibrosis.[119]

Reduction in oxidative stress

Vitamin E is an antioxidant that can lead to significant improvement in NASH by improving steatosis, lobular inflammation, and ballooning without any significant decrease in fibrosis.[110,120] Although a small study showed that a combination of vitamins E and C can lead to reduction in fibrosis,[121] a meta-analyses of various randomized controlled trials failed to show this benefit.[119]

Modification of Risk Factors for the Metabolic Syndrome

Statins

Although the hepatic safety of statins has been accepted in NAFLD patients,[122] their beneficial effects are limited to improvement in liver enzymes and steatosis.[123]

Although there is a dearth of randomized controlled trials involving statins, smaller studies lacked histologic analysis[123] or did not show any significant improvement in histology in NASH patients.[124]

Fibrates

Similar to statins, fibrates such as fenofibrate and gemfibrozil have been studies in small studies and they have shown a biochemical response in NASH patients without any significant histologic improvement.[125,126]

Niemann–Pick C1-like 1 inhibitor

Recent studies have linked the role of dietary cholesterol in causing liver inflammation in hyperlipidemic mice models.[127] This inflammation leads to NASH and ezetimibe can potentially reverse NAFLD in these mice.[128] Ezetimibe has been shown to lead to both biochemical and histologic regression of NASH in small studies without significant change in fibrosis.[129,130] However, a recent open-label randomized controlled trials has shown concerning results. This Japanese study showed improvement in liver fibrosis and ballooning scores, but concurrently led to increase in hepatic long-chain fatty acids and hemoglobin A1c.[131] Moreover, the hepatic gene expression analysis was worrisome for oxidative stress, although there was inhibition of fibrogenesis.

Antihypertensive medications

Recent work has described the role of RAS pathway inhibition in reversal of fibrogenesis.[132] This prompted researchers to study RAS inhibitors such as angiotensin receptor blockers as a potential therapeutic option in NASH. In 1 randomized controlled trial, both telmisartan and valsartan caused significant biochemical improvement. However, the telmisartan group had a significantly greater improvement in the Homeostasis Model Assessment of IR, steatosis, necroinflammation, and fibrosis, possibly related to its peroxisome proliferator activated receptor-γ–regulating activity.[133] Another recent study evaluated 290 NAFLD hypertensive patients treated with or without RAS blockers. It showed that patients on RAS blockers had significantly lower fibrosis and ballooning scores.[134]

PROGNOSIS

Overall, mortality in NAFLD patients is significantly higher than general population and is significantly more likely to be liver related. Presence of impaired fasting glucose, advanced age, and cirrhosis are associated with increased risk of death in the NAFLD population.[135] Data from NHANES III (1988–1994) was used in a study to show that MetS, IR, obesity, and diabetes mellitus are independent predictors of liver related mortality in NAFLD.[136] Another study used the NHANES III data and evaluated the long-term mortality of NAFLD patients with and without MetS. The study showed that presence of MetS in NAFLD was an independent predictor of all-cause, liver-related, and cardiovascular mortality.[137] Moreover, the prognosis of NAFLD patients without MetS was similar to patients without liver disease. Among NAFLD patients, NASH patients have a significantly higher risk of liver-related mortality as compared with non-NASH patients.[138]

SUMMARY

There is high prevalence of MetS and NASH in Western countries and the gap in prevalence between the industrialized and the third world is narrowing progressively. Although the pathogenesis of these 2 disease processes is closely linked to IR, other mechanisms such as genetic polymorphisms are definitely at play because not all patients with MetS and hepatic steatosis develop NASH. Further evaluation of the potential role of innate immunity along with the gut microbiome is needed to clarify the pathophysiology of NASH. The association between MetS, its risk factors, IR, and NASH is well-documented, but prospective studies to explain whether one leads to the other or whether they work in a vicious cycle are needed. Although current treatment involves a management strategy, which primarily involves reduction in IR through lifestyle changes, there is a lack of highly effective pharmacologic agents. Apart from identifying the complete mechanism of development of NASH, further research into the role of primary prevention strategies and early diagnostic workup may be needed in patients at high risk of developing NASH owing to the significant mortality associated with this disease.

REFERENCES

1. Ford ES. Risks for all-cause mortality, cardiovascular disease, and diabetes associated with the metabolic syndrome: a summary of the evidence. Diabetes Care 2005;28(7):1769–78.
2. Reaven GM. Banting lecture 1988. Role of insulin resistance in human disease. Diabetes 1988;37(12):1595–607.
3. Reaven GM. Banting lecture 1988. Role of insulin resistance in human disease. 1988. Nutrition 1997;13(1):65 [discussion: 64, 66].
4. Machado M, Cortez-Pinto H. Non-alcoholic steatohepatitis and metabolic syndrome. Curr Opin Clin Nutr Metab Care 2006;9(5):637–42.
5. Chalasani N, Younossi Z, Levine JE, et al. The diagnosis and management of non-alcoholic fatty liver disease: practice guideline by the American Association for the Study of Liver Diseases, American College of Gastroenterology, and the American Gastroenterological Association. Hepatology 2012;55(6):2005–23.
6. Wong RJ, Ahmed A. Obesity and non-alcoholic fatty liver disease: disparate associations among Asian populations. World J Hepatol 2014;6(5):263–73.
7. Neuschwander-Tetri BA. Nonalcoholic steatohepatitis and the metabolic syndrome. Am J Med Sci 2005;330(6):326–35.
8. Kleiner DE, Brunt EM, Van Natta M, et al. Design and validation of a histological scoring system for nonalcoholic fatty liver disease. Hepatology 2005;41(6):1313–21.
9. Marchesini G, Bugianesi E, Forlani G, et al. Nonalcoholic fatty liver, steatohepatitis, and the metabolic syndrome. Hepatology 2003;37(4):917–23.
10. Alberti KG, Eckel RH, Grundy SM, et al. Harmonizing the metabolic syndrome: a joint interim statement of the international diabetes federation task force on epidemiology and prevention; national heart, lung, and blood institute; American heart association; World heart federation; International atherosclerosis society; and International association for the study of obesity. Circulation 2009;120(16):1640–5.
11. Brunt EM, Kleiner DE, Wilson LA, et al, NASH Clinical Research Network (CRN). Nonalcoholic fatty liver disease (NAFLD) activity score and the histopathologic diagnosis in NAFLD: distinct clinicopathologic meanings. Hepatology 2011;53(3):810–20.
12. Beltrán-Sánchez H, Harhay MO, Harhay MM, et al. Prevalence and trends of metabolic syndrome in the adult U.S. population, 1999-2010. J Am Coll Cardiol 2013;62(8):697–703.
13. Ford ES, Li C, Zhao G. Prevalence and correlates of metabolic syndrome based on a harmonious definition among adults in the US. J Diabetes 2010;2(3):180–93.

14. Smits MM, Ioannou GN, Boyko EJ, et al. Non-alcoholic fatty liver disease as an independent manifestation of the metabolic syndrome: results of a US national survey in three ethnic groups. J Gastroenterol Hepatol 2013;28(4):664–70.
15. Cameron AJ, Shaw JE, Zimmet PZ. The metabolic syndrome: prevalence in worldwide populations. Endocrinol Metab Clin North Am 2004;33(2):351–75.
16. Vernon G, Baranova A, Younossi ZM. Systematic review: the epidemiology and natural history of non-alcoholic fatty liver disease and non-alcoholic steatohepatitis in adults. Aliment Pharmacol Ther 2011;34(3):274–85.
17. Farrell GC, Larter CZ. Nonalcoholic fatty liver disease: from steatosis to cirrhosis. Hepatology 2006;43(2 Suppl 1):S99–112.
18. McCullough AJ. The clinical features, diagnosis and natural history of nonalcoholic fatty liver disease. Clin Liver Dis 2004;8:521–33.
19. Mohan V, Farooq S, Deepa M, et al. Prevalence of non-alcoholic fatty liver disease in urban south Indians in relation to different grades of glucose intolerance and metabolic syndrome. Diabetes Res Clin Pract 2009;84(1):84–91.
20. Lee K, Sung JA, Kim JS, et al. The roles of obesity and gender on the relationship between metabolic risk factors and non-alcoholic fatty liver disease in Koreans. Diabetes Metab Res Rev 2009;25(2):150–5.
21. Akahoshi M, Amasaki Y, Soda M, et al. Correlation between fatty liver and coronary risk factors: a population study of elderly men and women in Nagasaki, Japan. Hypertens Res 2001;24(4):337–43.
22. Duseja A, Singh SP, Saraswat VA, et al. Non-alcoholic fatty liver disease and metabolic syndrome-position paper of the Indian National Association for the Study of the Liver, Endocrine Society of India, Indian College of Cardiology and Indian Society of Gastroenterology. J Clin Exp Hepatol 2015;5(1):51–68.
23. Reaven GM. Insulin resistance, the insulin resistance syndrome, and cardiovascular disease. Panminerva Med 2005;47(4):201–10.
24. Abate N, Garg A, Peshock RM, et al. Relationship of generalized and regional adiposity to insulin sensitivity in men with NIDDM. Diabetes 1996;45(12):1684–93.
25. Gallagher EJ, Leroith D, Karnieli E. The metabolic syndrome–from insulin resistance to obesity and diabetes. Med Clin North Am 2011;95(5):855–73.
26. Bugianesi E, Gastaldelli A, Vanni E, et al. Insulin resistance in non-diabetic patients with non-alcoholic fatty liver disease: sites and mechanisms. Diabetologia 2005;48(4):634–42.
27. Yamaguchi K, Yang L, McCall S, et al. Inhibiting triglyceride synthesis improves hepatic steatosis but exacerbates liver damage and fibrosis in obese mice with nonalcoholic steatohepatitis. Hepatology 2007;45(6):1366–74.
28. Feldstein AE, Werneburg NW, Canbay A, et al. Free fatty acids promote hepatic lipotoxicity by stimulating TNF-alpha expression via a lysosomal pathway. Hepatology 2004;40(1):185–94.
29. Pessayre D, Fromenty B. NASH: a mitochondrial disease. J Hepatol 2005;42(6):928–40.
30. Charlton M, Krishnan A, Viker K, et al. Fast food diet mouse: novel small animal model of NASH with ballooning, progressive fibrosis, and high physiological fidelity to the human condition. Am J Physiol Gastrointest Liver Physiol 2011;301(5):G825–34.
31. Kohli R, Kirby M, Xanthakos SA, et al. High-fructose, medium chain trans fat diet induces liver fibrosis and elevates plasma coenzyme Q9 in a novel murine model of obesity and nonalcoholic steatohepatitis. Hepatology 2010;52(3):934–44.

32. Tetri LH, Basaranoglu M, Brunt EM, et al. Severe NAFLD with hepatic necroin-flammatory changes in mice fed trans fats and a high-fructose corn syrup equivalent. Am J Physiol Gastrointest Liver Physiol 2008;295(5):G987–95.
33. Neuschwander-Tetri BA, Ford DA, Acharya S, et al. Dietary trans-fatty acid induced NASH is normalized following loss of trans-fatty acids from hepatic lipid pools. Lipids 2012;47(10):941–50.
34. Mells JE, Fu PP, Kumar P, et al. Saturated fat and cholesterol are critical to inducing murine metabolic syndrome with robust nonalcoholic steatohepatitis. J Nutr Biochem 2015;26(3):285–92.
35. Musso G, Gambino R, De Michieli F, et al. Dietary habits and their relations to insulin resistance and postprandial lipemia in nonalcoholic steatohepatitis. Hepatology 2003;37(4):909–16.
36. Petersen KF, Dufour S, Hariri A, et al. Apolipoprotein C3 gene variants in nonalcoholic fatty liver disease. N Engl J Med 2010;362(12):1082–9.
37. Romeo S, Kozlitina J, Xing C, et al. Genetic variation in PNPLA3 confers susceptibility to nonalcoholic fatty liver disease. Nat Genet 2008;40(12):1461–5.
38. Karpe F, Dickmann JR, Frayn KN. Fatty acids, obesity, and insulin resistance: time for a reevaluation. Diabetes 2011;60(10):2441–9.
39. Boden G, Lebed B, Schatz M, et al. Effects of acute changes of plasma free fatty acids on intramyocellular fat content and insulin resistance in healthy subjects. Diabetes 2001;50(7):1612–7.
40. Kelley DE, Mokan M, Simoneau JA, et al. Interaction between glucose and free fatty acid metabolism in human skeletal muscle. J Clin Invest 1993;92(1):91–8.
41. LeRoith D, Cohen DH. Obesity, type 2 diabetes, and cancer: the insulin and IGF connection. Endocr Relat Cancer 2012;19(5):F27–45.
42. Donnelly KL, Smith CI, Schwarzenberg SJ, et al. Sources of fatty acids stored in liver and secreted via lipoproteins in patients with nonalcoholic fatty liver disease. J Clin Invest 2005;115(5):1343–51.
43. Zarember KA, Godowski PJ. Tissue expression of human Toll-like receptors and differential regulation of Toll-like receptor mRNAs in leukocytes in response to microbes, their products, and cytokines. J Immunol 2002;168(2):554–61.
44. Jialal I, Huet BA, Kaur H, et al. Increased toll-like receptor activity in patients with metabolic syndrome. Diabetes Care 2012;35(4):900–4.
45. Bhargava P, Lee CH. Role and function of macrophages in the metabolic syndrome. Biochem J 2012;442(2):253–62.
46. Tsukumo DM, Carvalho-Filho MA, Carvalheira JB, et al. Loss-of-function mutation in Toll-like receptor 4 prevents diet-induced obesity and insulin resistance. Diabetes 2007;56(8):1986–98.
47. Miura K, Kodama Y, Inokuchi S, et al. Toll-like receptor 9 promotes steatohepatitis by induction of interleukin-1beta in mice. Gastroenterology 2010;139(1):323–34.
48. Miura K, Seki E, Ohnishi H, et al. Role of toll-like receptors and their downstream molecules in the development of nonalcoholic fatty liver disease. Gastroenterol Res Pract 2010;2010:362847.
49. Roth CL, Elfers CT, Figlewicz DP, et al. Vitamin D deficiency in obese rats exacerbates nonalcoholic fatty liver disease and increases hepatic resistin and Toll-like receptor activation. Hepatology 2012;55(4):1103–11.
50. Buettner C, Muse ED, Cheng A, et al. Leptin controls adipose tissue lipogenesis via central, STAT3-independent mechanisms. Nat Med 2008;14(6):667–75.
51. Shimabukuro M, Koyama K, Chen G, et al. Direct antidiabetic effect of leptin through triglyceride depletion of tissues. Proc Natl Acad Sci U S A 1997;94(9):4637–41.

52. Kalra SP. Disruption in the leptin-NPY link underlies the pandemic of diabetes and metabolic syndrome: new therapeutic approaches. Nutrition 2008;24(9): 820–6.

53. Münzberg H, Myers MG Jr. Molecular and anatomical determinants of central leptin resistance. Nat Neurosci 2005;8(5):566–70.

54. Rabe K, Lehrke M, Parhofer KG, et al. Adipokines and insulin resistance. Mol Med 2008;14(11–12):741–51.

55. Chiturri S, Farrell G, Frost L, et al. Serum leptin in NASH correlates with hepatic steatosis but not fibrosis: a manifestation of lipotoxicity? Hepatology 2002;36(2): 403–9.

56. Yamauchi T, Kamon J, Waki H, et al. The fat-derived hormone adiponectin reverses insulin resistance associated with both lipoatrophy and obesity. Nat Med 2001;7(8):941–6.

57. Kondo H, Shimomura I, Matsukawa Y, et al. Association of adiponectin mutation with type 2 diabetes: a candidate gene for the insulin resistance syndrome. Diabetes 2002;51(7):2325–8.

58. Musso G, Gambino R, Biroli G, et al. Hypoadiponectinemia predicts the severity of hepatic fibrosis and pancreatic Beta-cell dysfunction in nondiabetic nonobese patients with nonalcoholic steatohepatitis. Am J Gastroenterol 2005; 100(11):2438–46.

59. Musso G, Gambino R, Durazzo M, et al. Adipokines in NASH: postprandial lipid metabolism as a link between adiponectin and liver disease. Hepatology 2005; 42(5):1175–83.

60. Kaser S, Moschen A, Cayon A, et al. Adiponectin and its receptors in nonalcoholic steatohepatitis. Gut 2005;54(1):117–21.

61. Handa P, Maliken B, Nelson JE, et al. Reduced adiponectin signaling due to weight gain results in nonalcoholic steatohepatitis through impaired mitochondrial biogenesis. Hepatology 2014;60(1):133–45.

62. Musso G, Cassader M, De Michieli F, et al. Nonalcoholic steatohepatitis versus steatosis: adipose tissue insulin resistance and dysfunctional response to fat ingestion predict liver injury and altered glucose and lipoprotein metabolism. Hepatology 2012;56(3):933–42.

63. Tilg H, Diehl AM. Cytokines in alcoholic and nonalcoholic steatohepatitis. N Engl J Med 2000;343(20):1467–76.

64. Li Z, Yang S, Lin H, et al. Probiotics and antibodies to TNF inhibit inflammatory activity and improve nonalcoholic fatty liver disease. Hepatology 2003;37(2): 343–50.

65. Koves TR, Ussher JR, Noland RC, et al. Mitochondrial overload and incomplete fatty acid oxidation contribute to skeletal muscle insulin resistance. Cell Metab 2008;7(1):45–56.

66. Begricke K, Igoudjil A, Pessayre D, et al. Mitochondrial dysfunction in NASH: causes, consequences and possible means to prevent it. Mitochondrion 2006;6(1):1–28.

67. Asrih M, Jornayvaz FR. Metabolic syndrome and nonalcoholic fatty liver disease: is insulin resistance the link? Mol Cell Endocrinol 2015. [Epub ahead of print].

68. Gallagher EJ, Leroith D, Karnieli E. Insulin resistance in obesity as the underlying cause for the metabolic syndrome. Mt Sinai J Med 2010;77(5):511–23.

69. Muoio DM, Newgard CB. Mechanisms of disease: molecular and metabolic mechanisms of insulin resistance and beta-cell failure in type 2 diabetes. Nat Rev Mol Cell Biol 2008;9(3):193–205.

70. Tooke JE, Hannemann MM. Adverse endothelial function and the insulin resistance syndrome. J Intern Med 2000;247(4):425–31.

71. DeFronzo RA, Cooke CR, Andres R, et al. The effect of insulin on renal handling of sodium, potassium, calcium, and phosphate in man. J Clin Invest 1975;55(4): 845–55.

72. Barbato A, Cappuccio FP, Folkerd EJ, et al. Metabolic syndrome and renal sodium handling in three ethnic groups living in England. Diabetologia 2004;47(1): 40–6.

73. Massiera F, Bloch-Faure M, Ceiler D, et al. Adipose angiotensinogen is involved in adipose tissue growth and blood pressure regulation. FASEB J 2001;15(14): 2727–9.

74. Rahmouni K, Correia ML, Haynes WG, et al. Obesity-associated hypertension: new insights into mechanisms. Hypertension 2005;45(1):9–14.

75. Ginsberg HN, Stalenhoef AF. The metabolic syndrome: targeting dyslipidaemia to reduce coronary risk. J Cardiovasc Risk 2003;10(2):121–8.

76. Lewis GF, Uffelman KD, Szeto LW, et al. Interaction between free fatty acids and insulin in the acute control of very low density lipoprotein production in humans. J Clin Invest 1995;95(1):158–66.

77. Kirk EP, Klein S. Pathogenesis and pathophysiology of the cardiometabolic syndrome. J Clin Hypertens (Greenwich) 2009;11(12):761–5.

78. Hopkins GJ, Barter PJ. Role of triglyceride-rich lipoproteins and hepatic lipase in determining the particle size and composition of high density lipoproteins. J Lipid Res 1986;27(12):1265–77.

79. Tilg H, Moschen AR. Evolution of inflammation in nonalcoholic fatty liver disease: the multiple parallel hits hypothesis. Hepatology 2010;52(5):1836–46.

80. Ley RE, Bäckhed F, Turnbaugh P. Obesity alters gut microbial ecology. Proc Natl Acad Sci U S A 2005;102(31):11070–5.

81. Ley RE, Turnbaugh PJ, Klein S, et al. Microbial ecology: human gut microbes associated with obesity. Nature 2006;444(7122):1022–3.

82. Vrieze A, Van Nood E, Holleman F, et al. Transfer of intestinal microbiota from lean donors increases insulin sensitivity in individuals with metabolic syndrome. Gastroenterology 2012;143(4):913–6.

83. Mattace Raso G, Simeoli R, Russo R, et al. Effects of sodium butyrate and its synthetic amide derivative on liver inflammation and glucose tolerance in an animal model of steatosis induced by high fat diet. PLoS One 2013;8(7):e68626.

84. Marceau P, Biron S, Hould FS. 1999 Liver pathology and the metabolic syndrome X in severe obesity. J Clin Endocrinol Metab 1999;84(5):1513–7.

85. Marchesini G, Brizi M, Bianchi G, et al. Nonalcoholic fatty liver disease: a feature of the metabolic syndrome. Diabetes 2001;50(8):1844–50.

86. Shen YH, Yang WS, Lee LT, et al. Bright liver and alanine aminotransferase are associated with metabolic syndrome in adults. Obes Res 2005;13(7): 1238–45.

87. Bedogni G, Miglioli L, Masutti F, et al. Prevalence of and risk factors for nonalcoholic fatty liver disease: the dionysos nutrition and liver study. Hepatology 2005;42(1):44–52.

88. Jung KY, Cho SY, Kim HJ, et al. Nonalcoholic steatohepatitis associated with metabolic syndrome: relationship to insulin resistance and liver histology. J Clin Gastroenterol 2014;48(10):883–8.

89. Patton HM, Yates K, Unalp-Arida A, et al. Association between metabolic syndrome and liver histology among children with nonalcoholic Fatty liver disease. Am J Gastroenterol 2010;105(9):2093–102.

90. Manco M, Marcellini M, Devito R, et al. Metabolic syndrome and liver histology in paediatric non-alcoholic steatohepatitis. Int J Obes (Lond) 2008;32(2):381-7.
91. Uslusoy HS, Nak SG, Gülten M, et al. Liver histology according to the presence of metabolic syndrome in nonalcoholic fatty liver disease cases. World J Gastroenterol 2009;15(9):1093-8.
92. Huang HL, Lin WY, Lee LT, et al. Metabolic syndrome is related to nonalcoholic steatohepatitis in severely obese subjects. Obes Surg 2007;17(11):1457-63.
93. Ong JP, Elariny H, Collantes R, et al. Predictors of nonalcoholic steatohepatitis and advanced fibrosis in morbidly obese patients. Obes Surg 2005;15(3): 310-5.
94. Kroh M, Liu R, Chand B. Laparoscopic bariatric surgery: what else are we uncovering? Liver pathology and preoperative indicators of advanced liver disease in morbidly obese patients. Surg Endosc 2007;21(11):1957-60.
95. Anty R, Iannelli A, Patouraux S, et al. A new composite model including metabolic syndrome, alanine aminotransferase and cytokeratin-18 for the diagnosis of non-alcoholic steatohepatitis in morbidly obese patients. Aliment Pharmacol Ther 2010;32(11-12):1315-22.
96. Wang Y, Li YY, Nie YQ, et al. Association between metabolic syndrome and the development of non-alcoholic fatty liver disease. Exp Ther Med 2013;6(1):77-84.
97. García-Monzón C, Martín-Pérez E, Iacono OL, et al. Characterization of pathogenic and prognostic factors of nonalcoholic steatohepatitis associated with obesity. J Hepatol 2000;33(5):716-24.
98. Dixon JB, Bhathal PS, O'Brien PE. Nonalcoholic fatty liver disease: predictors of nonalcoholic steatohepatitis and liver fibrosis in the severely obese. Gastroenterology 2001;121(1):91-100.
99. Puljiz Z, Stimac D, Kovac D, et al. Predictors of nonalcoholic steatohepatitis in patients with elevated alanine aminotransferase activity. Coll Antropol 2010; 34(Suppl 1):33-7.
100. Ulitsky A, Ananthakrishnan AN, Komorowski R, et al. A noninvasive clinical scoring model predicts risk of nonalcoholic steatohepatitis in morbidly obese patients. Obes Surg 2010;20(6):685-91.
101. Campos GM, Bambha K, Vittinghoff E, et al. A clinical scoring system for predicting nonalcoholic steatohepatitis in morbidly obese patients. Hepatology 2008;47(6):1916-23.
102. Haukeland JW, Konopski Z, Linnestad P, et al. Abnormal glucose tolerance is a predictor of steatohepatitis and fibrosis in patients with non-alcoholic fatty liver disease. Scand J Gastroenterol 2005;40(12):1469-77.
103. Love-Osborne KA, Nadeau KJ, Sheeder J, et al. Presence of the metabolic syndrome in obese adolescents predicts impaired glucose tolerance and nonalcoholic fatty liver disease. J Adolesc Health 2008;42(6):543-8.
104. Zelber-Sagi S, Lotan R, Shibolet O, et al. Non-alcoholic fatty liver disease independently predicts prediabetes during a 7-year prospective follow-up. Liver Int 2013;33(9):1406-12.
105. Kasturiratne A, Weerasinghe S, Dassanayake AS, et al. Influence of nonalcoholic fatty liver disease on the development of diabetes mellitus. J Gastroenterol Hepatol 2013;28(1):142-7.
106. Marchesini G, Marzochhi R. Metabolic syndrome and NASH. Clin Liver Dis 2007;11(1):105-17.
107. Eckard C, Cole R, Lockwood J, et al. Prospective histopathologic evaluation of lifestyle modification in nonalcoholic fatty liver disease: a randomized trial. Therap Adv Gastroenterol 2013;6(4):249-59.

108. Sun WH, Song MQ, Jiang CQ, et al. Lifestyle intervention in non-alcoholic fatty liver disease in Chengyang District, Qingdao, China. World J Hepatol 2012;4(7): 224–30.

109. Promrat K, Kleiner DE, Neimeier HM, et al. Randomized controlled trial testing the effects of weight loss on nonalcoholic steatohepatitis. Hepatology 2010; 51(1):121–9.

110. Sanyal AJ, Chalasani N, Kowdley KV, et al. Pioglitazone, vitamin E, or placebo for nonalcoholic steatohepatitis. N Engl J Med 2010;362(18): 1675–85.

111. Belfort R, Harrison SA, Brown K, et al. A placebo-controlled trial of pioglitazone in subjects with nonalcoholic steatohepatitis. N Engl J Med 2006;355(22): 2297–307.

112. Aithal GP, Thomas JA, Kaye PV, et al. Randomized, placebo-controlled trial of pioglitazone in nondiabetic subjects with nonalcoholic steatohepatitis. Gastroenterology 2008;135(4):1176–84.

113. Neuschwander-Tetri BA, Brunt EM, Wehmeier KR, et al. Improved nonalcoholic steatohepatitis after 48 weeks of treatment with the PPAR-gamma ligand rosiglitazone. Hepatology 2003;38(4):1008–17.

114. Torres D, Jones F, Shaw J, et al. Rosiglitazone versus rosiglitazone and metformin versus rosiglitazone and losartan in the treatment of nonalcoholic steatohepatitis in humans: a 12-month randomized, prospective, open- label trial. Hepatology 2011;54(5):1631–9.

115. Musso G, Cassader M, Rosina F, et al. Impact of current treatments on liver disease, glucose metabolism and cardiovascular risk in non-alcoholic fatty liver disease (NAFLD): a systematic review and meta-analysis of randomised trials. Diabetologia 2012;55(4):885–904.

116. Rakoski MO, Singal AG, Rogers MA, et al. Meta-analysis: insulin sensitizers for the treatment of non-alcoholic steatohepatitis. Aliment Pharmacol Ther 2010; 32(10):1211–21.

117. Furuya CK Jr, de Oliveira CP, de Mello ES, et al. Effects of bariatric surgery on nonalcoholic fatty liver disease: preliminary findings after 2 years. J Gastroenterol Hepatol 2007;22(4):510–4.

118. Mathurin P, Hollebecque A, Arnalsteen L, et al. Prospective study of the long-term effects of bariatric surgery on liver injury in patients without advanced disease. Gastroenterology 2009;137(2):532–40.

119. Mummadi RR, Kasturi KS, Chennareddygari S, et al. Effect of bariatric surgery on nonalcoholic fatty liver disease: systematic review and meta-analysis. Clin Gastroenterol Hepatol 2008;6(12):1396–402.

120. Vilar Gomez E, Rodriguez de Miranda A, Gra Oramas B, et al. Clinical trial: a nutritional supplement Viusid, in combination with diet and exercise, in patients with nonalcoholic fatty liver disease. Aliment Pharmacol Ther 2009;30(10): 999–1009.

121. Harrison SA, Torgerson S, Hayashi P, et al. Vitamin E and vitamin C treatment improves fibrosis in patients with nonalcoholic steatohepatitis. Am J Gastroenterol 2003;98(11):2485–90.

122. Cohen DE, Anania FA, Chalasani N, National Lipid Association Statin Safety Task Force Liver Expert Panel. An assessment of statin safety by hepatologists. Am J Cardiol 2006;97(8A):77C–81C.

123. Athyros VG, Mikhailidis DP, Didangelos TP, et al. Effect of multifactorial treatment on non-alcoholic fatty liver disease in metabolic syndrome: a randomised study. Curr Med Res Opin 2006;22(5):873–83.

124. Hyogo H, Ikegami T, Tokushige K, et al. Efficacy of pitavastatin for the treatment of non-alcoholic steatohepatitis with dyslipidemia: an open-label, pilot study. Hepatol Res 2011;41(11):1057–65.
125. Fernandez-Miranda C, Perez-Carreras M, Colina F, et al. A pilot trial of fenofibrate for the treatment of non-alcoholic fatty liver disease. Dig Liver Dis 2008; 40(3):200–5.
126. Basaranoglu M, Acbay O, Sonsuz A. A controlled trial of gemfibrozil in the treatment of patients with nonalcoholic steatohepatitis. J Hepatol 1999;31(2):384.
127. Wouters K, van Gorp PJ, Bieghs V, et al. Dietary cholesterol, rather than liver steatosis, leads to hepatic inflammation in hyperlipidemic mouse models of nonalcoholic steatohepatitis. Hepatology 2008;48(2):474–86.
128. Zheng S, Hoos L, Cook J, et al. Ezetimibe improves high fat and cholesterol diet-induced non-alcoholic fatty liver disease in mice. Eur J Pharmacol 2008;584(1): 118–24.
129. Yoneda M, Fujita K, Nozaki Y, et al. Efficacy of ezetimibe for the treatment of non-alcoholic steatohepatitis: an open-label, pilot study. Hepatol Res 2010;40(6): 566–73.
130. Park H, Shima T, Yamaguchi K, et al. Efficacy of long-term ezetimibe therapy in patients with nonalcoholic fatty liver disease. J Gastroenterol 2011;46(1):101–7.
131. Takeshita Y, Takamura T, Honda M, et al. The effects of ezetimibe on non-alcoholic fatty liver disease and glucose metabolism: a randomised controlled trial. Diabetologia 2014;57(5):878–90.
132. Zvibel I, Bar-Zohar D, Kloog Y, et al. The effect of Ras inhibition on the proliferation, apoptosis and matrix metalloproteases activity in rat hepatic stellate cells. Dig Dis Sci 2008;53(4):1048–53.
133. Georgescu EF, Ionescu R, Niculescu M, et al. Angiotensin-receptor blockers as therapy for mild-to-moderate hypertension-associated non-alcoholic steatohepatitis. World J Gastroenterol 2009;15(8):942–54.
134. Goh GB, Pagadala MR, Dasarathy J, et al. Renin-angiotensin system and fibrosis in non-alcoholic fatty liver disease. Liver Int 2015;35(3):979–85.
135. Adams LA, Lymp JF, St Sauver J, et al. The natural history of nonalcoholic fatty liver disease: a population-based cohort study. Gastroenterology 2005;129(1): 113–21.
136. Stepanova M, Rafiq N, Younossi ZM. Components of metabolic syndrome are independent predictors of mortality in patients with chronic liver disease: a population-based study. Gut 2010;59(10):1410–5.
137. Younossi ZM, Otgonsuren M, Venkatesan C, et al. In patients with non-alcoholic fatty liver disease, metabolically abnormal individuals are at a higher risk for mortality while metabolically normal individuals are not. Metabolism 2013; 62(3):352–60.
138. Stepanova M, Rafiq N, Makhlouf H, et al. Predictors of all-cause mortality and liver-related mortality in patients with non-alcoholic fatty liver disease (NAFLD). Dig Dis Sci 2013;58(10):3017–23.

Empty

Nonalcoholic Fatty Liver Disease

Lipids and Insulin Resistance

Paul D. Berk, MD[a,b],*, Elizabeth C. Verna, MD, MS[a]

KEYWORDS

- Facilitated transport • Leptin • Lipotoxicity • Spexin • Weight regain

KEY POINTS

- Obesity is the increased accumulation of fat (ie, triglycerides [TG]), which are synthesized from glycerol and long chain fatty acids (LCFA) throughout the body.
- LCFA enter adipocytes, hepatocytes, and cardiomyocytes via specific, facilitated transport processes, which are regulated in obesity at least in part by insulin, leptin, and spexin.
- In obesity, metabolism of the increased cellular TG content may lead to cell-specific lipotoxicity, contributing to comorbidities such as nonalcoholic fatty liver disease (NAFLD) and cardiomyopathy.
- Dietary control and bariatric surgery can achieve major weight loss in many patients, but persistent upregulation of LCFA transport contributes to weight regain.
- Better understanding of these transport processes and their regulation may be a key to successful future strategies for treatment of obesity and NAFLD.

INTRODUCTION

Nonalcoholic fatty liver disease (NAFLD) is frequently described as encompassing a histologic spectrum from simple hepatic steatosis (SHS) or nonalcoholic fatty liver (NAFL) to SHS plus a characteristic pattern of steatohepatitis (nonalcoholic steatohepatitis [NASH]), to steatosis or steatohepatitis associated with fibrosis, cirrhosis,

Disclosure: The authors have nothing to disclose.
Funding: Supported by grant #5U01DK066667-11 Revised, Bariatric Surgery: Outcomes and Impact on Pathophysiology, from the National Institute of Diabetes and Digestive and Kidney Diseases of the National Institutes of Health.
[a] Division of Digestive and Liver Diseases, Department of Medicine, Columbia College of Physicians and Surgeons, Columbia University Medical Center, 650 West 168 Street, New York, NY 10032, USA; [b] Division of Preventive Medicine, Department of Medicine, Columbia College of Physicians and Surgeons, Columbia University Medical Center, William Black Building, 650 West 168 Street, Room 1006, Box 57A, New York, NY 10032, USA
* Corresponding author. Columbia University Medical Center, William Black Building, 650 West 168 Street, Room 1006, Box 57A, New York, NY 10032.
E-mail address: pb2158@cumc.columbia.edu

Clin Liver Dis 20 (2016) 245–262
http://dx.doi.org/10.1016/j.cld.2015.10.007
1089-3261/16/$ – see front matter © 2016 Elsevier Inc. All rights reserved.

and/or hepatocellular carcinoma (HCC).[1–5] Its various features have widely been considered to reflect hepatic manifestations of the metabolic syndrome (Met-Syn).[6–8] Although worldwide prevalence and incidence rates of NAFLD/NASH are not known precisely,[7] it is thought to have become the world's most prevalent liver disease.[9] NAFLD is linked to obesity and insulin resistance in Western cultures, but histologically similar NAFL and NASH both occur at lower body mass indices (BMIs) in Asian countries, where many patients also lack the insulin resistance typical in the west.[10,11] Genome-wide association studies and other approaches to studying NAFLD genomics are helping to understand both geographic differences and an increasing number of genetic differences within the Western NAFLD population (eg, Refs.[12,13]). This article focuses on obesity and NAFLD in the Western world.

The earlier literature indicated that NAFL and NASH were part of a clinical as well as a histologic continuum, in which SHS progressed to NASH, which could progress further to NASH with fibrosis, cirrhosis, and/or HCC.[4,5] However, although progression from NASH to NASH with fibrosis, cirrhosis, and/or HCC is by now well documented, the frequency of evolution from SHS to NASH is unclear.[5,7] Absent reliable surrogate markers, serial liver biopsies might be expected to be the gold standard for making this determination, but their invasiveness and issues with regard to their interpretation[5] have limited their deployment for this purpose. As of mid-2015, our literature searches identified only 16 articles, including less than or equal to 500 of a world-wide population of millions of patients with NAFLD, that examined the histologic evolution of steatosis, steatohepatitis, and fibrosis in NAFLD via paired liver biopsies (eg, Refs.[14–24]). Collectively, these articles suggested that development and progression of fibrosis in NAFL was uncommon, whereas fibrosis in NASH occurred and progressed more frequently. However, the most recent studies have challenged even this, suggesting that NAFL can occasionally evolve all the way to NASH with advanced fibrosis, implying that NAFL may not be the benign entity it is often considered.[23,24] A useful editorial summarizes the current data.[25] The view of NAFLD as an evolving continuum has also been challenged by claims that NAFL and NASH are distinct disease entities rather than points on a continuum.[9,26,27]

FATTY ACIDS, TRIGLYCERIDES, AND NONALCOHOLIC FATTY LIVER DISEASE PATHOPHYSIOLOGY

Most NAFLD in the Western world evolves on a background of obesity. Obesity is the increased accumulation of fat (ie, triglycerides [TG]), synthesized from glycerol and long-chain fatty acids (LCFA), throughout the body. TG are stored in large lipid droplets in adipocytes and smaller droplets in parenchymal cells, notably hepatocytes[28,29] and cardiomyocytes.[30] In obesity, metabolism of increased TG in parenchymal cells leads to cell-specific lipotoxicity. This article therefore concentrates on regulation of LCFA uptake and TG deposition and metabolism in adipocytes and hepatocytes, which are key to the understanding of NAFLD pathogenesis.

Until ~30 years ago it was thought that LCFA entered cells solely by passive diffusion. However, selective TG accumulation at specific sites in obesity clearly indicated that something other than unregulated, passive diffusion was involved.

Uptake of LCFA into hepatocytes, adipocytes, and cardiac myocytes consists of 2 distinct processes, each a function of the unbound LCFA concentration.[31–36] LCFA uptake velocity at any unbound LCFA concentration ([LCFAu]) is the arithmetical sum of a saturable and a nonsaturable function of the corresponding [LCFAu], according to the equation:

$$UT([LCFAu]) = V_{max} \times [LCFAu]/(Km + [LCFAu]) + k \times [LCFAu]$$

where $UT([LCFAu])$ is the experimental measurement of uptake (picomoles per second per 50,000 cells) at the stated concentration of unbound LCFA ([LCFAu]); V_{max} (picomoles per second per 50,000 cells) and Km (nanomolar) are the maximal velocity of saturable LCFA uptake and [LCFAu] at half the maximal uptake velocity, respectively; and k (milliliters per second per 50,000 cells) is the rate constant for nonsaturable uptake. In human studies, V_{max} has been shown to increase as an exponential function of patient BMI (**Fig. 1**).

At normal between-meal LCFA concentrations in mammals ~95% of total cellular LCFA uptake is via the saturable pathway.[34,35] Typical LCFA have a pKi of ~6.5, existing in plasma as a roughly equal mixture of fatty acid anions and uncharged, protonated fatty acids. Studies with the acidic LCFA analogue $\alpha_2,\beta_2,\omega_3$-heptaflourostearate[36] established (1) that saturable uptake reflected protein-mediated, regulatable transport of LCFA anions, whereas nonsaturable uptake represented passive transmembrane diffusion of protonated LCFA; and (2) that the rate of transmembrane LCFA movement by the former process was ~10 times faster than by the latter.[34,35] Subsequently multiple techniques have confirmed that cellular LCFA uptake involves, at least in part, regulatable, facilitated, protein-mediated transport (eg, Refs.[37–42]).

At least 4 proteins or protein families have been proposed as LCFA transporters: plasma membrane fatty acid binding protein (FABPpm)[43,44]; fatty acid translocase (or CD36)[45]; the fatty acid transporting polypeptide (FATP) family,[46,47] and caveolin-1.[48,49] Many reports suggest that additional transporters await discovery.[50,51]

FABPpm, the first LCFA transporter to be identified, proved similar or identical to the mitochondrial isoform of aspartate aminotransferase (mAspAT).[52] Molecular modeling, site-directed mutagenesis, transfection, and intracellular trafficking studies

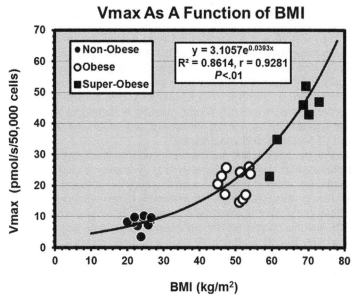

Fig. 1. Relationship of V_{max} for LCFA uptake by isolated human omental adipocytes to patient BMI. Cells were isolated from intraoperative fat biopsies obtained during clinically indicated abdominal surgical procedures in 10 nonobese patients, and during bariatric operations in 10 obese and 7 superobese patients who were participants in a 2-stage bariatric surgical protocol.[67] V_{max} increases as an exponential function of BMI.

proved that mAspAT contained a hydrophobic cleft of proper size to be an LCFA binding site, and that it was capable of facilitating cellular LCFA uptake.[53]

For most metabolic processes, LCFA are activated by esterification to an acyl coenzyme A (CoA) before they are used.[54] LCFA can be activated by 3 related protein families: the long-chain acyl-CoA synthetases, FATPs, and the so-called bubblegum family.[55] Among FATPs, some that are themselves candidate LCFA transporters[46,47] also have CoA enzymatic activity,[56–58] leading to several different models of how FATPs might facilitate LCFA uptake[55]: (1) FATPs could be classic plasma membrane transporters[47]; (2) because FATPs, either individually or in recently described heteromultimers (discussed later), have both transport and esterification activity, the driving force for LCFA transport could come from their enzyme activity via vectorial acylation[58]; (3) FATPs are enzymes, and could enhance uptake indirectly by depleting intracellular LCFA.[59]

LCFA uptake into HepG2 cells was found to be mediated by a heterotetrameric protein complex comprising FABPpm, Cav-1, CD36, and the Ca^{++}-independent membrane phospholipase A_2 ($iPLA_2\beta$).[60] Blocking $iPLA_2\beta$ with a bile acid–phospholipid conjugate dissociated the complex and inhibited LCFA uptake. Use of the same bile acid conjugate in a mouse hepatocyte cell line that showed both steatosis and inflammation decreased LCFA uptake by 56.5% and essentially abolished both steatosis and inflammation. Its role as a potential therapy for NASH is under investigation.

LCFA uptake clearly involves specific transport processes the regulation of which, in adipocytes and hepatocytes, is a key element in the pathogenesis of obesity per se and NAFLD. This recognition has driven a steady increase in PubMed citations about fatty acids and obesity from fewer than 100 per year from the 1960s to mid-1980s to 1200 or more per year by 2014.

LONG-CHAIN FATTY ACID TRANSPORT IN SPECIFIC DISEASE MODELS

At least in the Western world, there is a strong association between obesity and NAFLD. As just described, alterations in adipose tissue LCFA sequestration play an important role in the pathogenesis of obesity, and analogous alterations in hepatocellular LCFA uptake play a similar role in the excess hepatic TG accumulation characterizing SHS. However, in contrast with adipocyte LCFA transport, which has been extensively studied in both rodent and readily available human fat samples, the limited availability of appropriate samples of human liver has largely restricted studies of hepatocellular LCFA uptake to animal tissues.

LCFA uptake by adipocytes, hepatocytes, and cardiac myocytes from rodent models of obesity and obesity-associated fatty liver and cardiomyopathy has been extensively studied, starting with obese, leptin receptor–deficient Zucker fatty (*fa/fa*) and Zucker diabetic fatty (*ZDF*) rats and extending to analogous mouse models.[61–64] The V_{max} for saturable LCFA uptake was dramatically increased in adipocytes from the *fa/fa* and *ZDF* animals compared with nonobese Zucker heterozygous (*fa/+*) or wild-type Wistar strains (**Fig. 2**). Furthermore, V_{max} in rat adipocytes was highly correlated with messenger RNA (mRNA) expression for the LCFA transporter FABPpm. In contrast, there were only minor differences among rat groups in the V_{max} for LCFA uptake into hepatocytes and cardiac myocytes (see **Fig. 2**). Initially surprising, this became an instructive finding, as described later.

Although short-term regulation of adipocyte LCFA uptake in response to meals remains to be better defined, its chronic upregulation characterizes all studied rodent models of obesity, as well as obese humans. Thus, the V_{max} for adipocyte LCFA uptake is markedly increased in genetically obese (*ob/ob*), diabetic (*db/db*), fat (*fat*) and

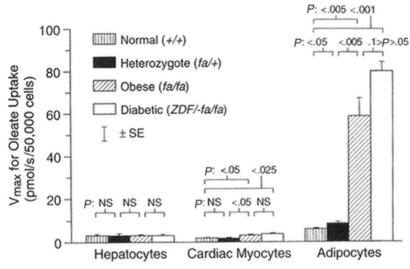

Fig. 2. Computed values of the V_{max} for saturable [^{3}H]-oleate uptake by isolated hepatocytes, cardiac myocytes, and adipocytes from 4 groups of adult male Zucker rats: +/+, fa/+, fa/fa, and ZDF. Saturable adipocyte LCFA uptake is appreciably increased compared with normal controls in the obese *fa/fa* and ZDF animals, despite their defective leptin signaling. There is little change in hepatocyte LCFA uptake in the different groups. Very similar findings have been reported in hepatocytes from obese, leptin signaling–deficient *ob/ob* and *db/db* mice, compared with C57BL6J control mice rendered obese by high-fat diets. (*From* Berk PD, Zhou SL, Bradbury M, et al. Regulated membrane transport of free fatty acids in adipocytes: role in obesity and non–insulin dependent diabetes mellitus. Trans Am Clin Climatol Assoc 1997;108:26–40; with permission.)

tubby (*tub*) mice; in both Wistar and Sprague-Dawley rats and C57BL6/J mice on high-fat diets,[65] and in omental[66,67] and subcutaneous[67] adipocytes from obese patients having bariatric surgery.

In some circumstances, upregulation of adipocyte LCFA uptake precedes onset of obesity,[61] whereas downregulation precedes weight loss.[68] These data support the hypothesis that upregulation of adipocyte LCFA uptake contributes to both regulation of adiposity and the pathogenesis of obesity. Further observations of consistent, tissue-specific upregulation of adipocyte LCFA uptake in association with weight gain have led to speculation that this could also contribute to and regulate LCFA partitioning. Partitioning might serve a protective function. By sequestering LCFA and TG in large droplets and protecting them from oxidative processes, adipocytes serve as a buffer. They protect downstream nonadipose cells, such as pancreatic beta cells, cardiac myocytes, skeletal muscle cells, and hepatocytes, from the lipotoxic consequences of their excessive LCFA and TG accumulation and metabolism to lipotoxic species, including diacylglycerols, ceramides, reactive oxygen species (ROS), and cholesterol.[69,70]

Several diverse lines of evidence thus suggest that regulation of adipocyte LCFA uptake may have a role in controlling body adiposity (eg, Refs.[61,63–66,69,71]). Although primary genetic defects in obesity models[63,64,71] can be expressed either in the central nervous system (CNS) (db mouse, Zucker fatty rat)[72,73] or peripheral tissues (ob mouse),[74] all such defects, rodent models of dietary obesity, and typical examples of human obesity result in selective upregulation of facilitated adipocyte LCFA uptake.

This finding suggests that such regulation may represent a final common pathway for control of adiposity resulting from diverse primary causes in multiple mammalian species, including humans (**Fig. 3**).

Obesity has serious consequences. Available treatments, including diet and lifestyle modifications and bariatric surgery, can achieve significant weight loss in many patients. However, posttreatment weight regain is common, often to levels exceeding the pretreatment value within 5 years.[75,76] Despite both extensive theoretic and clinical studies in humans and the recognized prolonged postoperative persistence of weight gain–promoting hormonal patterns; increased insulin sensitivity, rates of glucose transport, and lipoprotein lipase (LPL) activity; and other metabolic abnormalities,[75,76] these patients are often considered treatment failures, for which they may be blamed. However, in a recent study,[67] [³H]-LCFA uptake kinetics were determined in adipocytes isolated from intraoperative omental and subcutaneous fat biopsies from 10 nonobese, 10 obese, and 10 superobese (SO) patients. The obese and SO patients were undergoing bariatric surgical operations (sleeve gastrectomies); the nonobese patients were having other, clinically indicated, nonbariatric operations. By nonlinear regression, V_{max} for LCFA uptake by omental adipocytes increased exponentially as a function of BMI (r = 0.93; P<.01) in the 3 groups, from 5.1 ± 0.95 to 21.3 ± 3.20 to 68.7 ± 9.45 pmol/s/50,000 cells (see **Fig. 1**). Results in subcutaneous adipocytes were similar. The SO patients returned for second biopsies 16 ± 2 months later, after

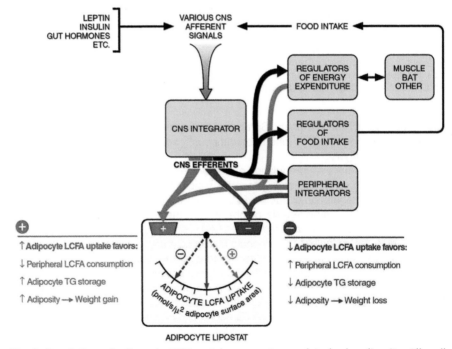

Fig. 3. Regulation of adipocyte LCFA uptake seems to regulate body adiposity. All well-studied genetic and dietary animal models of obesity, as well as obese humans, show selective upregulation of facilitated LCFA by adipocytes. This finding suggests that regulation of adipocyte LCFA uptake represents a final, common pathway for control of body adiposity resulting from a diversity of primary causes. BAT, brown adipose tissue. (*From* Bradbury MW, Berk PD. Lipid metabolism in hepatic steatosis. Clin Liver Dis 2004;8:639–71; with permission.)

losing 51.26 ± 5.9 kg (113 ± 13 lb). Their mean BMI had fallen from 62.6 ± 2.8 to 44.4 ± 2.5 kg/m^2 ($P<.01$), and had become similar to the obese group. However, V_{max} (42.1 ± 6.4 pmol/s/50,000 cells) in the weight-reduced SO group remained upregulated more than 2-fold ($P<.01$) from that predicted for their new BMI by the original BMI:V_{max} regression. Because upregulation of LCFA uptake strongly predicts weight gain, this suggests a biological process rather than failure of patient willpower as contributing to any weight regain.[75,77] These SO patients were a subset of a larger cohort of 2458, treated mainly with either Roux-en-Y gastric bypass or laparoscopic gastric banding in the Longitudinal Assessment of Bariatric Surgery-2 (LABS-2) protocol. Most patients achieved maximum weight loss in the first postoperative year, based on which they were assigned to one of 5 weight trajectory groups. By the end of year 3, all weight trajectory groups showed some degree of weight regain.[78]

Lipotoxicity, Leptin, and Spexin

In severe obesity, excessive LCFA availability can exceed the LCFA storage capacity of adipose tissue. This excess leads to ectopic accumulation of LCFA, TG, and their lipotoxic metabolites in nonadipose cells, and can result in the cellular injury now designated as lipotoxicity. Many obesity comorbidities result from disordered LCFA disposition and/or lipotoxicity.

Leptin is widely considered the principal liporegulatory hormone, exerting profound antisteatotic effects.[79–81] When caloric intake chronically exceeds energy expenditure, TG accumulate throughout the body. This accumulation is amplified by the hyperinsulinemia associated with the excess caloric intake, which also upregulates enzymes involved in lipogenesis. Intermediates in the lipogenic pathway inhibit LCFA oxidation, further increasing the LCFA available for storage as TG. Much of this increase is restricted to adipose tissue, which reflects that, as adipose tissue TG increases, it stimulates an increased release of leptin.[82–84] In some situations, leptin functions as an insulin counter-regulatory hormone,[85] exerting an antilipogenic, pro-oxidative program on peripheral, nonadipose cells.[80,81] In one rodent model of diet-induced obesity, when total body fat had increased 150-fold, with a significant weight regain and increased plasma LCFA, the lipid content of pancreatic islets, liver, heart, and skeletal muscle had increased by no more than 10-fold.[79] With further increases in total body fat, these effects of leptin diminish despite markedly increased plasma leptin concentrations, indicating a state of leptin resistance. The mechanisms underlying leptin resistance remain unclear,[86] but may involve inhibition of brain leptin uptake by circulating n-3 polyunsaturated fatty acids.[87] A total lack of leptin effect occurs in various lipodystrophies, as well as in situations in which leptin signaling is abolished because of either an absence of leptin (*ob/ob* mouse)[74] or an absence or functional mutations of its receptor (*db/db* mouse, Zucker *fa/fa* rat).[72,73] The result is a progressive, generalized steatosis, with ectopic accumulation of TG in nonadipose tissues. The increased ectopic TG pool exchanges with an increased intracellular pool of LCFA, and these enter into nonoxidative pathways, of which the most studied, but not the only one,[88] leads to the accumulation of ceramides and other metabolites.[70,89,90] These metabolites cause extensive tissue damage and apoptosis, resulting in, for example, T2DM, cardiomyopathy, and liver injury, which can be ameliorated to varying degrees when there is a functioning leptin receptor by administration of recombinant leptin.[91] In rodents, lipotoxicity leads to several components of the rodent equivalent of MetSyn. Although evidence that true lipotoxic disease occurs in humans is limited, leptin resistance is characteristic of human obesity, and may permit TG accumulation in ectopic sites. Further studies of this phenomenon in humans are clearly indicated.[89,90]

Spexin

Probing whole human genome microarrays containing 55K genes and expressed sequence tags (EST) led to identification of ~3500 showing significant differences in expression between obese and nonobese human fat. Of these, the gene most extensively regulated was initially identified only as Ch12orf39. Its mRNA was underexpressed 14.9-fold in obese versus nonobese fat, in parallel with a similar decrease in the levels of its circulating gene product, which was subsequently recognized as being identical to spexin, a novel peptide identified by Mirabeau and colleagues[92] in 2007 using Markov modeling. Its regulation relative to BMI, and other observations, led to studies of a possible role in weight control. In mice with diet-induced obesity, spexin administration reduced food intake in the absence of generalized taste aversive effects or evident toxicity, increased energy expenditure (locomotor activity), and decreased the respiratory exchange ratio, favoring burning of fat compared with carbohydrate.[93] Similar effects were found in rats. These results are thought to be mainly centrally mediated. In addition, spexin directly and selectively inhibits LCFA uptake by rodent adipocytes, further contributing to weight loss. In sera from nonobese, obese, and SO patients, spexin concentrations showed a negative, nonlinear correlation with leptin ($r = -0.64$; $P<.01$). Spexin concentrations were also significantly negatively correlated with the V_{max} for omental adipocyte LCFA uptake in the same patient ($r = -0.71$; $P<.01$), whereas leptin was strongly positively correlated with V_{max} ($r = +0.81$; $P<.01$). These and other data indicate that spexin and leptin may play important, antagonistic roles in regulating adipocyte LCFA uptake (**Fig. 4**), which other studies suggest regulates overall adiposity.

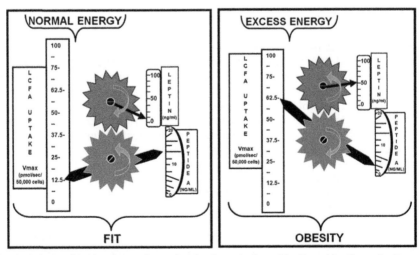

Fig. 4. Relationships between plasma levels of spexin (peptide A) and leptin and adipocyte LCFA uptake. (*Left*) These relationships in the presence of normal energy balance and physical fitness: low levels of leptin and LCFA uptake V_{max}, high levels of spexin. (*Right*) The situation in the presence of excessive energy, leading to obesity: higher levels of leptin and increased LCFA uptake V_{max}, low levels of spexin. The interlocking gears represent the strong, negative correlation between plasma spexin and leptin concentrations, and their respective relationships to the V_{max} for adipocyte LCFA uptake.

OBESITY-RELATED LIVER DISEASE: HEPATIC STEATOSIS AND STEATOHEPATITIS
Hepatic Steatosis

SHS and other stages of NAFLD commonly accompany obesity. More than half of all obese patients have some form of NAFLD; ~ 25% have NASH, with or without significant hepatic fibrosis (eg, Refs.[7–9,94]).

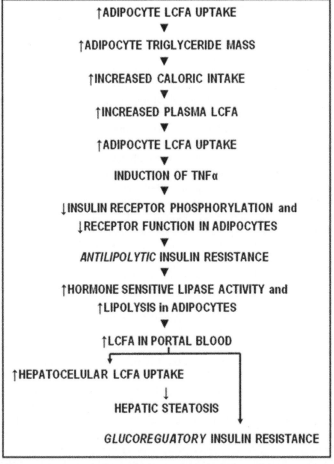

Fig. 5. The road to insulin resistance and hepatic steatosis in obesity. Ten discrete and identifiable steps leading to insulin resistance and hepatic steatosis are initiated by an increase in caloric intake and consequent increase in the plasma concentration of LCFA. TNFα, tumor necrosis factor alpha. (*Adapted from* Bradbury MW, Berk PD. Lipid metabolism in hepatic steatosis. Clin Liver Dis 2004;8:639–71; with permission.)

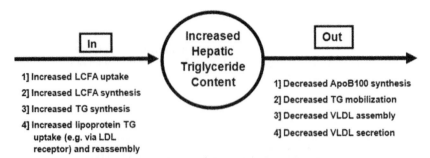

Fig. 6. Processes that could contribute to the increased hepatic TG content that characterizes hepatic steatosis and NASH. Those on the left potentially contribute to an increased input to the hepatocellular pool of TG. Those on the right increase hepatic TG content by decreasing normal levels of TG output, principally in very-low-density lipoprotein (VLDL). LDL, low-density lipoprotein. (*From* Bradbury MW, Berk PD. Lipid metabolism in hepatic steatosis. Clin Liver Dis 2004;8:639–71; with permission.)

Mechanisms of hepatic steatosis

The basis for the development of insulin resistance and SHS in the setting of obesity is clear (**Fig. 5**). Not every case of SHS results from obesity. SHS can potentially result from many different processes. Virtually all of those listed in **Fig. 6** reportedly play a role in one or another model of hepatic steatosis, increasing the hepatocyte TG pool either by ultimately increasing TG input or decreasing output from the pool. Very few studies have assessed several of these processes simultaneously, especially in humans, so their relative contributions remain largely unclear.

Increased hepatocellular LCFA uptake is a major contributor to both obesity-related and ethyl alcohol (EtOH)–related hepatic steatosis in rat and mouse models and human-derived HepG2 cells.[28,95,96] In a mouse study[28] involving C57BL6J controls, similar mice on a high-fat diet or consuming 10%, 14%, or 18% EtOH, designated the functional leptin signaling groups (FLSGs), and leptin signaling–deficient homozygous *ob/ob* and *db/db* animals, the V_{max} for hepatocellular LCFA uptake was significantly increased in all FLSGs, but not in the *ob/ob* and *db/db* animals, which had the heaviest, greasiest livers. There was a highly significant linear correlation between the V_{max} for hepatocellular LCFA uptake and hepatic TG content in the FLSGs, but hepatic TG content in the *ob/ob* and *db/db* animals was considerably above the FLSG regression line, suggesting that a significant part of the hepatic TG content in the *ob/ob* and *db/db* animals was not derived from LCFA uptake.[28]

In FLSGs, despite variably increased expression of single transporter genes in individual EtOH and HFD (high fat diet) groups, the mean expression ratio for FABPpm, FATP1, FATP2, FATP4, FATP5, and CD36 in each group was highly correlated with both V_{max} for hepatocellular LCFA uptake and hepatic TG. V_{max} was also highly correlated with the corresponding expression ratios for Srebp-1c ($r = 0.99$) and NfkB ($r = 0.94$). Increased hepatic TG in *ob/ob* and *db/db* mice did not relate to hepatic LCFA uptake, but instead was highly correlated with increased expression of lipogenic enzymes involved in LCFA synthesis (SCD-1 (stearoyl coenzyme A desaturase-1), FASN [fatty acid synthase]). Thus, hepatic TG is seemingly regulated by the same factors that control a wide array of hepatic lipid metabolic pathways.

Individual FABPpm, *Slc27a2*, Slc27a4, *Slc27a5*, CD36 gene expression ratios were significantly upregulated in a dose-dependent fashion in the EtOH groups, and the mean values for their expression ratios in the different groups were closely correlated with the V_{max} for hepatocellular LCFA uptake. The V_{max} data, in turn, were highly correlated with hepatic TG content. However, these expression ratios were not significantly increased in any of the obesity groups (HFD, *ob/ob*, or *db/db*), whether or not they had functional leptin signaling. *CD36* was the most widely upregulated individual transporter, being significantly increased in the 14% and 18% EtOH, HFD, *ob/ob,* and *db/db* groups. These data suggest that regulation of hepatic LCFA transporter expression and participation of individual transporters in LCFA uptake are far more complex than was previously thought. Correlations between transcription factor expression and mean expression of multiple transporter genes suggests possible regulatory interaction, and may support reports postulating that a complex of FABPpm, CAV-1, CD36 and FATP4, and possibly FATP5 mediates hepatic LCFA uptake.[55,60]

Steatohepatitis

SHS is the most common form of NAFLD and is, in its earliest stages, largely reversible. Despite some controversy, the most common fates of SHS are either regression, maintenance of status quo, or progression to NASH.

Mechanisms leading to nonalcoholic steatohepatitis

In NASH, inflammatory processes are superimposed on SHS, resulting in a well-described histologic picture[97–99] similar to that of alcoholic hepatitis. Although a two-hit model of the progression from SHS to NASH, in which the first hit is the development of SHS,[100] had become widely accepted 2 decades ago, it has subsequently become clear that the second hit is, itself, multifactorial.[101] Rather than a sequential series of hits, many of the now multiple hits are pathways that act on the increased TG mass more or less simultaneously, and in recent widely accepted models involve oxidative stress, resulting in hepatocellular injury and apoptosis; inflammation and cytokine cascades (eg, Refs.[102–105]); stellate cell activation; fibrosis; and, ultimately, progression to cirrhosis. HCC is an increasingly recognized outcome of NASH,[106,107] evolving often, and almost uniquely, in noncirrhotic livers.[108]

Insulin Resistance

Early SHS may develop in the absence of insulin resistance. However, a critical step in the progression of NAFLD is the virtually universal development of insulin resistance, which plays an important role in adipocyte LCFA disposition. Under normal circumstances adipocytes are intermittent importers of LCFA, sequestering them postprandially as TG and then releasing them via lipolysis as required to meet metabolic needs. Insulin resistance, by derepressing adipocyte hormone-sensitive lipase, converts these cells into virtually continuous net LCFA exporters. LCFA released from the intra-abdominal, visceral fat depots enter the portal vein and are translocated directly to the liver. Hepatocellular LCFA oxidation at both mitochondrial and extramitochondrial sites is a major source of the ROS that initiate the processes of hepatocellular injury that characterize steatohepatitis (**Fig. 7**). In particular, ROS lead to mitochondrial injury, including both morphologic changes and defective ATP repletion; lipid peroxidation with production of malondialdehyde (MDA) and hydroxynonenal (HNE); activation of the FAS system; and the release of specific cytokines, in particular tumor necrosis factor alpha, transforming growth factor beta, and interleukin-6.[69] Together these result in several of the characteristic features of NASH that are recognizable histologically: apoptotic cell death, development of Mallory hyaline, polymorphonuclear leukocyte infiltration, and fibrosis. ROS generated from ethanol oxidation lead to many of the same metabolites, which may explain histologic similarities between alcoholic steatohepatitis and NASH. However, because alcoholic steatohepatitis also

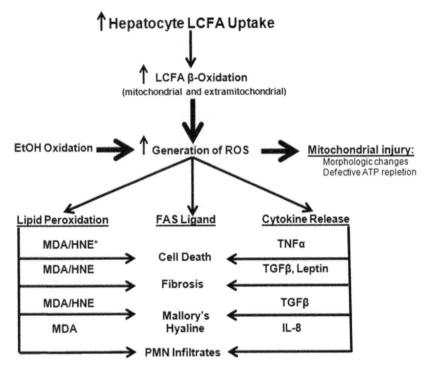

*MDA: malondialdehyde; HNE: hydroxynonenal

Fig. 7. Consequences of increased hepatocellular uptake and oxidation of LCFA in obesity. Many of the features of NASH follow logically from the increase in hepatocellular LCFA uptake and subsequent increase in the generation of ROS by mitochondrial and extramitochondrial LCFA oxidation. These processes in turn lead to generation of intracellular mediators such as malondialdehyde (MDA), hydroxynonenal (HNE), TNFα, transforming growth factor beta (TGFβ), leptin, and interleukin-8 (IL-8), which in turn cause several of the characteristic histologic features of NASH including infiltration with polymorphonuclear neutrophils (PMNs). ROS resulting from EtoH oxidation lead to generation of some of the same mediators, potentially explaining the histologic similarity between NASH and alcoholic hepatitis. (*Adapted from* Bradbury MW, Berk PD. Lipid metabolism in hepatic steatosis. Clin Liver Dis 2004;8:639–71; with permission.)

develops on a background of simple steatosis, oxidation of fatty acids may also contribute to that condition. Although numerous processes have been identified as contributing to the development of NASH,[109] all typically operate against a background of SHS, which is the sine qua non of NAFLD.

FUTURE PROSPECTS

NAFLD has sparked a dramatic expansion of the literature. From mid-1995 to mid-2015, more than 8200 articles about NAFLD entered major databases. Despite improved understanding of its pathophysiology, the prevalences of NAFLD and NASH continue to increase worldwide, and the long-term effectiveness of most currently available therapies is limited,[110,111] in part because of the frequency of weight regain. For additional reviews about current and future therapies see Ganesh S, Rustgi VK: Current Pharmacologic Therapy for Nonalcoholic Fatty Liver Disease and Hameed B, Terrault N: Emerging Therapies for Nonalcoholic Fatty Liver Disease, in this issue. Although several drugs are under advanced clinical development and testing for patients with early stage disease, as well as those with advanced liver fibrosis,[112,113] there are as this is written, no US Food and Drug Administration–approved therapeutic agents for the treatment of NAFLD and NASH.

The ultimate goal should be the development of effective prevention strategies and therapies for NAFLD. However, this has not yet been achieved.

REFERENCES

1. Ludwig J, Viggiano TR, McGill DB, et al. Nonalcoholic steatohepatitis: Mayo clinic experiences with a hitherto unnamed disease. Mayo Clin Proc 1980;55: 434–8.
2. Diehl AM, Goodman Z, Ishak KG. Alcohol-like liver disease in non-alcoholics. Gastroenterology 1988;95:1056–62.
3. Clain DJ, Lefkowitch JH. Fatty liver disease in morbid obesity. Gastroenterol Clin North Am 1987;16:239–52.
4. Chalasani N, Younossi Z, Lavine JE, et al, American Gastroenterological Association, American Association for the Study of Liver Diseases, American College of Gastroenterology. The diagnosis and management of non-alcoholic fatty liver disease: practice guideline by the American Gastroenterological Association, American Association for the Study of Liver Diseases, and American College of Gastroenterology. Gastroenterology 2012;142(7):1592–609.
5. Burt AD, Lackner C, Tiniakos DG. Diagnosis and assessment of NAFLD: definitions and histopathological classification. Semin Liver Dis 2015;35(3):207–20.
6. Vanni E, Bugianesi E, Kotronen A, et al. From the metabolic syndrome to NAFLD or vice versa. Dig Liver Dis 2010;42(5):320–30.
7. Satapathy SK, Sanyal AJ. Epidemiology and natural history of non-alcoholic fatty liver disease. Semin Liver Dis 2015;35(3):221–35.
8. Vanni E, Marengo A, Mezzabotta L, et al. Systemic complications of nonalcoholic fatty liver disease: when the liver is not an innocent bystander. Semin Liver Dis 2015;35(3):236–49.
9. Moore JB. Non-alcoholic fatty liver disease: the hepatic consequence of obesity and the metabolic syndrome. Proc Nutr Soc 2010;69:211–20.
10. Farrell GC, Wong VW, Chitturi S. NAFLD in Asia–as common and as important as in the West. Nat Rev Gastroenterol Hepatol 2013;10:307–18.
11. Loomba R, Sanyal AJ. The global NAFLD epidemic. Nat Rev Gastroenterol Hepatol 2013;10:686–90.
12. Speliotes EK, Yerges-Armstrong LM, Wu J, et al. Genome-wide association analysis identifies variants associated with nonalcoholic fatty liver disease that have distinct effects on metabolic traits. PLoS Genet 2011;7(3):e1001324.
13. Anstee QM, Day CP. The genetics of nonalcoholic fatty liver disease; spotlight on PNPLA3 & TM6SF2. Semin Liver Dis 2015;35(5):270–90.
14. Powell EE, Cooksley WG, Hanson R, et al. The natural history of nonalcoholic steatohepatitis: a follow-up study of forty-two patients for up to 21 years. Hepatology 1990;11(1):74–80.
15. Teli MR, James OF, Burt AD, et al. The natural history of nonalcoholic fatty liver: a follow-up study. Hepatology 1995;22(6):1714–9.
16. Harrison SA, Torgerson S, Hayashi PH. The natural history of nonalcoholic fatty liver disease: a clinical histopathological study. Am J Gastroenterol 2003;98:2042–7.
17. Fassio E, Alvarez E, Dominguez N, et al. Natural history of nonalcoholic steatohepatitis: a longitudinal study of repeat liver biopsies. Hepatology 2004;40(4):820–6.

18. Adams LA, Sanderson S, Lindor K, et al. The histological course of nonalcoholic fatty liver: a longitudinal study of 103 patients with sequential liver biopsies. J Hepatol 2005;42(1):132–8.
19. Ekstedt M, Franzén LE, Mathiesen UL, et al. Long-term follow-up of patients with NAFLD and elevated liver enzymes. Hepatology 2006;44(4):865–73.
20. Merriman RB, Ferrell LD, Patti MG, et al. Correlation of paired liver biopsies in morbidly obese patients with suspected nonalcoholic fatty liver disease. Hepatology 2006;44(4):874–80.
21. Wong VW, Wong GL, Choi PC, et al. Disease progression of non-alcoholic fatty liver disease: a prospective study with paired liver biopsies at 3 years. Gut 2010; 59(7):969–74.
22. Pais R, Charlotte F, Fedchuk L, et al, LIDO Study Group. A systematic review of follow-up biopsies reveals disease progression in patients with non-alcoholic fatty liver. J Hepatol 2013;59(3):550–6.
23. McPherson S, Hardy T, Henderson E, et al. Evidence of NAFLD progression from steatosis to fibrosing-steatohepatitis using paired biopsies: implications for prognosis and clinical management. J Hepatol 2015;62(5):1148–55.
24. Singh S, Allen AM, Wang Z, et al. Fibrosis progression in nonalcoholic fatty liver vs. nonalcoholic steatohepatitis: a systematic review and meta-analysis of paired-biopsy studies. Clin Gastroenterol Hepatol 2015;13(4):643–54.
25. Harrison SA. Nonalcoholic fatty liver disease and fibrosis progression: the Good, the Bad, and the Unknown. Clin Gastroenterol Hepatol 2015;13(4): 655–7.
26. Yilmaz Y. Review article: is non-alcoholic fatty liver disease a spectrum, or are steatosis and non-alcoholic steatohepatitis distinct conditions? Aliment Pharmacol Ther 2012;36:815–23.
27. Fielding C, Angulo P. Hepatic steatosis and steatohepatitis: are they really two distinct entities? Curr Hepatol Rep 2014;13(2):151–8.
28. Ge F, Zhou S, Hu C, et al. Increased insulin- and leptin-regulated fatty acid uptake plays a key causal role in hepatic steatosis in mice with intact leptin signaling, but not in those lacking leptin or its receptor. Am J Physiol Gastrointest Liver Physiol 2010;299:855–66.
29. Ge F, Lobdell H IV, Zhou S, et al. Digital analysis of hepatic sections accurately quantitates triglycerides and selected properties of lipid droplets. Exp Biol Med 2010;235(11):1282–6.
30. Ge F, Hu C, Hyodo E, et al. Cardiomyocyte triglyceride accumulation and reduced ventricular function occurs in mice with obesity and hepatic steatosis from many causes and reflects increased long chain fatty acid uptake and de novo fatty acid synthesis. J Obes 2012;2012:205648.
31. Stremmel W, Berk PD. Hepatocellular influx of [14C]oleate reflects membrane transport rather than intracellular metabolism or binding. Proc Natl Acad Sci U S A 1986;83(10):3086–90.
32. Schwieterman W, Sorrentino D, Potter BJ, et al. Uptake of oleate by isolated rat adipocytes is mediated by a 40-kDa plasma membrane fatty acid binding protein closely related to that in liver and gut. Proc Natl Acad Sci U S A 1988;85(2): 359–63.
33. Stump DD, Nunes RM, Sorrentino D, et al. Characteristics of oleate binding to liver plasma membranes and its uptake by isolated hepatocytes. J Hepatol 1992;16(3):304–15.
34. Berk PD, Stump DD. Mechanisms of cellular uptake of long chain free fatty acids. Mol Cell Biochem 1999;192(1–2):17–31.

35. Stump DD, Fan X, Berk PD. Oleic acid uptake and binding by rat adipocytes define dual pathways for cellular fatty acid uptake. J Lipid Res 2001;42(4):509–20.

36. Schmider W, Fahr A, Blum HE, et al. Transport of heptafluorostearate across model membranes: membrane transport of long-chain fatty acid anions. J Lipid Res 2000;41(5):775–87.

37. Abumrad NA, Park JH, Park CR. Permeation of long-chain fatty acid into adipocytes: kinetics, specificity, and evidence for involvement of a membrane protein. J Biol Chem 1984;259(14):8945–53.

38. Weisiger RA, Fitz JG, Scharschmidt BF. Hepatic oleate uptake: electrochemical driving forces in intact rat liver. J Clin Invest 1989;83(2):411–20.

39. Glatz JF, van Nieuwenhoven FA, Luiken JJ, et al. Role of membrane-associated and cytoplasmic fatty acid-binding proteins in cellular fatty acid metabolism. Prostaglandins Leukot Essent Fatty Acids 1997;57(4–5):373–8.

40. Luiken JJ, Glatz JF, Bonen A. Fatty acid transport proteins facilitate fatty acid uptake in skeletal muscle. Can J Appl Physiol 2000;25(5):333–52.

41. Kampf JP, Kleinfeld AM. Fatty acid transport in adipocytes monitored by imaging intracellular free fatty acid levels. J Biol Chem 2004;279(34):35775–80.

42. Kleinfeld AM, Kampf JP, Lechene C. Transport of 13C-oleate in adipocytes measured using multi imaging mass spectrometry. J Am Soc Mass Spectrom 2004;15(11):1572–80.

43. Stremmel W, Strohmeyer G, Borchard F, et al. Isolation and partial characterization of a fatty acid binding protein in rat liver plasma membranes. Proc Natl Acad Sci U S A 1985;82(1):4–8.

44. Bradbury MW, Berk PD. Cellular uptake of long chain free fatty acids: the structure and function of plasma membrane fatty acid binding protein. Adv Mol Cell Biol 2004;33:47–81.

45. Abumrad NA, el-Maghrabi MR, Amri EZ, et al. Cloning of a rat adipocyte membrane protein implicated in binding or transport of long-chain fatty acids that is induced during preadipocyte differentiation: homology with human CD36. J Biol Chem 1993;268(24):17665–8.

46. Schaffer JE, Lodish HF. Expression cloning and characterization of a novel adipocyte long chain fatty acid transport protein. Cell 1994;79(3):427–36.

47. Stahl A, Gimeno RE, Tartaglia LA, et al. Fatty acid transport proteins: a current view of a growing family. Trends Endocrinol Metab 2001;12(6):266–73.

48. Trigatti BL, Anderson RG, Gerber GE. Identification of caveolin-1 as a fatty acid binding protein. Biochem Biophys Res Commun 1999;255(1):34–9.

49. Pohl J, Ring A, Stremmel W. Uptake of long-chain fatty acids in HepG2 cells involves caveolae: analysis of a novel pathway. J Lipid Res 2002;43(9):1390–9.

50. Kampf JP, Parmley D, Kleinfeld AM. Free fatty acid transport across adipocytes is mediated by an unknown membrane protein pump. Am J Physiol Endocrinol Metab 2007;293(5):E1207–14.

51. Kampf JP, Kleinfeld AM. Is membrane transport of FFA mediated by lipid, protein, or both? An unknown protein mediates free fatty acid transport across the adipocyte plasma membrane. Physiology (Bethesda) 2007;22:7–14.

52. Berk PD, Wada H, Horio Y, et al. Plasma membrane fatty acid-binding protein and mitochondrial glutamic-oxaloacetic transaminase of rat liver are related. Proc Natl Acad Sci U S A 1990;87(9):3484–8.

53. Bradbury MW, Stump D, Guarnieri F, et al. Molecular modeling and functional confirmation of a predicted fatty acid binding site in mitochondrial aspartate aminotransferase. J Mol Biol 2011;412(3):412–22.

54. Watkins PA. Fatty acid activation. Prog Lipid Res 1997;36:55–83.
55. Digel M, Ehehalt R, Stremmel W, et al. Acyl-CoA synthetases: fatty acid uptake and metabolic channeling. Mol Cell Biochem 2009;326:23–8.
56. Hall AM, Smith AJ, Bernlohr DA. Characterization of the acyl-CoA synthetase activity of purified murine fatty acid transport protein 1. J Biol Chem 2003;278: 43008–13.
57. Hall AM, Wiczer BM, Herrmann T, et al. Enzymatic properties of purified murine fatty acid transport protein 4 and analysis of acyl CoA synthetase activities in tissues from FATP4 null mice. J Biol Chem 2005;280:11948–54.
58. Black PN, DiRusso CC. Transmembrane movement of exogenous long-chain fatty acids: proteins, enzymes, and vectorial esterification. Microbiol Mol Biol Rev 2003;67:4544–72.
59. Kalant D, Cianflone K. Regulation of fatty acid transport. Curr Opin Lipidol 2004; 15:309–14.
60. Stremmel W, Staffer S, Wannhoff A, et al. Plasma membrane phospholipase A2 controls hepatocellular fatty acid uptake and is responsive to pharmacologic modulation: implications for nonalcoholic steatohepatitis. FASEB J 2014;28: 3159–70.
61. Berk PD, Zhou SL, Kiang CL, et al. Uptake of long chain free fatty acids is selectively up-regulated in adipocytes of Zucker rats with genetic obesity and non-insulin-dependent diabetes mellitus. J Biol Chem 1997;272(13):8830–5.
62. Chua SC Jr, Chung WK, Wu-Peng XS, et al. Phenotypes of mouse *diabetes* and rat *fatty* due to mutations in the OB (leptin) receptor. Science 1996;271(5251): 994–6.
63. Wang B, Charukeshi-Chandrasekera P, Pippin JJ. Leptin- and leptin receptor-deficient rodent models: relevance for human type 2 diabetes. Curr Diabetes Rev 2014;10:131–45.
64. Sanches SC, Ramalho LN, Augusto MJ, et al. Nonalcoholic steatohepatitis: a search for factual animal models. Biomed Res Int 2015;2015:574832.
65. Berk PD, Zhou S, Kiang C, et al. Selective up-regulation of fatty acid uptake by adipocytes characterizes both genetic and diet-induced obesity in rodents. J Biol Chem 1999;274(40):28626–31.
66. Petrescu O, Fan X, Gentileschi P, et al. Long-chain fatty acid uptake is upregulated in omental adipocytes from patients undergoing bariatric surgery for obesity. Int J Obes (Lond) 2005;29(2):196–203.
67. Ge F, Walewski JL, Torghabeh MH, et al. Facilitated long chain fatty acid uptake by adipocytes remains upregulated relative to BMI for more than a year after major bariatric surgical weight loss. Obesity (Silver Spring) 2016;24(1):113–22.
68. Fan X, Bradbury MW, Berk PD. Leptin and insulin modulate nutrient partitioning and weight loss in ob/ob mice through regulation of long-chain fatty acid uptake by adipocytes. J Nutr 2003;133(9):2707–15.
69. Vacca M, Allison M, Griffin JL, et al. Fatty acid and glucose sensors in hepatic lipid metabolism: implications for NAFLD. Semin Liver Dis 2015;35(5):250–61.
70. Schaffer JE. Lipotoxicity: when tissues overeat. Curr Opin Lipidol 2003;14: 281–7.
71. Bradbury MW, Berk PD. Lipid metabolism in hepatic steatosis. Clin Liver Dis 2004;8(3):639–71.
72. Lee GH, Proenca R, Montez JM, et al. Abnormal splicing of the leptin receptor in diabetic mice. Nature 1996;379(6566):632–5.
73. Phillips MS, Liu Q, Hammond HA, et al. Leptin receptor missense mutation in the fatty Zucker rat. Nat Genet 1996;13(1):18–9.

74. Zhang Y, Proenca R, Maffei M, et al. Positional cloning of the mouse obese gene and its human homologue. Nature 1994;372(6505):425–32.
75. Maclean PS, Bergouignan A, Cornier MA, et al. Biology's response to dieting: the impetus for weight regain. Am J Physiol Regul Integr Comp Physiol 2011; 301(3):R581–600.
76. Blomain ES, Dirhan DA, Valentino MA, et al. Mechanisms of weight regain following weight loss. ISRN Obes 2013;2013:210524.
77. Greenway FL. Physiological adaptations to weight loss and factors favouring weight regain. Int J Obes (Lond) 2015;39(8):1188–96.
78. Courcoulas AP, Christian NJ, Belle SH, et al, Longitudinal Assessment of Bariatric Surgery (LABS) Consortium. Weight change and health outcomes at 3 years after bariatric surgery among individuals with severe obesity. JAMA 2013; 310(22):2416–25.
79. Lee Y, Wang MY, Kakuma T, et al. Liporegulation in diet induced obesity: the antisteatotic role of hyperleptinemia. J Biol Chem 2001;276(8):5629–35.
80. Unger RH. Lipotoxic diseases. Annu Rev Med 2002;53:319–36.
81. Unger RH. The physiology of cellular liporegulation. Annu Rev Physiol 2003;65: 333–47.
82. Halaas JL, Gajiwala KS, Maffei M, et al. Weight-reducing effects of the plasma protein encoded by the obese gene. Science 1995;269(5223):543–6.
83. Pelleymounter MA, Cullen MJ, Baker MB, et al. Effects of the obese gene product on body weight regulation in ob/ob mice. Science 1995;269(5223): 540–3.
84. Campfield LA, Smith FJ, Guisez Y, et al. Recombinant mouse OB protein: evidence for a peripheral signal linking adiposity and central neural networks. Science 1995;269(5223):546–9.
85. Remesar X, Rafecas I, Fernandez-Lopez JA, et al. Is leptin an insulin counter-regulatory hormone? FEBS Lett 1997;402(1):9–11.
86. Myers MG, Cowley MA, Munzberg H. Mechanisms of leptin action and leptin resistance. Annu Rev Physiol 2008;70:537–56.
87. Oh-I S, Shimizu H, Sato T, et al. Molecular mechanisms associated with leptin resistance: n-3 polyunsaturated fatty acids induce alterations in the tight junction of the brain. Cell Metab 2005;1(5):331–41.
88. Listenberger LL, Ory DS, Schaffer JE. Palmitate-induced apoptosis can occur through a ceramide-independent pathway. J Biol Chem 2001;276(18):14890–5.
89. Unger RH, Orci L. Diseases of liporegulation: new perspective on obesity and related disorders. FASEB J 2001;15(2):312–21.
90. Unger RH. Minireview: weapons of lean body mass destruction—the role of ectopic lipids in the metabolic syndrome. Endocrinology 2003;144(12):5159–65.
91. Shimomura I, Hammer RE, Ikemoto S, et al. Leptin reverses insulin resistance and diabetes mellitus in mice with congenital lipodystrophy. Nature 1999; 401(6748):73–6.
92. Mirabeau O, Perlas E, Severini C, et al. Identification of novel peptide hormones in the human proteome by hidden Markov model screening. Genome Res 2007; 17:320–7.
93. Walewski JL, Ge F, Lobdell H 4th, et al. Spexin is a novel human peptide that reduces adipocyte uptake of long chain fatty acids and causes weight loss in rodents with diet-induced obesity. Obesity (Silver Spring) 2014;22(7): 1643–52.
94. Haynes P, Liangpunsakul S, Chalasani N. Nonalcoholic fatty liver disease in individuals with severe obesity. Clin Liver Dis 2004;8(3):535–47.

95. Zhou SL, Gordon RE, Bradbury M, et al. Ethanol up-regulates fatty acid uptake and plasma membrane expression and export of mitochondrial aspartate aminotransferase in HepG2 cells. Hepatology 1998;27(4):1064–74.
96. Berk PD, Zhou S, Bradbury MW. Increased hepatocellular uptake of long chain fatty acids occurs by different mechanisms in fatty livers due to obesity or excess ethanol use, contributing to development of steatohepatitis in both settings. Trans Am Clin Climatol Assoc 2005;116:335–44.
97. Yeh MM, Brunt EM. Pathological features of fatty liver disease. Gastroenterol 2014;147(4):754–64.
98. Kleiner DE, Berk PD, Hsu JY, et al, LABS Consortium. Hepatic pathology among patients without known liver disease undergoing bariatric surgery: observations and a perspective from the Longitudinal Assessment of Bariatric Surgery (LABS) study. Semin Liver Dis 2014;34(1):98–107.
99. Neuschwander-Tetri BA, Clark JM, Bass NM, et al, NASH Clinical Research Network. Clinical, laboratory and histological associations in adults with nonalcoholic fatty liver disease. Hepatology 2010;52(3):913–24.
100. Day CP, James OF. Steatohepatitis: a tale of two "hits"? Gastroenterology 1998; 114(4):842–5.
101. Charlton M. Noninvasive indices of fibrosis in NAFLD: starting to think about a three-hit (at least) phenomenon. Am J Gastroenterol 2007;102(2):409–11.
102. McCullough AJ. Pathophysiology of nonalcoholic steatohepatitis. J Clin Gastroenterol 2006;40(3 Suppl 1):S17–29.
103. Mantena SK, King AL, Andringa KK, et al. Mitochondrial dysfunction and oxidative stress in the pathogenesis of alcohol- and obesity-induced fatty liver diseases. Free Radic Biol Med 2008;44(7):1259–72.
104. Mahli H, Gores G. Molecular mechanisms of lipotoxicity in nonalcoholic fatty liver disease. Semin Liver Dis 2008;28(4):360–9.
105. Diehl A. Mechanisms of disease and progression in NAFLD. Semin Liver Dis 2008;28(4):370–9.
106. Bugianesi E, Leone N, Vanni E, et al. Expanding the natural history of nonalcoholic steatohepatitis: from cryptogenic cirrhosis to hepatocellular carcinoma. Gastroenterology 2002;123(1):134–40.
107. Pocha C, Kolly P, Dufour J-F. Nonalcoholic fatty liver disease-related hepatocellular carcinoma – a problem of growing magnitude. Semin Liver Dis 2015;35(3): 304–17.
108. Torres DM, Harrison SA. Nonalcoholic steatohepatitis and noncirrhotic hepatocellular carcinoma: fertile soil. Semin Liver Dis 2012;32(1):30–8.
109. Ponziani FR, Pecere S, Gasbarrini A, et al. Physiology and pathophysiology of liver lipid metabolism. Expert Rev Gastroenterol Hepatol 2015;9(8):1055–67.
110. Nguyen V, George J. Nonalcoholic fatty liver disease management: dietary and lifestyle modifications. Semin Liver Dis 2015;35(3):318–37.
111. Gawrieh S, Chalasani N. Pharmacotherapy for non-alcoholic fatty liver disease. Semin Liver Dis 2015;35(3):338–48.
112. Filozof C, Goldstein BJ, Williams RN, et al. Non-alcoholic steatohepatitis: limited available treatment options but promising drugs in development and recent progress towards a regulatory approval pathway. Drugs 2015;75(12):1373–92.
113. Takahashi Y, Sugimoto K, Inui H, et al. Current pharmacological therapies for nonalcoholic fatty liver disease/nonalcoholic steatohepatitis. World J Gastroenterol 2015;21(13):3777–85.

Nonalcoholic Fatty Liver Disease and the Gut Microbiome

Jerome Boursier, MD, PhD[a,b,*], Anna Mae Diehl, MD[c]

KEYWORDS

- Nonalcoholic fatty liver disease • Fatty liver • Steatohepatitis • Fibrosis
- Liver cirrhosis • Hepatocellular carcinoma • Gut microbiota

KEY POINTS

- As observed in other chronic metabolic diseases, nonalcoholic fatty liver disease (NAFLD) is associated with gut dysbiosis.
- At the interface between diet and the liver, gut microbiota can induce liver steatosis through its metabolic functions and endotoxemia.
- Gut microbiota can also drive the severity of NAFLD through increased endogenous production of alcohol, activation of liver inflammation, or altering the bile acid profile.
- Modulation of the gut microbiota, such as pre/probiotic use, for the treatment of NAFLD needs to be evaluated further.

INTRODUCTION

The human gastrointestinal tract hosts about one hundred trillion commensal organisms that represent 10 times more cells than the whole body cell count.[1] Approximately 800 to 1000 different bacterial species and more than 7000 different strains inhabit the gut.[2] These commensal bacteria are grouped into phyla, which are dominated by the Gram-negative Bacterioidetes and Proteobacteria, and the Gram-positive Firmicutes and Actinobacteria. The taxonomic composition of gut microbial community varies between individuals, even between those who are closely related.[3] Consequently, all genes of microbes that make up the gut microbiome has recently been referred as our "second genome" that outnumbers human genes by more

The authors have nothing to disclose.
[a] Hepato-Gastroenterology Department, University Hospital, 4 Larrey street, 49933 Angers Cedex 09, France; [b] HIFIH Laboratory, UPRES 3859, SFR 4208, LUNAM University, Angers, France; [c] Division of Gastroenterology, Department of Medicine, Duke University Medical Center, 595 LaSalle Street, Snyderman Building, Suite 1073, Durham, NC 27710, USA
* Corresponding author. Hepato-Gastroenterology Department, University Hospital, 4 Larrey street, 49933 Angers Cedex 09, France.
E-mail address: JeBoursier@chu-angers.fr

than 100-fold. Gut microbiota participates in health maintenance and helps to balance vital functions for the host, including immunity, nutritional status, and metabolic functions.[4–6]

It is now well-established that gut flora and chronic liver diseases are closely inter-related. This association is the most evident at late stages of the disease: cirrhosis and impaired liver function are associated with intestinal bacterial overgrowth, small bowel dysmotility, increased gut permeability, and decreased immunologic de-fenses, all promoting bacterial translocation from the gut to the systemic circulation and leading to infections that in turn aggravate liver dysfunction in a vicious circle.[7] For a long time, the implication of gut flora in the pathophysiology of less-advanced chronic liver diseases has been underestimated because technical limita-tions allow only for the culture of a small fraction of gut bacteria. Recent technological progress and next-generation DNA sequencing has allowed for more sophisticated analysis and sampling of the gut microbiota by culture-independent methods.[8] Thanks to these recent technological advances, the knowledge about the role of gut microbiota disruption (dysbiosis) in gut diseases such as colon cancer, inflamma-tory bowel diseases, or irritable bowel syndrome has greatly increased with possible new therapeutic strategies. More surprisingly, gut dysbiosis has been implicated in chronic metabolic disorders, such as obesity, metabolic syndrome, diabetes, and cardiovascular diseases.[5] Nonalcoholic fatty liver disease (NAFLD) is the liver mani-festation of the metabolic syndrome and thus evolves in the same context as these metabolic diseases.[9] It is thus not surprising that recent literature emphasizes a po-tential role for gut dysbiosis in the pathophysiology of NAFLD.

NAFLD encompasses a spectrum of hepatic pathology (ie, liver phenotypes). Accu-mulation of triglycerides in hepatocytes (hepatic steatosis) is the most common liver phenotype in NAFLD. Some individuals with hepatic steatosis develop nonalcoholic steatohepatitis (NASH), a more severe type of liver damage characterized by hepatic inflammation and liver cell death. In some individuals with the NASH phenotype, liver regeneration cannot keep pace with the increased rate of hepatocyte death, and liver scarring (fibrosis) ensues. Over time, some of these individuals accumulate sufficient fibrosis to develop cirrhosis. Liver cirrhosis is the NAFLD phenotype that has the worst prognosis because cirrhosis dramatically increases the risk for both primary liver can-cer and overall liver-related mortality.[10,11] Epidemiologic studies indicate that NAFLD is now the most common cause of liver disease in many countries, including the United States.[12] It is estimated that at least 25% of American adults have some form of NAFLD, with about 6% of the general adult population having NASH and 2% to 3% having NAFLD-related cirrhosis.

GUT MICROBIOTA PROMOTES THE ONSET OF NONALCOHOLIC FATTY LIVER DISEASE

By using fecal transplantation, recent animal studies have demonstrated that gut microbiota can itself directly induce NAFLD. Conventional C57BL/6J mice fed 16 weeks with a high-fat diet (HFD) generally display liver steatosis, hyperglycemia, and systemic inflammation (responders), but some mice are nonresponders, devel-oping no metabolic disorder with this dietary manipulation.[13] To explore the potential role of gut microbiota in these discrepant responses, gut microbiota from a responder or from a nonresponder mouse were transplanted into germ-free mice (ie, responder or nonresponder receivers) that were then fed HFD for another 16 weeks. Despite similar weight gain, food consumption, and epididymal fat, responder–receiver mice developed a higher level of liver steatosis, glycemia, and insulin resistance than nonresponder receivers. Level of the transcription factors SREBP and ChREBP were increased in responder mice indicating enhancement of de novo lipogenesis. These data support the concept that interindividual differences in the intestinal microbiome modulate the metabolic and hepatic consequences of consumption of a HFD. Interestingly, isobutyrate and isovalerate were significantly greater in the caecum of responder mice. Isobutyrate and isovalerate are branched-chain fatty acids known to result from the bacterial fermentation of leucine and valine. Protein fermentation also produces branched-chain amino acids that have been associated with insulin resistance and the development of metabolic disease.[14]

Potential mechanisms for enhanced liver steatosis were demonstrated in earlier studies. Small intestinal bacterial overgrowth (SIBO) has been described in NAFLD patients.[15–19] In 2 studies, SIBO correlated with the severity of steatosis[18] and was an independent predictor of severe steatosis,[17] without any association with liver inflammation, fibrosis, or NASH. In the study from Miele and associates,[18] NAFLD patients with SIBO had increased intestinal permeability, which is itself associated with a greater prevalence of moderate or severe steatosis. Another work showed that SIBO observed in NASH patients is associated with expression of Toll-like receptor (TLR)4 and release of interleukin-8.[19] Taken together, these results suggest that SIBO contribute to liver steatosis through enhanced inflammation. Indeed, the activation of liver inflammatory pathways causes impairment of the insulin signaling with subsequent increase in free fatty acid afflux.[20] However, other studies failed to demonstrate a higher prevalence of SIBO[21] or increased intestinal permeability[15] in NAFLD patients. Finally, because all these studies used different protocols for SIBO or intestinal permeability assessment, their results should be interpreted with caution.

Other potential mechanisms are emerging rapidly. Gut bacteria can increase the efflux of free fatty acids to the liver by suppressing the intestinal expression of the lipoprotein lipase inhibitor Fiaf (fasting-induced adipose factor, also known as angiopoietin-like protein-4).[22,23] In a very recent study conducted in mice fed an HFD, the suppression of gut microbiota turned the gut bile acid composition with an increase in tauro-β-muricholic acid that was associated with inhibition of intestinal FXR signaling.[24] This FXR inhibition elicited an improvement in mitochondrial function with a decrease in serum ceramide levels that downregulated hepatic SREBP1C and CIDEA expression, finally resulting in decreased hepatic steatosis. There was no effect on liver FXR signaling in this study, suggesting a direct link between gut microbiota, bile acids/intestinal FXR, and NAFLD. Colonic bacteria also ferment nondigestible carbohydrates to short chain fatty acids (SCFA). SCFA have been proposed to contribute to obesity and liver steatosis because they provide approximately 10% of daily caloric consumption and may enhance nutrient absorption by promoting expression of glucagon-like peptide 2.[25,26] However, it has also been shown that SCFA improve lipid and glucose metabolism and maintain intestinal homeostasis.[25,27] A recent human study has randomized 16 treatment-naïve subjects with the metabolic syndrome to receive either an allogenic (from lean donor) or an autologous gut microbiota infusion after a bowel lavage through a duodenal tube.[28] Six weeks after the allogenic gut microbiota infusion, there was a significant improvement in insulin sensitivity along with levels of butyrate-producing intestinal microbiota. Hence, the role of SCFA seems to be complex and further studies are required to decipher their net effect on NAFLD pathogenesis. Choline deficiency is well-known to cause NAFLD with NASH and fibrosis in rodents.[29] The intestinal microbiome seems to play an important role in regulating the availability of dietary choline and the gene cluster responsible for anaerobic choline degradation has been discovered recently.[30] A metabolomic study in

C129S6 mice showed that feeding HFD shifts the gut microbiota into a "choline-degradation" profile, resulting in low circulating levels of plasma phosphatidylcholine and high urinary excretion of methylamines.[31] The reduced bioavailability of choline in the HFD-fed mice mimicked the effect of choline-deficient diets that cause NAFLD. This information is relevant clinically because a recent human study demonstrated increased hepatic steatosis in 15 women who ate low-choline diets for 42 days.[32] Sequencing gut microbiota before the diet identified 2 classes of bacteria that predicted choline deficiency-induced fatty liver: Firmicutes/Erysipelotrichi and Proteobacteria/Gammaproteobacteria. Interestingly, taking into account microbiota profile and the polymorphism of phosphatidylethanolamine N-methyltransferase, which encodes an enzyme in the choline biosynthetic pathway, improved the prediction of liver steatosis occurrence. These findings demonstrate that host genetic background, diet, and the gut microbiota interact to influence NAFLD pathogenesis in humans, as is now known to occur in rodent models. Finally, new concepts are emerging thanks to experience with bariatric surgery. Within 1 year, bariatric surgery remarkably suppresses NASH in 85% of patients and reduces fibrosis stage in 35%.[33] In mice undergoing Roux-en-Y gastric bypass, surgery is rapidly followed by significant changes in the gut microbiota composition.[34] Interestingly, inoculation of cecal content from Roux-en-Y gastric bypass or sham donors to germ-free mice showed that mice receiving the gut microbiota from Roux-en-Y gastric bypass donors lost significantly more weight and fat mass than mice receiving fecal content from sham donors. The mechanisms that link gut microbiota and weight loss after bariatric surgery are under investigation.

Few works have evaluated the taxonomic composition of gut microbiota in NAFLD patients.[35–39] By comparison with to the controls, they all show the presence of gut dysbiosis in NAFLD (**Table 1**). However, results are conflicting; the differences observed in taxonomic composition were not the same among the different works. These discrepancies may be explained by the small sample sizes and several differences among the cohorts studied: countries (North America, Asia, and Europe), manner of patient selection, age (adults or children), insufficient documentation of liver disease with liver biopsy performed only in a subset of patients, methods for gut microbiota analysis (quantitative polymerase chain reaction vs pyrosequencing). Nevertheless, by showing gut dysbiosis in NAFLD patients, these works support the results obtained in animal studies suggesting a potential role of gut microbiota in the pathogenesis of NAFLD. Munukka and colleagues[39] evaluated gut microbiota and adipose tissue inflammation in 10 patients having high hepatic fat content as determined by ^{1}H MR spectroscopy versus 21 patients with low hepatic fat content. They found that dysbiotic gut microbiota correlated with parameters of insulin resistance and liver fat content. In addition, the expression level of inflammatory genes in adipose tissue correlated with the hepatic fat content and dysbiotic gut microbiota. These authors made the interesting hypothesis that gut dysbiosis induces macrophage infiltration and inflammation in adipose tissue, thus leading to the adipose tissue insulin resistance that further promotes hepatic steatosis.

GUT MICROBIOTA PARTICIPATES TO THE SEVERITY OF NONALCOHOLIC FATTY LIVER DISEASE

There are thousands of bacterial species in the gut and they all display an incredibly wide range of metabolic functions. Now that we realize that gut microbiota modulate NAFLD-related pathophysiology, the challenge is to decipher the mechanisms by

Table 1
Cross-sectional studies that have evaluated gut dysbiosis in human NAFLD

Reference	Patients	Sample Size	Method	Results
Raman et al,[35] 2013	Adults (Canada)	30 healthy controls 30 NAFLD	16S ribosomal RNA pyrosequencing (Roche GS Junior platform)	In NAFLD vs controls: ↑ Proteobacteria/Alphaproteobacteria/Kiloniellales/Kiloniellaceae ↑ Proteobacteria/Gammaproteobacteria/Pasteurellales/Pasteurellaceae ↑ Firmicutes/Bacilli/Lactobacillales/Lactobacillaceae/Lactobacillus ↑ Firmicutes/Clostridia/Clostridiales/Veillonellaceae ↑ Firmicutes/Clostridia/Clostridiales/Lachnospiraceae/Robinsoniella ↑ Firmicutes/Clostridia/Clostridiales/Lachnospiraceae/Roseburia ↑ Firmicutes/Clostridia/Clostridiales/Lachnospiraceae/Dorea ↓ Firmicutes/Clostridia/Clostridiales/Ruminococcaceae ↓ Firmicutes/Clostridia/Clostridiales/Oscillospiraceae/Oscillibacter ↓ Bacteroidetes/Bacteroidia/Bacteroidales/Porphyromonadaceae
Mouzaki et al,[36] 2013	Adults (Canada)	17 healthy controls 11 simple steatosis[a] 22 NASH[a]	Quantitative polymerase chain reaction	In NASH vs simple steatosis: ↑ Firmicutes/Clostridia/Clostridiales/Lachnospiraceae/Clostridium coccoides In NASH patients vs both simple steatosis and controls: ↓ Bacteroidetes

(continued on next page)

Table 1
(continued)

Reference	Patients	Sample Size	Method	Results
Zhu et al,[37] 2013	Children (USA)	16 healthy controls 25 obese 22 NASH[a]	16S ribosomal RNA pyrosequencing (454-FLX-Titanium Genome Sequencer)	In NASH vs obeses or controls ↑ Proteobacteria/ Gammaproteobacteria/ Enterobacteriales/ Enterobacteriaceae/Escherichia
Wong et al,[38] 2013	Adults (China)	22 healthy controls 16 NASH[a]	16S ribosomal RNA pyrosequencing (GS FLX system)	In NASH vs controls: ↑ Bacteroidetes/Bacteroidia/ Bacteroidales/Porphyromonadaceae/ Parabacteroides ↑ Firmicutes/Negativicutes/ Selenomonadales/Veillonellaceae/ Allisonella ↓ Firmicutes/Clostridia/Clostridiales/ Ruminococcaceae/Faecalibacterium ↓ Firmicutes/Clostridia/Clostridiales/ Clostridiaceae/Anaerosporobacter
Munukka et al,[39] 2014	Adults (Finland)	21 low hepatic fat content 10 high hepatic fat content	Oligonucleotide probe targeting 16S RNA	In patients with high vs low hepatic fat content: ↓ Firmicutes/Clostridia/Clostridiales/ Ruminococcaceae/Faecalibacterium prausnitzii

Abbreviations: NAFLD, nonalcoholic fatty liver disease; NASH, nonalcoholic steatohepatitis.
[a] As determined by histologic examination of liver biopsy.

which they exacerbate NAFLD severity.[40] In addition to directly inducing NAFLD, several works have suggested that gut microbiota can drive the severity of NAFLD and promote NASH, liver fibrosis, or liver cancer.

Steatohepatitis

Targeted disruption of the NLRP3 or NLRP6 inflammasome altered the gut microbiota, and was associated with enhanced colonic inflammation and NASH in mice fed methionine choline–deficient diets.[41] By studying several knockout models, the researchers discovered that more severe diet-induced NASH resulted from influx of intestinally derived TLR4 and TLR9 agonists into the portal circulation which, in turn, activated tumor necrosis factor (TNF)-α in the liver. Wild-type mice that were cohoused with inflammasome-deficient mice also exhibited worsened NASH. Antibiotic treatment with ciprofloxacin and metronidazole reduced the severity of NASH in inflammasome-deficient mice and abolished transmission of the phenotype to wild-type animals, showing that gut microbiota drive NASH progression in this model. These findings have clinical relevance because human studies have demonstrated that NASH patients have greater endotoxemia and higher liver TNF-α levels than patients with simple hepatic steatosis.[42–44] However, endotoxemia does not seem to be an absolute requirement for NASH development; it was absent in a majority of patients in another NASH cohort.[45]

Other possible mechanisms involving gut microbiota in NASH development have raised from cross-sectional studies performed in humans (see **Table 1**). Using quantitative polymerase chain reaction for selected bacteria in a small cohort of 50 patients (17 controls, 11 patients with hepatic steatosis, and 22 patients with NASH), Mouzaki and colleagues[36] showed that NASH patients had decreased fecal Bacteroidetes and increased *Clostridium coccoides*. The negative association between NASH and Bacteroidetes persisted after adjustment for body mass index and daily fat intake. The authors suggested that the low prevalence of Bacteroidetes could affect energy balance by facilitating metabolic dominance of other bacteria that are more efficient in extracting energy from the diet. Zhu and colleagues[37] screened the whole gut microbiota using 16S ribosomal RNA pyrosequencing in a pediatric cohort of 63 children including 16 healthy controls, 25 obese subjects without known liver disease, and 22 patients with biopsy-proven NASH. They found that fecal species richness was diminished in obese subjects and NASH patients compared with controls. Most samples clustered by health status but not by age, gender, or ethnicity, indicating a specific connection between the liver phenotype and gut microbiome. At the phylum level, obese and NASH patients had a similar increase in Bacteroidetes and decrease in Firmicutes compared with controls. Proteobacteria exhibited a progressive increase from the control to the obese and the NASH groups, and was the only phylum with significant difference between obese and NASH patients. The increase in Proteobacteria was mainly explained by an increase abundance of Enterobacteriaceae, especially Escherichia, which was the only abundant genus within the whole bacteria domain exhibiting a significant difference between the obese and the NASH groups. Interestingly, Escherichia are known alcohol-producing bacteria and the serum alcohol concentration was significantly higher in NASH patients compared with obese or control groups. Further studies including larger and well-characterized cohorts are required to better identify the associations between gut microbiota and the various liver phenotypes observed in NAFLD.

Liver Fibrosis

Gut microbiota can also promote liver fibrosis, a known risk factor for NAFLD-related cirrhosis. In a recent study, mice fed HFD before bile duct ligation (BDL) developed more severe liver fibrosis than control mice that were fed a standard chow diet before BDL.[46] HFD-related increases in liver fibrosis were associated with gut dysbiosis, especially an increase in Proteobacteria. To establish the causal link between the gut dysbiosis and worsened liver fibrosis, gut microbiota transplantation was performed before BDL. Control mice that received the gut microbiota from HFD mice demonstrated more severe liver fibrosis after BDL than HFD mice that were transplanted with gut microbiota from chow-fed mice. Selective transplantation of Gram-negative or Gram-positive bacteria showed that Gram-negative bacteria were responsible for the observed enhancement of liver fibrosis. In another animal study, intestinal decontamination with rifaximin decreased hepatic stellate cells activation, liver fibrosis and portal pressure in BDL mice.[47] The same experiment conducted in TLR4-mutant mice showed the beneficial effect of antibiotics was mediated by TLR4. In vivo and in vitro experiments demonstrated that the bacterial lipopolysaccharide promoted hepatic stellate cells mediated fibronectin production through TLR4, and that fibronectin further promoted liver endothelial cells migration and angiogenesis. This work provides rationale for the participation of gut microbiota in both liver fibrosis and portal hypertension. To date, no study has addressed specifically the association between gut dysbiosis and liver fibrosis in human NAFLD. The discovery of mechanisms that link gut bacteria with liver fibrogenesis in human NAFLD would of great interest by offering the possibility of new therapeutic targets.

Hepatocellular Carcinoma

A recent study established a link between the gut microbiota and NAFLD-related hepatocellular carcinoma.[48] Neonatal mice were treated with a single application of the carcinogenic agent dimethylbenz(a)antracene, and then fed HFD or standard chow diet for 30 weeks. HFD-fed mice developed more hepatocellular carcinoma, and intestinal decontamination with antibiotics reduced liver cancer formation. Metabolomic analysis showed that HFD feeding increased deoxycholic acid, a secondary bile acid generated solely by gut bacterial strains that 7α-dehydroxylate primary bile acids (eg, Clostridium cluster XI and XIVa). Oral antibiotics decreased deoxycholic acid levels in HFD-fed mice. Moreover, deoxycholic acid administration restored liver cancer development in HFD fed mice despite concomitant treatment with antibiotics. These results demonstrate the importance of the gut microbiome in modulating bile acid homeostasis. The relationship between bile acids and severity of NAFLD is very complex, however, with deleterious or beneficial effects probably depending on the type of bile acid and/or the particular bile acid-sensitive signaling pathway targeted. Bile acids are ligands for the nuclear receptor FXR and the G-protein–coupled receptor TGR5, both having been implicated in metabolic syndrome pathobiology.[49,50] In a recent randomized double-blind placebo-controlled phase II clinical trial, obeticholic acid, a semisynthetic FXR agonist derived from the primary human bile acid chenodeoxycholic acid, significantly improved markers of liver inflammation and fibrosis in NAFLD patients.[51] Thus, both harmful and beneficial hepatic effects of bile acids have been demonstrated in NAFLD, and further research is necessary to clarify the basis for the discrepant outcomes.

HOW TO MODULATE GUT MICROBIOTA TO IMPROVE NONALCOHOLIC FATTY LIVER DISEASE

Gut microbial ecosystem is strongly linked to diet. A very recent study evaluated whether gut microbial communities are altered by 2 dietary interventions: a "plant-based diet" rich in grains, legumes, fruits and vegetables, and an "animal diet" composed of meats, egg, and cheese.[52] Both diets induced rapid changes in the gut microbiota composition that were more pronounced with the animal diet. The animal diet turned the metabolic functions of gut microbiota toward a decreased production of SCFA and an increased production of branched-chain fatty acids and deoxycholic acid. In addition, the expression of genes for vitamin biosynthesis, degradation of polycyclic aromatic hydrocarbons (which are carcinogenic compounds), and β-lactamase were increased. Diet is also an important contributor to the pathogenesis of NAFLD. Particularly, saturated fat and fructose are more likely to stimulate hepatic lipid accumulation and progression into NASH.[53] Because it is at the interface between nutrients and the liver, gut microbiota probably contributes to the diet-induced liver lesions through the products it delivers in the portal circulation. In this setting, a high-fructose diet in mice induces gut-derived portal endotoxemia that promotes liver steatosis through the activation of TLR4 and TNF-α,[54,55] and such fructose-induced steatosis is markedly reduced by antibiotic intestinal decontamination.[56] Global lifestyle modification, including healthy feeding with weight loss, is the main objective to improve the metabolic syndrome and NAFLD. However, whether modulation of gut microbiota by specific dietary intervention can improve liver lesions of NAFLD remains still unclear and needs further evaluation.

Considering that gut microbiota has a role in NAFLD, a logical approach would be to modulate and redirect it in the right way by using probiotics and/or prebiotics. Probiotics are live microorganisms that, when consumed in appropriate amounts in food, confer a health benefit on the host; *prebiotics* is a general term to refer to chemicals that induce the growth or activity of microorganisms that contribute to the well-being of their host. Several studies have evaluated probiotics and prebiotics in animal models of NAFLD.[57,58] As an example, in mice fed a methionine choline–deficient diet, administration of *Lactobacillus casei* reduced serum lipopolysaccharide concentration and significantly improved liver parameters of inflammation and fibrosis.[59] In another mice experiment, cranberry extract increased the gut relative abundance of the mucin-degrading bacteria *Akkermansia,* and improved endotoxemia, insulin sensitivity, liver steatosis, liver inflammation, and liver oxidative stress induced by high-fat/high-sucrose feeding.[60] Only a few clinical studies with small sample sizes, heterogeneous populations, and various preparations have evaluated probiotics in NAFLD patients.[61,62] In a recent metaanalysis that pooled 4 randomized controlled trials for a total of 134 patients included, probiotics were shown to decrease significantly serum aminotransferases, total and high-density lipoprotein cholesterol, TNF-α, and insulin resistance as assessed by the Homeostasis Model Assessment index.[63] There was no effect on body mass index, glucose, or low-density lipoprotein cholesterol. Another recent randomized controlled trial conducted in 48 obese children with biopsy-proven NAFLD showed that VSL#3 during 4 months significantly improved liver steatosis, as well as body mass index and glucagon-like peptide 1.[64] There was no effect on serum transaminases, triglycerides, or Homeostasis Model Assessment in this work. Finally, more evidence is required before recommending the use of probiotics or prebiotics for NAFLD patients in clinical practice.

SUMMARY

NAFLD is an extremely common, complex disease that results from interactions between susceptible polygenic backgrounds and environmental factors. Recent evidence has introduced the gut microbiota as a new and crucial player in this complex story. The gut microbiota is like a big and complex factory that produces many compounds that are further delivered to the liver with activation of numerous pathways. We

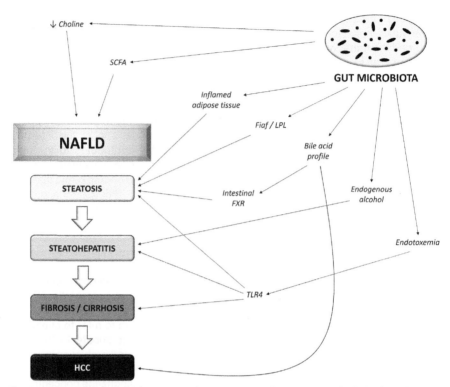

Fig. 1. Mechanisms by which gut microbiota can contributes to nonalcoholic fatty liver disease (NAFLD) and its severity. HCC, hepatocellular carcinoma; LPL, lipoprotein lipase; SCFA, short-chain fatty acids.

are only starting to decipher the numerous mechanisms linking gut microbiota to NAFLD (**Fig. 1**). This research will advance the understanding of the disease's pathogenesis, thereby identifying new therapeutic targets that will ultimately improve the outcome of patients with this disease.

REFERENCES

1. Gill SR, Pop M, Deboy RT, et al. Metagenomic analysis of the human distal gut microbiome. Science 2006;312:1355–9.
2. Backhed F, Ley RE, Sonnenburg JL, et al. Host-bacterial mutualism in the human intestine. Science 2005;307:1915–20.
3. Turnbaugh PJ, Hamady M, Yatsunenko T, et al. A core gut microbiome in obese and lean twins. Nature 2009;457:480–4.
4. Cerf-Bensussan N, Gaboriau-Routhiau V. The immune system and the gut microbiota: friends or foes? Nat Rev Immunol 2010;10:735–44.
5. Nicholson JK, Holmes E, Kinross J, et al. Host-gut microbiota metabolic interactions. Science 2012;336:1262–7.
6. Janssen AW, Kersten S. The role of the gut microbiota in metabolic health. FASEB J 2015;29(8):3111–23.
7. Wiest R, Garcia-Tsao G. Bacterial translocation (BT) in cirrhosis. Hepatology 2005;41:422–33.

8. Weinstock GM. Genomic approaches to studying the human microbiota. Nature 2012;489:250–6.

9. Cusi K. Role of obesity and lipotoxicity in the development of nonalcoholic steatohepatitis: pathophysiology and clinical implications. Gastroenterology 2012; 142:711–25.e6.

10. Angulo P, Kleiner DE, Dam-Larsen S, et al. Liver fibrosis, but no other histologic features, associates with long-term outcomes of patients with nonalcoholic fatty liver disease. Gastroenterology 2015;149(2):389–97.e10.

11. Ekstedt M, Hagstrom H, Nasr P, et al. Fibrosis stage is the strongest predictor for disease-specific mortality in NAFLD after up to 33 years of follow-up. Hepatology 2015;61:1547–54.

12. Younossi ZM, Stepanova M, Afendy M, et al. Changes in the prevalence of the most common causes of chronic liver diseases in the United States from 1988 to 2008. Clin Gastroenterol Hepatol 2011;9:524–30.

13. Le Roy T, Llopis M, Lepage P, et al. Intestinal microbiota determines development of non-alcoholic fatty liver disease in mice. Gut 2013;62:1787–94.

14. Newgard CB. Interplay between lipids and branched-chain amino acids in development of insulin resistance. Cell Metab 2012;15:606–14.

15. Wigg AJ, Roberts-Thomson IC, Dymock RB, et al. The role of small intestinal bacterial overgrowth, intestinal permeability, endotoxaemia, and tumour necrosis factor alpha in the pathogenesis of non-alcoholic steatohepatitis. Gut 2001;48: 206–11.

16. Sajjad A, Mottershead M, Syn WK, et al. Ciprofloxacin suppresses bacterial overgrowth, increases fasting insulin but does not correct low acylated ghrelin concentration in non-alcoholic steatohepatitis. Aliment Pharmacol Ther 2005;22:291–9.

17. Sabate JM, Jouet P, Harnois F, et al. High prevalence of small intestinal bacterial overgrowth in patients with morbid obesity: a contributor to severe hepatic steatosis. Obes Surg 2008;18:371–7.

18. Miele L, Valenza V, La Torre G, et al. Increased intestinal permeability and tight junction alterations in nonalcoholic fatty liver disease. Hepatology 2009;49: 1877–87.

19. Shanab AA, Scully P, Crosbie O, et al. Small intestinal bacterial overgrowth in nonalcoholic steatohepatitis: association with toll-like receptor 4 expression and plasma levels of interleukin 8. Dig Dis Sci 2011;56:1524–34.

20. Caricilli AM, Saad MJ. The role of gut microbiota on insulin resistance. Nutrients 2013;5:829–51.

21. Volynets V, Kuper MA, Strahl S, et al. Nutrition, intestinal permeability, and blood ethanol levels are altered in patients with nonalcoholic fatty liver disease (NAFLD). Dig Dis Sci 2012;57:1932–41.

22. Backhed F, Ding H, Wang T, et al. The gut microbiota as an environmental factor that regulates fat storage. Proc Natl Acad Sci U S A 2004;101:15718–23.

23. Backhed F, Manchester JK, Semenkovich CF, et al. Mechanisms underlying the resistance to diet-induced obesity in germ-free mice. Proc Natl Acad Sci U S A 2007;104:979–84.

24. Jiang C, Xie C, Li F, et al. Intestinal farnesoid X receptor signaling promotes nonalcoholic fatty liver disease. J Clin Invest 2015;125:386–402.

25. den Besten G, van Eunen K, Groen AK, et al. The role of short-chain fatty acids in the interplay between diet, gut microbiota, and host energy metabolism. J Lipid Res 2013;54:2325–40.

26. Zhu L, Baker RD, Baker SS. Gut microbiome and non-alcoholic fatty liver diseases. Pediatr Res 2015;77(1–2):245–51.

27. Puertollano E, Kolida S, Yaqoob P. Biological significance of short-chain fatty acid metabolism by the intestinal microbiome. Curr Opin Clin Nutr Metab Care 2014; 17:139–44.

28. Vrieze A, Van Nood E, Holleman F, et al. Transfer of intestinal microbiota from lean donors increases insulin sensitivity in individuals with metabolic syndrome. Gastroenterology 2012;143:913–6.e7.

29. Maher JJ. New insights from rodent models of fatty liver disease. Antioxid Redox Signal 2011;15:535–50.

30. Craciun S, Balskus EP. Microbial conversion of choline to trimethylamine requires a glycyl radical enzyme. Proc Natl Acad Sci U S A 2012;109:21307–12.

31. Dumas ME, Barton RH, Toye A, et al. Metabolic profiling reveals a contribution of gut microbiota to fatty liver phenotype in insulin-resistant mice. Proc Natl Acad Sci U S A 2006;103:12511–6.

32. Spencer MD, Hamp TJ, Reid RW, et al. Association between composition of the human gastrointestinal microbiome and development of fatty liver with choline deficiency. Gastroenterology 2011;140:976–86.

33. Lassailly G, Caiazzo R, Buob D, et al. Bariatric surgery reduces features of non-alcoholic steatohepatitis in morbidly obese patients. Gastroenterology 2015; 149(2):379–88.

34. Liou AP, Paziuk M, Luevano JM Jr, et al. Conserved shifts in the gut microbiota due to gastric bypass reduce host weight and adiposity. Sci Transl Med 2013; 5:178ra141.

35. Raman M, Ahmed I, Gillevet PM, et al. Fecal microbiome and volatile organic compound metabolome in obese humans with nonalcoholic fatty liver disease. Clin Gastroenterol Hepatol 2013;11:868–75.e1–3.

36. Mouzaki M, Comelli EM, Arendt BM, et al. Intestinal microbiota in patients with nonalcoholic fatty liver disease. Hepatology 2013;58:120–7.

37. Zhu L, Baker SS, Gill C, et al. Characterization of gut microbiomes in nonalcoholic steatohepatitis (NASH) patients: a connection between endogenous alcohol and NASH. Hepatology 2013;57:601–9.

38. Wong VW, Tse CH, Lam TT, et al. Molecular characterization of the fecal micro-biota in patients with nonalcoholic steatohepatitis–a longitudinal study. PLoS One 2013;8:e62885.

39. Munukka E, Pekkala S, Wiklund P, et al. Gut-adipose tissue axis in hepatic fat accumulation in humans. J Hepatol 2014;61:132–8.

40. Schnabl B, Brenner DA. Interactions between the intestinal microbiome and liver diseases. Gastroenterology 2014;146:1513–24.

41. Henao-Mejia J, Elinav E, Jin C, et al. Inflammasome-mediated dysbiosis regulates progression of NAFLD and obesity. Nature 2012;482:179–85.

42. Farhadi A, Gundlapalli S, Shaikh M, et al. Susceptibility to gut leakiness: a possible mechanism for endotoxaemia in non-alcoholic steatohepatitis. Liver Int 2008;28:1026–33.

43. Ruiz AG, Casafont F, Crespo J, et al. Lipopolysaccharide-binding protein plasma levels and liver TNF-alpha gene expression in obese patients: evidence for the potential role of endotoxin in the pathogenesis of non-alcoholic steatohepatitis. Obes Surg 2007;17:1374–80.

44. Alisi A, Manco M, Devito R, et al. Endotoxin and plasminogen activator inhibitor-1 serum levels associated with nonalcoholic steatohepatitis in children. J Pediatr Gastroenterol Nutr 2010;50:645–9.

45. Yuan J, Baker SS, Liu W, et al. Endotoxemia unrequired in the pathogenesis of pediatric nonalcoholic steatohepatitis. J Gastroenterol Hepatol 2014;29:1292–8.

46. De Minicis S, Rychlicki C, Agostinelli L, et al. Dysbiosis contributes to fibrogenesis in the course of chronic liver injury. Hepatology 2014;59:1738–49.
47. Zhu Q, Zou L, Jagavelu K, et al. Intestinal decontamination inhibits TLR4 dependent fibronectin-mediated cross-talk between stellate cells and endothelial cells in liver fibrosis in mice. J Hepatol 2012;56:893–9.
48. Yoshimoto S, Loo TM, Atarashi K, et al. Obesity-induced gut microbial metabolite promotes liver cancer through senescence secretome. Nature 2013;499:97–101.
49. Calkin AC, Tontonoz P. Transcriptional integration of metabolism by the nuclear sterol-activated receptors LXR and FXR. Nat Rev Mol Cell Biol 2012;13:213–24.
50. Chiang JY. Bile acid metabolism and signaling. Compr Physiol 2013;3:1191–212.
51. Neuschwander-Tetri BA, Loomba R, Sanyal AJ, et al. Farnesoid X nuclear receptor ligand obeticholic acid for non-cirrhotic, non-alcoholic steatohepatitis (FLINT): a multicentre, randomised, placebo-controlled trial. Lancet 2015;385:956–65.
52. David LA, Maurice CF, Carmody RN, et al. Diet rapidly and reproducibly alters the human gut microbiome. Nature 2014;505:559–63.
53. de Wit NJ, Afman LA, Mensink M, et al. Phenotyping the effect of diet on non-alcoholic fatty liver disease. J Hepatol 2012;57:1370–3.
54. Spruss A, Kanuri G, Wagnerberger S, et al. Toll-like receptor 4 is involved in the development of fructose-induced hepatic steatosis in mice. Hepatology 2009;50:1094–104.
55. Kanuri G, Spruss A, Wagnerberger S, et al. Role of tumor necrosis factor alpha (TNFalpha) in the onset of fructose-induced nonalcoholic fatty liver disease in mice. J Nutr Biochem 2011;22:527–34.
56. Bergheim I, Weber S, Vos M, et al. Antibiotics protect against fructose-induced hepatic lipid accumulation in mice: role of endotoxin. J Hepatol 2008;48:983–92.
57. Abenavoli L, Scarpellini E, Rouabhia S, et al. Probiotics in non-alcoholic fatty liver disease: which and when. Ann Hepatol 2013;12:357–63.
58. Parnell JA, Raman M, Rioux KP, et al. The potential role of prebiotic fibre for treatment and management of non-alcoholic fatty liver disease and associated obesity and insulin resistance. Liver Int 2012;32:701–11.
59. Okubo H, Sakoda H, Kushiyama A, et al. Lactobacillus casei strain Shirota protects against nonalcoholic steatohepatitis development in a rodent model. Am J Physiol Gastrointest Liver Physiol 2013;305:G911–8.
60. Anhe FF, Roy D, Pilon G, et al. A polyphenol-rich cranberry extract protects from diet-induced obesity, insulin resistance and intestinal inflammation in association with increased Akkermansia spp. population in the gut microbiota of mice. Gut 2015;64:872–83.
61. Ferolla SM, Armiliato GN, Couto CA, et al. The role of intestinal bacteria overgrowth in obesity-related nonalcoholic fatty liver disease. Nutrients 2014;6:5583–99.
62. Tarantino G, Finelli C. Systematic review on intervention with prebiotics/probiotics in patients with obesity-related nonalcoholic fatty liver disease. Future Microbiol 2015;10:889–902.
63. Ma YY, Li L, Yu CH, et al. Effects of probiotics on nonalcoholic fatty liver disease: a meta-analysis. World J Gastroenterol 2013;19:6911–8.
64. Alisi A, Bedogni G, Baviera G, et al. Randomised clinical trial: the beneficial effects of VSL#3 in obese children with non-alcoholic steatohepatitis. Aliment Pharmacol Ther 2014;39:1276–85.

Clinical Presentation and Patient Evaluation in Nonalcoholic Fatty Liver Disease

Vaishali Patel, MBBS, Arun J. Sanyal, MBBS, MD,
Richard Sterling, MD, MSc*

KEYWORDS

- Nonalcoholic fatty liver • Steatohepatitis • Evaluation

KEY POINTS

- Nonalcoholic fatty liver disease (NAFLD) is a spectrum of liver disease ranging from simple steatosis to cirrhosis.
- Although identifying people with advanced fibrosis is important for monitoring of cirrhosis and its complications, currently there are no treatment options available to arrest or reverse disease progression.
- To date, noninvasive investigations help in diagnosing steatosis and excluding or definitively diagnosis advanced fibrosis; however, people with early or intermediate degree of fibrosis are often not identified by serologic or radiological noninvasive tests.
- Transient elastography is the most widely used of these tests; but the reliability of the results, even by experienced providers, has been questioned.
- As of 2015, nonalcoholic steatohepatitis remains a histologic diagnosis; until the methods are further developed for diagnosing NAFLD by noninvasive methods, liver biopsies, although flawed, remain our gold standard.

DEFINITIONS
Nonalcoholic Fatty Liver Disease

Nonalcoholic fatty liver disease (NAFLD) is defined as presence of fat in the liver in the absence of alcohol use for which no cause can be found after a thorough clinical and

Disclosure statement: Dr A.J. Sanyal has served as a consultant to AbbVie, Astra Zeneca, Nitto Denko, Nimbus, Salix, Tobira, Takeda, Fibrogen, Immuron, Exhalenz, and Genfit. His institution has received grant support from Gilead, Salix, Tobira, and Novartis. Drs V. Patel and R. Sterling have nothing to disclose.
Section of Hepatology, Department of Gastroenterology, Hepatology and Nutrition, Virginia Commonwealth University, 1200 East Broad Street, West Hospital, Room 1478, Richmond, VA 23298-0341, USA
* Corresponding author.
E-mail address: rksterli@vcu.edu

Clin Liver Dis 20 (2016) 277–292
http://dx.doi.org/10.1016/j.cld.2015.10.006
1089-3261/16/$ – see front matter © 2016 Elsevier Inc. All rights reserved.

laboratory evaluation. NAFLD is currently thought to be a hepatic manifestation of metabolic syndrome. The term represents a spectrum of liver disease, ranging from hepatic steatosis to nonalcoholic steatohepatitis (NASH) cirrhosis.

Nonalcoholic Fatty Liver

Fat in the liver without significant inflammation or fibrosis is referred to as nonalcoholic fatty liver (NAFL) and represents the more benign end of the disease spectrum.

Nonalcoholic Steatohepatitis

NASH requires inflammation in addition to steatosis in the presence of ballooned hepatocytes, usually in the presence of pericellular fibrosis. As fibrosis progresses, the amount of fat and inflammation can decrease. Hence, most people diagnosed with cryptogenic cirrhosis may have evolved from NASH.[1] One in 5 people with NAFLD have NASH on liver biopsies.

WHY DO WE NEED TO DIAGNOSE NONALCOHOLIC FATTY LIVER DISEASE?

NAFLD is usually associated with the metabolic syndrome (**Fig. 1**). It can also be associated with certain medications, hormonal disturbances, and nutritional disturbances. Overall patients with NAFLD had a 34% to 69% increased chance of dying over 15 years compared with the general population. The most common cause of mortality from NAFLD is due to cardiovascular disease, followed by extrahepatic malignancy. Liver-related mortality occurs in less than 5% of patients and is the third leading cause of death in these patients.[2] NAFLD is now the second most common cause for listing for liver transplant. However, people with NAFLD were less likely to receive a transplant and had a higher mortality on the transplant list when compared with patients with hepatitis C virus (HCV), alcohol, or liver disease from both alcohol and HCV combined.[3]

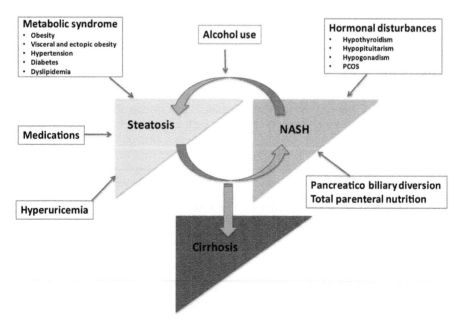

Fig. 1. Spectrum and risk factors of NALFD. PCOS, polycystic ovary syndrome.

FIBROSIS AS A PREDICTOR OF MORTALITY: WHO WITH NONALCOHOLIC FATTY LIVER DISEASE IS AT RISK OF DYING?

Before initiating tests, it is important to determine who with NAFLD has the highest mortality from NAFLD and the predictors thereof. NASH itself is a histologic diagnosis. MRI-based techniques are being investigated in the diagnosis of inflammation. But these need further validation. Until then, short of a liver biopsy, NASH can only be diagnosed on by a liver biopsy. But the need to diagnose NASH has been challenged. Data from multiple long-term studies suggest that patients with NAFLD with advanced fibrosis have 60% liver-related mortality compared with 9% in NAFLD without advanced fibrosis.[2] In a study of 118 patients with NAFLD with a follow-up over a median duration of 21 years, there was no difference in mortality in patients with biopsy-proven NASH compared with those without NASH.[4] Another study from the United States whereby 209 patients with NAFLD were followed over 12 years showed that grade 3 fibrosis was independently associated with liver-related mortality with a hazard ratio of 5.68 and confidence interval (CI) 1.5 to 21.5. NASH only corelated with mortality when fibrosis was included in the analysis.[5] People with NAFLD, thus, have an increased mortality compared with the general population. Advanced fibrosis and not inflammation is a predictor of NAFLD-related mortality. Hence, although NASH is a histologic diagnosis, to identify an individual patient's risk of mortality based on current evidence, identifying the degree of fibrosis in the liver is required.

The Evaluation of Suspected Nonalcoholic Fatty Liver Disease

There are 3 general pathways whereby the clinical suspicion of NAFLD arises (**Fig. 2**). Patients who are diagnosed with NAFLD can initially present with abnormal liver enzymes or abnormalities on imaging performed for other reasons or are identified based on clinical features of the metabolic syndrome. Regardless of how they are identified, the evaluation process is similar.

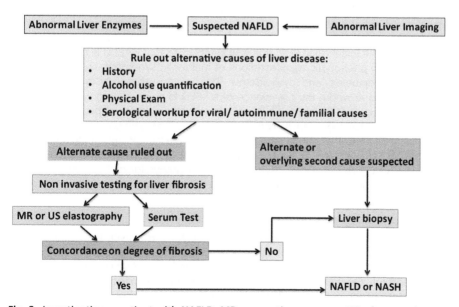

Fig. 2. Investigating a patient with NAFLD. MR, magnetic resonance; US, ultrasound.

The office visit

History Most people with NAFLD are diagnosed incidentally when liver enzymes are noted to be abnormal or when imaging done for unrelated purposes shows hepatic steatosis. People are usually asymptomatic until they develop signs/symptoms of decompensated liver disease. Early diagnosis is possible if a high index of suspicion is maintained in those with risk factors for metabolic syndrome. Often, however, subtle elevations of liver enzymes go unnoticed because most laboratories report the upper limit of alanine transaminase (ALT) to be much higher than what is now known to be normal, that is, 19 and 32 for women and men, respectively. The prevalence of NAFLD is estimated to be approximately 30% in the general population.[6,7] The reported prevalence of NAFLD varies depending on the modality used to diagnose NAFLD and the population under study.[8] By ultrasound (US), 46% of the general population in United States may have NAFLD.[9] However, about a 30% incidence is reported with magnetic resonance (MR) spectroscopy. However, most people in the community with NALFD are not currently recognized by their primary care physician. NASH is rarer and present in about 5% of the general population.[10]

Demographic features

Sex When Ludwig and colleagues[11] first described NAFLD in 1980 in a series of 20 patients, they reported that the disease might be more common in women. However, several more recent studies have since reported a higher prevalence in men when compared with women.[8,12]

Age The prevalence of NAFLD and advanced fibrosis in people with NAFLD increases with age.[10,13]

Race Depending on the population being studied, the prevalence of histologically proven NAFLD also varies. A prevalence of 20% was reported in Korean living donors versus in 51% of donors in the United States.[14,15] NAFLD is less common in African Americans, whereas the prevalence is higher in age- and body mass index (BMI)–matched Hispanic patients.[9]

Associated medical problems

A detailed history of medical problems known to coexist with NAFLD should be obtained during the initial clinic visit. It is well established that NAFLD is more common in patients with phenotypic manifestations of metabolic syndrome, such as obesity, hypertension, diabetes, and dyslipidemia. This is true, especially in patients with type 2 diabetes in whom the prevalence of NAFLD is much higher, with a reported prevalence of up to 69% by US.[10,16] Patients with dyslipidemia, especially with high triglycerides and low high-density lipoprotein, also have a higher prevalence of hepatic steatosis.[17] Several other chronic medical problems are increasingly being recognized to be associated with NAFLD, such as sleep apnea, polycystic ovarian disease, hypopituitarism, vitamin D deficiency, hypopituitarism, hypothyroidism, hyperuricemia, and pancreaticoduodenal resection. Hyperuricemia is associated with advanced fibrosis in patients with biopsy-proven NAFLD.[18–20]

Physical examination

NAFLD is typically common in people with higher BMIs. However, the distribution of fat is more important than just the amount of fat. Individuals who expand their stores of visceral fat in an overfed state tend to develop NAFLD and other features of metabolic syndrome. On the other hand, there are individuals, currently referred to as the metabolically healthy obese (MHO), who have a higher BMI but their subcutaneous fat stores are able to expand in a state of overfeeding.[21] In NAFLD, the liver is the organ in which there is ectopic distribution of body fat. Other such areas where metabolically active visceral fat is distributed is the pericardium, within skeletal muscles, and the pancreas. Visceral fat is more inflammatory than peripheral fat, which explains the fact that a higher waist to hip ratio is more important than BMI in identifying patients with NAFLD.[22] In NAFLD, dorsocervical fat correlates with the degree of inflammation and fibrosis.[23] Whether MHO is a unique entity or whether it represents the proximal end of the spectrum before decompensating to develop visceral adiposity, then adiposopathy, or the unhealthy visceral fat is yet to be determined in longitudinal studies.[21]

In lean patients, NAFLD represents a unique disease entity and a diagnostic challenge. People with NAFLD in the setting of normal BMIs usually have had a recent, rapid weight gain and often have increased visceral adipose tissue.[24,25] Most of the data on the so-called lean NAFLD is, however, not reliable as it is described in Asian populations in whom the standard BMI definitions do not hold and several features of metabolic syndrome are seen at lower BMIs. Nevertheless, lean NAFLD remains a challenge to manage, as the patients tend to be younger and often without a clear association with insulin resistance and dyslipidemia.[26] On physical examination, findings such as asymptomatic hepatomegaly may be noted. In patients with cirrhosis, stigmata of chronic liver disease can be seen. None of these findings on physical examination are in itself specific to NAFLD.

Differential diagnosis to consider

Chronic liver diseases associated with steatosis Before narrowing down the diagnosis, it is important to consider and rule out other diseases that may lead to or worsen hepatic steatosis and steatohepatitis. Certain chronic liver diseases, such as Wilson disease and HCV genotype 3, and certain inborn errors of metabolism, such as abetalipoproteinemia and lipodystrophy, are associated with varying degrees of hepatic steatosis. Hence, to identify these it is crucial to maintain a high degree of clinical suspicion and perform targeted tests in select individuals.

Drugs associated with steatosis and steatohepatitis The process of history taking should include details on current prescription and nonprescription medications (eg, nonsteroidal antiinflammatory drugs), herbs, and natural remedies. Certain cancer treatments, such as prednisone for lymphovascular malignancies, tamoxifen for breast cancer, and colon cancer chemotherapeutic agents, are associated with steatohepatitis. Depending on the drug under consideration, the steatosis may be predominantly caused by the drug as in the case of patients with long-term amiodarone use. Other drugs like tamoxifen or prednisone may simply be unmasking an individual's predisposition to NAFLD.[27-29]

Alcoholic liver disease A key portion of the history in making the diagnosis of NAFLD involves excluding those with heavy alcohol intake (more than 210 g of per week in men and 140 g per week in women). This amount translates to more than 2 drinks per day in women and 3 drinks per day in men. NAFLD may be indistinguishable from alcoholic liver disease on liver biopsy. Alcohol to nonalcohol index has been proposed with an online calculator to help distinguish the two.[30] In clinical practice, however, an objective assessment of alcohol consumption as assessed by using scores, such as the CAGE (cut down, annoyed, guilty, eye opener) questionnaire or preferably the World Health Organization's Alcohol Use Disorders Identification Test (AUDIT), is more likely to be useful. Although the CAGE is more sensitive and fast, its results depend on an individual's personal sense of how much they drink. On the other hand, the AUDIT is more likely to identify those with harmful alcohol intake regardless of whether they perceive it as excessive. Quantifying the amount of alcohol consumed is important as obesity and alcohol have a synergistic effect in the progression of liver disease, including the risk of hepatocellular carcinoma.[31] However, interestingly, a recent meta-analysis identified that as seen in cardiovascular disease, modest alcohol consumption may protect from developing steatohepatitis and advanced fibrosis in patients with NAFLD.[32]

LIVER BIOPSY

Liver biopsy is the current gold standard for assessing liver fibrosis and to differentiate NAFL from NASH. A core of 2.5 cm in length obtained with 16-gauge cutting needle is required for adequate assessment of fibrosis. If fewer than 11 complete portal tracts are visualized, then the pathologist should deem the sample inadequate. Even an adequate sample is, however, a very small 1 in 50,000th fragment of the liver and, hence, may not be representative of the true severity of the disease and fibrosis.[33–35] Liver biopsies in NAFLD are discussed by Kleiner DE, Makhlouf HR: Histology of Nonalcoholic Fatty Liver Disease and Nonalcoholic Steatohepatitis in Adults and Children, in this issue. However, it is crucial to note that noninvasive methods of assessing fibrosis use a method parallel to the Metavir score to grade fibrosis. Hence, F3 and F4 fibrosis represent bridging fibrosis and cirrhosis, respectively, and denote advanced fibrosis.[36]

Noninvasive Tests for Diagnosing Hepatic Steatosis

In the absence of liver biopsy, liver US has been used to diagnose steatosis.[37] In those without other liver disease, such as HCV, it is fairly accurate to diagnose moderate to severe steatosis (>30%) with both high sensitivity (>80%) and specificity (>95%). In those with lesser degrees of steatosis (which are most patients), the sensitivity decreases to 50%. It is subject to significant intraobserver and interobserver variability[38,39] and may be affected by underlying fibrosis. Computed tomography is also accurate to diagnosis moderate to severe steatosis but again less accurate for those with mild disease (5%–30% fat). MRI and MR spectroscopy seem to perform much better, even at lower grades of steatosis. However, these imaging techniques come with a cost. To overcome this limitation, several serum models have been developed to identify hepatic steatosis.[40] Both the fatty liver index and the lipid accumulation product have been validated to identify greater than 5% steatosis with 80% accuracy.[41–43] However, their ability to quantify the amount of fat is poor, and these tests can also be affected by liver inflammation and fibrosis. Although not yet approved by the Food and Drug Administration, continuous attenuated parameter, which assesses severity of steatosis at the same time as transient elastography (TE) (see later discussion), has shown promise with area under the receiver operating characteristic curve (AUROC) of greater than 0.80 with a sensitivity of 80% and specificity of 80%[44,45] However, before incorporating these models into routine practice, additional data are needed.

SEROLOGIC TESTS FOR DIAGNOSING HEPATIC FIBROSIS IN NONALCOHOLIC FATTY LIVER DISEASE

Serologic tests include direct and indirect measurement of fibrosis. The direct serologic markers are molecules that are derived directly from the extracellular matrix or are produced by activated hepatic stellate cells. The indirect markers of fibrosis attempt to capture an overall deterioration of hepatic function. Direct and indirect markers may be used alone or in combination to produce composite scores for estimating fibrosis.

Indirect Markers of Fibrosis

Clinical calculators: based on routine laboratory tests and vitals

These clinical calculators are predictive models based on indirect markers of fibrosis and often combine routine laboratory tests with certain clinical parameters, such as the BMI. The NASH fibrosis score, aspartate transaminase (AST)/ALT ratio, FIB-4, and BARD are commonly used calculators. Simplicity and cost are the two greatest advantages of these scores. Overall these scores are able to exclude those with no fibrosis and identify patients with advanced fibrosis.

Aspartate transaminase/alanine transaminase ratio Early in the course of the disease, AST and ALT are modestly elevated with ALT being higher than ALT. However, a normal ALT may fail to identify nearly half the patients with NASH.[46,47]

In normal people, the AST/ALT ratio is less than 0.8. With an increase in fibrosis, the ratio of AST to ALT increases.[13] In the absence of alcohol, a ratio is greater than 1 is commonly used in clinical practice to suggest cirrhosis. Although it is widely used and several scores incorporate the ratio of AST/ALT, by itself it is not reliable.[48]

BARD The BARD score was developed in NAFLD to predict fibrosis. It includes a BMI greater than or equal to 28 kg/m^2 = 1 point, AST/ALT ratio greater than or equal to 0.8 = 2 points, AST/ALT ratio less than 0.8 = 0 points, and freshly recognized or pre-existing diabetes = 1 point, with a score of 2 to 4 points suggestive of significant fibrosis. In a series of 126 patients with NAFLD, the positive and negative predictive values of the BARD score for advanced fibrosis were 69% and 96%, respectively, with an AUROC of 0.87.[49]

Nonalcoholic fatty liver disease fibrosis score The NAFLD fibrosis score was also developed specifically to determine the likelihood of fibrosis in patients with NAFLD. It consists of glucose intolerance, age, BMI, platelets, AST, ALT, and albumin. A high NAFLD fibrosis score cutoff (>0.676) is highly specific (96%) with a positive predictive value of 82% for detecting bridging fibrosis. The low cutoff value of less than −1.455 has a negative predictive value of 88% and sensitivity of 77% with a high specificity of 72%. This score remains the most studied of the clinical scores and has a simple online calculator for easy use in day-to-day practice (www.nafldscore.com/).[50] However, its utility in clinical practice is limited because most patients do not have all the characteristics that are required to get a low score.

FIB-4 The FIB-4 index combines platelet count, ALT, AST, and age. It was developed in human immunodeficiency virus/HCV and validated in those with HCV alone. At a cutoff of less than 1.45, the negative predictive value to exclude advanced fibrosis (stage 4–6) was 90%; a cutoff of greater than 3.25 had a positive predictive value of 65% and a specificity of 97%.[51] It has been validated in NAFLD. In a study of 541 adults with NAFLD, FIB-4 and 7 other markers were compared in their utility in predicting liver-related mortality. FIB-4 outperformed all other markers, including the AST/ALT ratio, AST to platelet ratio index (APRI), NAFLD fibrosis score, and the BARD score. The AUROC for FIB-4 was 0.802 (95% CI, 0.758–0.847), which was higher than that of the NAFLD fibrosis score (0.768; 95% CI, 0.720–0.816; P = .09), AST:ALT ratio (0.742; 95% CI, 0.690–0.794; P<.015), APRI (0.730; 95% CI, 0.681–0.779; P<.001), BMI, AST:ALT, and diabetes (BARD) score (0.70; P<.001).[52]

Propriety Panels of Clinical Parameters

Fibrotest and nonalcoholic fatty liver disease fibrometer

These two tests are proprietary tests that have been validated to have good negative predictive values for excluding fibrosis in NAFLD. Although these are more readily available compared with panels of direct markers, their cost and comparable performance with other calculators mentioned earlier limits their routine use. Comparative performance of indirect makers of hepatic fibrosis is summarized in **Table 1**.[50,52–56]

Direct markers of fibrosis In theory, panels that incorporate direct markers of matric turnover are more specific in identifying fibrosis. However, studies have shown that they are comparable with panels of indirect markers that include simple tests (such as FIB-4) in their accuracy in detecting fibrosis. The biggest limitation is concerns over cost and lack of availability. The direct markers validated in NAFLD are summarized in **Table 2**.[48,57–60]

Cytokeratin-18 Cytokeratin-18 (CK18) is an intermediate filament and has been studied extensively in NALFD. It comprises about 5% of total protein in epithelial and parenchymal cells. Caspases induce the apoptosis by cleaving CK18; hence, the resultant CK18 fragments (CK18Fs) serve as surrogate markers of apoptosis and fibrosis. CK18 are increased in the serum in NAFLD.[61,62] In NAFLD, levels of

Table 1
Panels of indirect markers of hepatic fibrosis

Test	Components of the Panel	Study (n)	Cutoff	AUROC	Reference
Clinical calculators					
FIB-4	AST, ALT, age, platelet count	541	<1.3	0.802 (advanced fibrosis)	52
		320	>2.67	0.81 (adverse liver related outcomes)	53
BARD	AST/ALT, BMI, age	126	2.0	0.87 (advanced fibrosis)	54
		541	—	0.70 (advanced fibrosis)	52
		320	—	0.73 (adverse liver related outcomes)	53
APRI	AST, platelets	320	1.0	0.73 (advanced fibrosis)	52
				0.80 (adverse liver related outcomes)	53
NFS	AST/ALT, IFG/DM, age, BMI, platelets, and albumin	733	<−1.455	0.768 (advanced fibrosis)	52
			>0.676	0.82–0.088 (adverse liver related outcomes)	50
Proprietary panels of indirect markers					
NAFLD Fibrometer	AST, ALT< weight, age, platelets, glucose, and ferritin	235	—	0.93–0.94 (advanced fibrosis)	55
Fibrotest	Age, sex, bilirubin, GGT, haptoglobin, apolipoprotein A1, and α2-microglobulin	267	>0.3 >0.7	0.84 (advanced fibrosis)	56

Abbreviations: DM, diabetes mellitus; GGT, γ-glutamyltransferase; IFG, impaired fasting glucose; NFS, NAFLD fibrosis score.

Table 2
Direct markers of fibrosis in NAFLD

Test	Components of the Panel	Study (n)	Cutoff	AUROC (for Advanced Fibrosis)
Hyaluronate	Hyaluronate	148	42 ng/mL	0.97
Type 4 collagen 7S	Type 4 collagen 7S	112	5 ng/mL	0.82
Enhanced liver fibrosis panel	Tissue inhibitors of matrix metaaloproteinases-1, hyaluronate, terminal peptide of procollagen III	192	0.3576	0.90
Hepascore	Age, sex, bilirubin, α2-microglobulin, GGT, and hyaluronate	242	0.37	0.81

Abbreviation: GGT, γ-glutamyltransferase.
Data from Refs.[47,55–58]

specific CK18Fs, M30 antigen and M65, have been shown to help distinguish between advanced fibrosis and early stage fibrosis.[63]

IMAGING TESTS FOR DIAGNOSING HEPATIC FIBROSIS IN NONALCOHOLIC FATTY LIVER DISEASE
Conventional Imaging

Conventional and Doppler US and MRI may help in identifying steatosis, but sensitivity and specificity for diagnosing advanced fibrosis is limited. With MRI the cost and availability is often the limiting factor.[64,65]

Elastography

Elastography measures the stiffness of the liver. Stiffness depends on the amount of scaring in the liver. The technology uses a force to displace the liver tissue, and the degree of displacement is then measured by US or MRI. The underlying principle is that fibrotic tissue offers less strain compared with normal liver. In other words, scar is stiffer and displaces. Because scars displace less, shear waves propagate faster through fibrotic tissue. Both US- and MRI-based techniques are now used to quantify the elasticity of the liver. Besides scaring, several factors can affect the liver stiffness and, hence, the accuracy of elastography (**Box 1**).[48,66]

Ultrasonography Elastography

Depending on the modality used to deform the liver tissue, elastography can be strain elastography, in which for example heart movements are used to deform the liver tissue or the more widely studied shear wave elastography (SWE). SWE in turn can be classified into Transient Elastography (TE) or acoustic radiation force imaging (ARFI). In TE, the force is a physical force used to displace the tissue, whereas in ARFI, a radiation force is used to generate the shear force. ARFI is referred to as point-SWE if measurements are made from one area (0.5 cm–1.0 cm) or 2-dimensional–SWE if multiple points are measured sequentially. Comparisons and contrasts between the two are summarized in **Table 3**.[58,66–70] TE, marketed as FibroScan (Echosens, Paris, France), has better accuracy than ARFI. A recent meta-analysis on FibroScan reported that it detects F3+ fibrosis with a sensitivity of 85% and specificity of 82% (AUROC 0.76–0.98). It is more accurate in cirrhosis with a sensitivity and specificity of 92% (AUROC 0.91–0.99).[71] The biggest limitation with US-based

---

Box 1
Factors that affect accuracy of elastography

Hepatic inflammation

Hepatic congestion

Cholestatic liver diseases

Focal liver lesions

Distance between skin and liver
- Obesity
- Ascites
- Musculoskeletal deformity

Recent food ingestion

Beta-blockers

Respiratory movements

Data from Castera L, Vilgrain V, Angulo P. Noninvasive evaluation of NAFLD. Nat Rev Gastroenterol Hepatol 2013;10:666–75; and Wong VW, Vergniol J, Wong GL, et al. Diagnosis of fibrosis and cirrhosis using liver stiffness measurement in nonalcoholic fatty liver disease. Hepatology 2010;51:454–62.

---

elastography techniques is unreliability of the results in people with a BMI greater than 35, even when using an XL probe in case of TE.[70]

Magnetic Resonance Elastography

MR elastography (MRE) uses a similar principle as TE to measure liver stiffness. It is also noninvasive and has several advantages when compared with TE, including assessing stiffness over a larger segment of liver and simultaneous imaging of liver parenchyma. The cost and inability to use contrast in patients with kidney failure are the limitations. When compared directly with TE, in a study of 141 patients with varying causes of chronic liver disease, the diagnostic accuracy of MRE was 94% compared

Table 3
Comparisons and contrasts between TE and ARFI

TE	ARFI
Shear force is mechanical.	Shear force is acoustic.
For detecting F2 or greater fibrosis: Sensitivity was 0.78 (95% CI: 0.72–0.83). Specificity was 0.84 (95% CI: 0.75–0.90).	For detecting F2 or greater fibrosis: Sensitivity was 0.74 (95% CI: 0.66–0.80). Specificity was 0.83 (95% CI: 0.75–0.89).
Pressure is reported in kPa.	Shear wave speed reported in m/s.
Larger measured segment is 5 cm.	Smaller measured segment is 1–2 cm.
There is no visualization of liver parenchyma.	There is visualization of the liver parenchyma.
It is affected by the distance of liver tissue from the skin; XL probe is available for people with elevated BMI.	It is not affected by the distance of liver tissue, but results are affected by the presence of hepatic fat and inflammation.
It is validated in posttransplant patients.	It is not studied in posttransplant patients.
It cannot be used in patients with ascites.	It can be used in patients with ascites.

Data from Refs.[58,66–70]

with 84% for TE for detecting fibrosis. Accuracy of MRE is significantly higher for cirrhosis and significant fibrosis. MRE can also be useful in distinguishing NAFL from NASH with fibrosis.[72,73] In 58 patients with NAFLD, the liver stiffness was 4.16 kPa in patients with fibrosis, 3.24 kPa with NASH, and 2.51 with steatosis. For diagnosis of NASH, the reported sensitivity and specificity were 94% and 73%, respectively.[74] MR spectroscopy is an MRI technique that allows measuring the chemical composition of a tissue and, hence, can be effectively used for quantifying hepatic fat. In preliminary studies it has been shown to correlate well with histologic fat quantification.[75]

Breath Tests for Diagnosis of Nonalcoholic Fatty Liver Disease and Degree of Fibrosis

The carbon-13 (^{13}C) breath tests are hepatic function tests in which the excretion of the ^{13}C isotope in the breath is measured after administering a labeled probe that is metabolized in the liver. Depending on the rate-limiting step needed in the metabolism of the probe molecule, a specific metabolic pathway can be studied. Several breath tests with molecules metabolized by cytosolic (eg, ketoiscaproic acid, aminopyrine), microsomal (methacetin), or mitochondrial (eg, methionine) pathways have been developed and are being studied in chronic liver diseases.[76] In NAFLD, ^{13}C caffeine breath tests have shown the most promising results. Excretion of ^{13}C is significantly lower in patients with NASH (1.59 ± 0.65, P = .005) and cirrhosis (1.00 ± 0.73, $P<.001$) when compared with controls. The AUROC for identifying cirrhosis was 0.86. No difference in the excretion of ^{13}C was found in normal subjects (2.31 ± 0.85, P = 1.0) and patients with simple steatosis (2.28 ± 0.71).[77] Similarly, the ^{13}C-labeled methionine breath test has been shown to identify NASH from normal subjects and, depending of the cutoff used, helps distinguish between early and advanced fibrosis in patients with NAFLD.[78] Although promising, these tests are still in the preliminary stages of being studied but provide a noninvasive and functional assessment of liver function.

Tiers of Investigating Nonalcoholic Fatty Liver Disease

The diagnosis of NAFLD is often based on the finding of abnormal liver enzymes and hepatic steatosis by imaging in asymptomatic individuals. The first approach should be performing a detailed history and physical examination to make a note of associated medical problems, medication and herbal product use, and quantifying alcohol use. This approach should be followed with laboratory tests to rule out alternative causes of chronic liver disease (see **Fig. 2**). If NALFD is suspected because of steatosis on imaging, abnormal enzymes, and negative serologic work-up for other liver diseases, then tests should be undertaken to assess the degree of fibrosis in the liver. If both serum and imaging tests agree, then liver biopsy can often be avoided. In patients with indeterminate results on noninvasive tests for fibrosis, a liver biopsy should be performed. This point is especially true in patients with diabetes who can have advanced fibrosis despite normal liver enzymes. Liver biopsy may be needed in additional cases, which includes patients in whom the diagnosis of NAFLD remains in doubt or a secondary cause of liver disease is suspected. In nondiabetic patients, differentiating NAFLD from NASH is important because those with NASH are the population targeted for therapy. Although the exact sequence or combination of these noninvasive tests that will give the highest accuracy in diagnosis fibrosis is NAFLD not clear, **Fig. 3** is a suggested algorithm for clinical practice. Those patients with a low probability of significant disease (low APRI and FIB-4) can be managed conservatively. Conversely, those with a high APRI and FIB-4 can have elastography for confirmation and should be managed by an experienced provider.

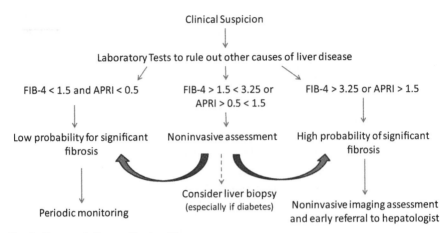

Fig. 3. Proposed diagnostic algorithm.

SUMMARY

NAFLD is not a single disease entity; rather it is a spectrum of liver disease ranging from simple steatosis to cirrhosis. Different modalities, laboratory tests, and imaging in combination often help in identifying different aspects of the disease. Fibrosis is a predictor of mortality from NAFLD. Although identifying people with advanced fibrosis is important for the monitoring of cirrhosis and its complications, currently there are no treatment options available to arrest or reverse disease progression. To date, noninvasive investigations help in diagnosing steatosis and excluding or definitively diagnosing advanced fibrosis. However, people with an early or intermediate degree of fibrosis are often not identified by serologic or radiological noninvasive tests. And it is these people who are in the greatest need of intervention to prevent further progression of scaring and, hence, NAFLD-related mortality. TE is the most widely used of these, but the reliability of the results even by an experienced provider has been questioned. Besides, the only approved treatment of NAFLD is vitamin E in patients who have NASH without diabetes. As of 2015, NASH remains a histologic diagnosis. Hence, until we finesse our methods for precisely diagnosing NAFLD by noninvasive methods, liver biopsies, although flawed, remain our gold standard.

REFERENCES

1. Chalasani N, Younossi Z, Lavine J, et al. The diagnosis and management of nonalcoholic fatty liver disease: practice guideline by the American Association for the Study of Liver Diseases, American College of Gastroenterology, and the American Gastroenterological Association. Hepatology 2012;55(6):2005–23.
2. Angulo P. The natural history of NAFLD. In: Farrell GC, McCullough AJ, Day CP, editors. Non-alcoholic fatty liver disease: a practical guide. London: Wiley Blackwell Press; 2013. p. 37–45.
3. Wong RJ, Aguilar M, Cheung R, et al. Nonalcoholic steatohepatitis is the second leading etiology of liver disease among adults awaiting liver transplantation in the United States. Gastroenterology 2015;148(3):547–55.
4. Soderberg C, Stal P, Askling J, et al. Decreased survival of subjects with elevated liver function tests during a 28-year follow-up. Hepatology 2010;51:595–602.

5. Younossi ZM, Stepanova M, Rafiq N, et al. Pathologic criteria for nonalcoholic steatohepatitis: interprotocol agreement and ability to predict liver-related mortality. Hepatology 2011;53:1874–82.
6. Browning J, Szczepaniak L, Dobbins R. Prevalence of hepatic steatosis in an urban population in the United States: impact of ethnicity. Hepatology 2004;40: 1387–95.
7. Lazo M, Clark J. The epidemiology of nonalcoholic fatty liver disease: a global perspective. Semin Liver Dis 2008;28(4):339–50.
8. Vernon G, Baranova A, Younossi ZM. Systematic review: the epidemiology and natural history of non-alcoholic fatty liver disease and non-alcoholic steatohepatitis in adults. Aliment Pharmacol Ther 2011;34:274–85.
9. Williams C, Stengel J, Asike M, et al. Prevalence of nonalcoholic fatty liver disease and nonalcoholic steatohepatitis among a largely middle-aged population utilizing ultrasound and liver biopsy: a prospective study. Gastroenterology 2011;140(1):124–31.
10. Leite N, Salles G, Araujo A, et al. Prevalence and associated factors of non-alcoholic fatty liver disease in patients with type-2 diabetes mellitus. Liver Int 2009;29:113–9.
11. Ludwig J, Viggiano T, McGill D, et al. Nonalcoholic steatohepatitis: Mayo Clinic experiences with a hitherto unnamed disease. Mayo Clin Proc 1980;55(7):434–8.
12. Adams L, Lymp J, St Sauver J, et al. The natural history of nonalcoholic fatty liver disease: a population-based cohort study. Gastroenterology 2005;129:113–21.
13. Noureddin M, Yates KP, Vaughn IA, et al, NASH CRN. Clinical and histological determinants of nonalcoholic steatohepatitis and advanced fibrosis in elderly patients. Hepatology 2013;58(5):1644–54.
14. Lee J, Kim K, Lee SG, et al. Prevalence and risk factors of non-alcoholic fatty liver disease in potential living liver donors in Korea: a review of 589 consecutive liver biopsies in a single center. J Hepatol 2007;47(2):239–44.
15. Marcos A, Fischer R, Ham JM. Selection and outcome of living donors for adult to adult right lobe transplantation. Transplantation 2000;69:2410–5.
16. Targher G, Bertolini L, Padovani R, et al. Prevalence of nonalcoholic fatty liver disease and its association with cardiovascular disease among type 2 diabetic patients. Diabetes Care 2007;30:1212–8.
17. Assy N, Kaita K, Mymin D, et al. Fatty infiltration of liver in hyperlipidemic patients. Dig Dis Sci 2000;45:1929–34.
18. Gambarin-Gelwan M, Kinkhabwala S, Schiano T, et al. Prevalence of nonalcoholic fatty liver disease in women with polycystic ovary syndrome. Clin Gastroenterol Hepatol 2007;5(4):496–501.
19. Chin K, Nakamura T, Takahashi K, et al. Effects of obstructive sleep apnea syndrome on serum aminotransferase levels in obese patients. Am J Med 2003; 114:370–6.
20. Singh H, Pollock R, Uhanova J. Symptoms of obstructive sleep apnea in patients with nonalcoholic fatty liver disease. Dig Dis Sci 2005;50(12):2338–43.
21. Moreli M, Gaggini M, Daniel G, et al. Ectopic fat: the true culprit linking obesity and cardiovascular disease? Thromb Haemost 2013;110:651–60.
22. Fracanzani A, Valenti L, Bugianesi E, et al. Risk of nonalcoholic steatohepatitis and fibrosis in patients with nonalcoholic fatty liver disease and low visceral adiposity. J Hepatol 2011;54:1244–9.
23. Cheung O, Kapoor A, Puri P, et al. The impact of fat distribution on the severity of nonalcoholic fatty liver disease and metabolic syndrome. Hepatology 2007;46: 1091–100.

24. Kechagias S, Ernersson A, Dahlqvist O, et al. Fast-food-based hyper-alimentation can induce rapid and profound elevation of serum alanine aminotransferase in healthy subjects. Gut 2008;57:649–54.

25. Wong V, Wong G, Yeung D, et al. Incidence of non-alcoholic fatty liver disease in Hong Kong: a population study with paired proton-magnetic resonance spectroscopy. J Hepatol 2015;62:182–9.

26. Younossi Z, Stepanova M, Negro F, et al. Nonalcoholic fatty liver disease in lean individuals in the United States. Medicine (Baltimore) 2012;91(6):319–27.

27. Farrell G. Drugs and steatohepatitis. Semin Liver Dis 2002;22(2):185–94.

28. Stravitz R, Sanyal A. Drug-induced steatohepatitis. Clin Liver Dis 2003;7(2): 435–51.

29. Patel V, Sanyal A. Drug-induced steatohepatitis. Clin Liver Dis 2013;17(4): 5333–46.

30. Dunn W, Angulo P, Sanderson S. Utility of a new model to diagnose an alcohol basis for steatohepatitis. Gastroenterology 2006;131(4):1057–63.

31. Loomba R, Yang HI, Su J, et al. Synergism between obesity and alcohol in increasing the risk of hepatocellular carcinoma: a prospective cohort study. Am J Epidemiol 2013;177(4):333–42.

32. Sookoian S, Castaño GO, Pirola CJ. Modest alcohol consumption decreases the risk of non-alcoholic fatty liver disease: a meta-analysis of 43 175 individuals. Gut 2014;63(3):530–2.

33. Poynard T, Munteanu M, Imbert-Bismut F, et al. Prospective analysis of discordant results between biochemical markers and biopsy in patients with chronic hepatitis C. Clin Chem 2004;50(8):1344–55.

34. Vuppalanchi R, Unalp A, Van Natta M, et al. Effects of liver biopsy sample length and number of readings on sampling variability in nonalcoholic fatty liver disease. Clin Gastroenterol Hepatol 2009;7(4):481–6.

35. Rockey D, Caldwell S, Goodman Z. Liver biopsy. Hepatology 2009;49(3):1017–44.

36. Bedossa P, Poynard T. An algorithm for the grading of activity in chronic hepatitis C. The METAVIR Cooperative Study Group. Hepatology 1996;24(2):289–93.

37. Lee SS, Park SH. Radiologic evaluation of nonalcoholic fatty liver disease. World J Gastroenterol 2014;20:7392–402.

38. Clark JM, Brancati FL, Diehl AM. Nonalcoholic fatty liver disease. Gastroenterology 2002;122(6):1649–57.

39. Strauss S, Gavish E, Gottlieb P, et al. Interobserver and intraobserver variability in the sonographic assessment of fatty liver. AJR Am J Roentgenol 2007;189(6): W320–3.

40. Fedchuk L, Nascimbeni F, Pais R, et al. Performance and limitations of steatosis biomarkers in patients with nonalcoholic fatty liver disease. Aliment Pharmacol Ther 2014;40:1209–22.

41. Bedogni G, Kahn HS, Bellentani S, et al. A simple index of lipid overaccumulation is a good marker of liver steatosis. BMC Gastroenterol 2010;10:98.

42. Koehler EM, Schouten JN, Hansen BE, et al. External validation of the fatty liver index for identifying nonalcoholic fatty liver disease in a population-based study. Clin Gastroenterol Hepatol 2013;11(9):1201–4.

43. Siddiqui MS, Patidar KR, Boyett S, et al. Validation of noninvasive methods for detecting hepatic steatosis in patients with human immunodeficiency virus infection. Clin Gastroenterol Hepatol 2015;13(2):402–5.

44. Shi J, Sun Q, Wang Y, et al. Comparison of microwave ablation and surgical resection for treatment of hepatocellular carcinomas conforming to Milan criteria. J Gastroenterol Hepatol 2014;29(7):1500–7.

45. de Lédinghen V, Vergniol J, Capdepont M, et al. Controlled attenuation parameter (CAP) for the diagnosis of steatosis: a prospective study of 5323 examinations. J Hepatol 2014;60(5):1026–31.
46. Mofrad P, Contos M, Haque M, et al. Clinical and histologic spectrum of nonalcoholic fatty liver disease associated with normal ALT values. Hepatology 2003; 37(6):1286–92.
47. Fracanzani AL, Valenti L, Bugianesi E, et al. Risk of severe liver disease in nonalcoholic fatty liver disease with normal aminotransferase levels: a role for insulin resistance and diabetes. Hepatology 2008;48:792–8.
48. Castera L, Vilgrain V, Angulo P. Noninvasive evaluation of NAFLD. Nat Rev Gastroenterol Hepatol 2013;10:666–75.
49. Harrison SA, Oliver D, Arnold HL, et al. Development and validation of a simple NAFLD clinical scoring system for identifying patients without advanced disease. Gut 2008;57(10):1441–7.
50. Angulo P, Hui JM, Marchesini G, et al. The NAFLD fibrosis score: a noninvasive system that identifies liver fibrosis in patients with NAFLD. Hepatology 2007; 45(4):846.
51. Sterling R, Lissen E, Clumeck N, et al. Development of a simple noninvasive index to predict significant fibrosis in patients with HIV/HCV coinfection. Hepatology 2006;43(6):1317–25.
52. Shah AG, Lydecker A, Murray K, et al. Comparison of noninvasive markers of fibrosis in patients with nonalcoholic fatty liver disease. Clin Gastroenterol Hepatol 2009;7(10):1104.
53. Angulo P, Bugianesi E, Bjornsson ES, et al. Simple noninvasive systems predict long-term outcomes of patients with nonalcoholic fatty liver disease. Gastroenterology 2013;145(4):782.
54. Cichoż-Lach H, Celiński K, Prozorow-Król B, et al. The BARD score and the NAFLD fibrosis score in the assessment of advanced liver fibrosis in nonalcoholic fatty liver disease. Med Sci Monit 2012;18(12):CR735–40.
55. Calès P, Lainé F, Boursier J, et al. Comparison of blood tests for liver fibrosis specific or not to NAFLD. J Hepatol 2009;50(1):165–73.
56. Poynard T, Morra R, Halfon P, et al. Meta-analyses of FibroTest diagnostic value in chronic liver disease. BMC Gastroenterol 2007;7:40.
57. Poynard T, Lassailly G, Diaz E, et al. Performance of biomarkers FibroTest, ActiTest, SteatoTest, and NashTest in patients with severe obesity: meta analysis of individual patient data. PLoS One 2012;7:e30325.
58. Kwok R, Tse YK, Wong GL, et al. Systematic review with meta-analysis: non-invasive assessment of non-alcoholic fatty liver disease–the role of transient elastography and plasma cytokeratin-18 fragments. Aliment Pharmacol Ther 2014;39(3): 254–69.
59. Rosenberg WM, Voelker M, Thiel R, et al. Serum markers detect the presence of liver fibrosis: a cohort study. Gastroenterology 2004;127(6):1704–13.
60. Guha IN, Parkes J, Roderick P, et al. Noninvasive markers of fibrosis in nonalcoholic fatty liver disease: validating the European Liver Fibrosis Panel and exploring simple markers. Hepatology 2008;47:455–60.
61. Wieckowska A, Zein NN, Yerian LM, et al. In vivo assessment of liver cell apoptosis as a novel biomarker of disease severity in nonalcoholic fatty liver disease. Hepatology 2006;44:27–33.
62. Feldstein A, Wieckowska A, Rocio Lopez A, et al. Cytokeratin-18 fragment levels as noninvasive biomarkers for nonalcoholic steatohepatitis: a multicenter validation study. Hepatology 2009;50(4):1072–8.

63. Yilmaz Y, Dolar E, Ulukaya E, et al. Soluble forms of extracellular cytokeratin 18 may differentiate simple steatosis from nonalcoholic steatohepatitis. World J Gastroenterol 2007;13:837–44.
64. Gaiani S, Gramantieri L, Venturoli N, et al. What is the criterion for differentiating chronic hepatitis from compensated cirrhosis? A prospective study comparing ultrasonography and percutaneous liver biopsy. J Hepatol 1997; 27(6):979–85.
65. Claudon M, Dietrich CF, Choi BI, et al. Guidelines and good clinical practice recommendations for contrast enhanced ultrasound (CEUS) in the liver–update 2012: a WFUMB-EFSUMB initiative in cooperation with representatives of AFSUMB, AIUM, ASUM, FLAUS and ICUS. Ultraschall Med 2013;34(1):11–29.
66. Wong VW, Vergniol J, Wong GL, et al. Diagnosis of fibrosis and cirrhosis using liver stiffness measurement in nonalcoholic fatty liver disease. Hepatology 2010;51:454–62.
67. Palmeri ML, Wang MH, Rouze NC, et al. Noninvasive evaluation of hepatic fibrosis using acoustic radiation force-based shear stiffness in patients with nonalcoholic fatty liver disease. J Hepatol 2011;55:666–72.
68. Bota S, Herkner H, Sporea I, et al. Meta-analysis: ARFI elastography versus transient elastography for the evaluation of liver fibrosis. Liver Int 2013;33(8): 1138–47.
69. Adebajo C, Talwalkar J, Poterucha J, et al. Ultrasound-based transient elastography for the detection of hepatic fibrosis in patients with recurrent hepatitis C virus after liver transplantation: a systematic review and meta-analysis. Liver Transpl 2012;18(3):323–31.
70. Bamber J, Cosgrove D, Dietrich CF, et al. EFSUMB guidelines and recommendations on the clinical use of ultrasound elastography. Part 1: basic principles and technology. Ultraschall Med 2013;34(2):169–84.
71. Myers RP, Pomier-Layrargues G, Kirsch R, et al. Feasibility and diagnostic performance of the FibroScan XL probe for liver stiffness measurement in overweight and obese patients. Hepatology 2012;55(1):199–208.
72. Huwart L, Sempoux C, Vicaut E, et al. Magnetic resonance elastography for the noninvasive staging of liver fibrosis. Gastroenterology 2008;135(1):32.
73. Loomba R, Wolfson T, Ang B, et al. Magnetic resonance elastography predicts advanced fibrosis in patients with nonalcoholic fatty liver disease: a prospective study. Hepatology 2014;60:1920–8.
74. Chen J, Talwalkar J, Yin M, et al. Early detection of nonalcoholic steatohepatitis in patients with nonalcoholic fatty liver disease by using MR elastography. Radiology 2011;259(3):749–56.
75. Szczepaniak LS, Nurenberg P, Leonard D, et al. Magnetic resonance spectroscopy to measure hepatic triglyceride content: prevalence of hepatic steatosis in the general population. Am J Physiol Endocrinol Metab 2005;288(2):E462–8.
76. Furnari M, Savarino V, Giannini E. Use of liver breath tests to assess severity of nonalcoholic fatty liver disease. Rev Recent Clin Trials 2014;9(3):178–84.
77. Park G, Wiseman E, George J, et al. Non-invasive estimation of liver fibrosis in non-alcoholic fatty liver disease using the 13 C-caffeine breath test. J Gastroenterol Hepatol 2011;26:1411–6.
78. Banasch M, Ellrichmann M, Tannapfel A, et al. The non-invasive (13)C-methionine breath test detects hepatic mitochondrial dysfunction as a marker of disease activity in non-alcoholic steatohepatitis. Eur J Med Res 2011;16:258–64.

Histology of Nonalcoholic Fatty Liver Disease and Nonalcoholic Steatohepatitis in Adults and Children

David E. Kleiner, MD, PhD[a],*, Hala R. Makhlouf, MD, PhD[b,c]

KEYWORDS

• Steatohepatitis • Liver biopsy • Steatosis • Histology • Scoring • Staging

KEY POINTS

- Nonalcoholic fatty liver disease (NAFLD) is a histologically complex disease with the potential to progress to cirrhosis.
- Nonalcoholic steatohepatitis is a specific progressive subtype of NAFLD, characterized by ballooning hepatocellular injury in zone 3, steatosis, inflammation, and often fibrosis.
- NAFLD in preadolescent children has an acinar zone 1 pattern of steatosis, inflammation, and fibrosis that usually lacks ballooning but may progress to advanced fibrosis.
- Liver biopsy remains the gold standard for confirmation of the diagnosis and definition of the severity of histologic findings.
- Paired biopsy-based natural history studies suggest that over the short term there may be fluctuation in disease severity and fibrosis.

INTRODUCTION

Nonalcoholic fatty liver disease (NAFLD) and its more severe subtype, nonalcoholic steatohepatitis (NASH), are steatotic liver diseases that develop in the absence of significant alcohol use. NAFLD is most often associated with obesity, specifically central obesity; insulin resistance and other insulin resistance syndromes; type II diabetes; and hyperlipidemia. Because of these associations, NAFLD is now recognized as

Disclosure: The authors have nothing to disclose.
[a] Laboratory of Pathology, Center for Cancer Research, National Cancer Institute, Building 10, Room 2S235, MSC 1500, 10 Center Drive, Bethesda, MD 20892, USA; [b] Cancer Diagnosis Program, Pathology Investigation and Resources Branch, Division of Cancer Treatment and Diagnosis, National Cancer Institute, 9609 Medical Center Drive, Room 4W438, Bethesda, MD 20892, USA; [c] Department of Pathology, Ain Shams University, Faculty of Medicine, 38 Al Abbassyah, Cairo, Greater Cairo 11566, Egypt
* Corresponding author.
E-mail address: kleinerd@mail.nih.gov

the hepatic manifestation of the metabolic syndrome. It shows a spectrum of liver disease characterized by the accumulation of lipid, mainly in the form of macrovesicular steatosis. The histologic manifestations range from mild steatosis in only 5% of hepatocytes to more severe forms with lobular and/or portal inflammation, ballooning hepatocyte injury, and fibrosis in varying patterns of distribution to the end stage of cirrhosis.[1] As with other chronic liver diseases, patients are at risk to develop hepatocellular or other primary liver carcinomas.[2]

There is a growing recognition of NAFLD as a serious disease. Even with the most conservative estimates, NAFLD is very common in the United States (it is probably more common than hepatitis C and alcoholic liver disease [ALD]) and is significantly more prevalent in patients who are obese or diabetics. The prevalence of NAFLD is higher than was previously estimated and is 5-fold to 6-fold higher than the estimated prevalence of chronic hepatitis C.[3,4] The prevalence of NAFLD has been estimated to range from 2.8% to 46% throughout the world depending on the study population and the diagnostic tool used to verify NAFLD (eg, serology, imaging, liver biopsy).[4,5]

Prevalence studies of NASH, the most clinically relevant subtype of NAFLD, depend on histologic evaluation. In an autopsy study from the late 1980s, the prevalence of steatohepatitis was significantly different between the markedly obese patients (18.5%) and the lean patients (2.7%).[6] In Marchesini and colleagues'[7] study of well-characterized NAFLD, 163 of 304 patients underwent liver biopsy and, of those, 74% had NASH. More recently, Dr Stephen Harrison and his team evaluated the prevalence of NAFLD and NASH in healthy US adults via ultrasonography followed by liver biopsy.[4] Of 328 patients who completed an ultrasonography and questionnaire, 156 (48%) had at least 5% steatosis on ultrasonography. In addition, nearly 30% of patients with NAFLD had NASH on histologic review. Moreover, 9 (3%) of the patients with NASH had significant fibrosis (more than stage 1). These patients were more insulin resistant than those with mild fibrosis.[4]

Nonetheless, it remains challenging to estimate the prevalence of a disease for which there are no serologic confirmatory tests and a liver biopsy is required for definite diagnosis.

IMPORTANCE OF LIVER BIOPSY IN NONALCOHOLIC FATTY LIVER DISEASE

The presumptive diagnosis of NAFLD is often made in the setting of persistently increased serum aminotransferase levels with a positive imaging study (often ultrasonography), no history of significant alcohol use, and absence of other congenital or chronic liver diseases. However, 4% to 5% of patients with other chronic liver diseases may have NASH[8] and autoantibodies may be present in significant titers in 20% of patients with NAFLD.[9,10] In order to correctly classify the liver disease and exclude other coincident liver diseases, a liver biopsy is required.[1,11,12] Although a liver biopsy can provide a wealth of information about the state of the liver, is it not practical to try to distinguish NAFLD from ALD by histopathologic examination only.[13]

Several retrospective and prospective studies have suggested that simple steatosis without inflammation carries a benign prognosis, whereas those with the lesions of NASH are more likely to progress to advanced fibrosis and cirrhosis.[14,15] NASH has also been the focus of clinical trials.[1] It is therefore important to try to distinguish those with steatosis alone from those with NASH. Steatosis can be detected by imaging, using ultrasonography, computed tomography, or MRI. Modern MRI methods can detect a fat fraction as low as 5%, making it useful for detecting clinically relevant steatosis.[16] However, the distinction between steatosis and steatohepatitis cannot be made by current imaging methods, nor can imaging detect the lobular arrangement of steatosis, which is useful to distinguish the pediatric pattern of NAFLD (described later).[17] Noninvasive serologic markers have had limited success at making the distinction between steatosis alone and NASH, although they may have value as screening tests to identify patients unlikely to have NASH.[18,19] Use of liver enzyme tests alone can lead to overdiagnosis of NASH. Serum aminotransferases correlate poorly with histologic activity. For example, in one early study, NASH was incorrectly diagnosed by clinical tests alone before biopsy in 17% of the cases (4 out of 24) studied by Sorbi and colleagues.[20] Liver biopsy changed the diagnosis in 4 patients with suspected NASH; 3 had normal histology and the fourth had primary sclerosing cholangitis (later confirmed by imaging). Normal levels of aminotransferases are also no guarantee that significant disease is absent. Some fraction of patients with metabolic syndrome who have features of NAFLD or NASH including fibrosis and cirrhosis have aminotransferase levels within the normal range; these patients therefore might not be identified by serologic screening tools.[20–22] Liver biopsy remains the only diagnostic tool that can distinguish steatosis from steatohepatitis, grade the severity of the liver disease, and correctly classify cases with more than one diagnosis.

PATHOLOGY OF NONALCOHOLIC FATTY LIVER DISEASE AND NONALCOHOLIC STEATOHEPATITIS

The term NAFLD is typically used to refer to the whole constellation of nonalcoholic steatotic disease, whereas NASH represents a histologically specific pattern of liver disease. NASH may be identified in the presence of other chronic liver diseases,[8] whereas, if only steatosis is present, it may not be related to the usual metabolic causes of NAFLD.[23] NASH is the most common form of histologically progressed NAFLD and is almost always associated with some degree of fibrosis. It is unclear whether patients with steatosis but without NASH can progress to cirrhosis, although children with the pediatric pattern of NAFLD (discussed later) can develop advanced fibrosis without the typical features of NASH.

By definition, NAFLD has steatosis that is more than 5%.[1] The presence of less than 5% of steatosis is not regarded as clinically significant. This degree of steatosis is present in almost all cases of NASH; exceptions include cases with advanced fibrosis/cirrhosis, and rare cases of steatohepatitis that are caused by exposure to the drug amiodarone. Steatosis from patients with NASH is most often of the macrovesicular type with both large droplets of fat that push the nucleus aside and small droplets of fat that leave the nucleus in the center of the cell. However, in both alcoholic liver disease and NAFLD, small patches of microvesicular steatosis may also be present (**Fig. 1**). Diffuse microvesicular steatosis is not a feature of NAFLD but rather a manifestation of acute liver injury resulting from severe acute mitochondrial injury from a variety of causes, including alcohol, drugs (tetracycline, zidovudine, cocaine, valproic acid, aspirin [Reyes syndrome]), acute fatty liver of pregnancy, and rare metabolic disorders like carnitine deficiency. In most cases, the steatosis is mild to moderate but may vary from minimal to marked.[18] The distribution of steatosis within the hepatic acinus is characteristic; steatosis is most intense around the central veins (predominantly in zones 2 and 3), and the periportal areas are often spared in early disease.[24,25]

The inflammatory changes in steatohepatitis are nonspecific and variable but are usually mild compared with chronic hepatitis or chronic cholestatic liver disease. Some degree of lobular inflammation is common in NAFLD (**Fig. 2**). It is typically mild mixed inflammation but is nearly always present in an adequate needle liver biopsy. Clusters of mononuclear cells, including T cells and macrophages, infiltrate

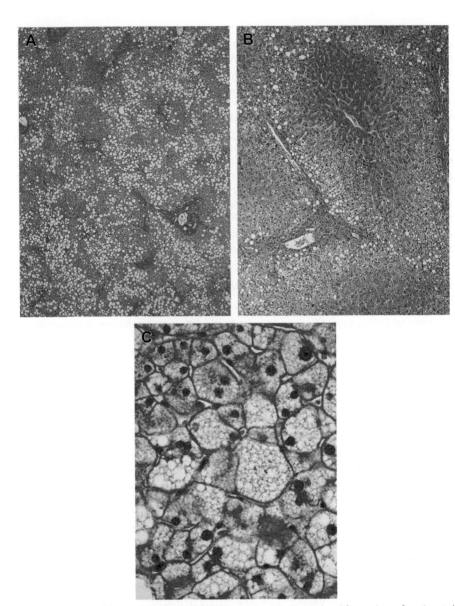

Fig. 1. Patterns of steatosis in NAFLD. (A) Zone 3 center steatosis with sparing of periportal areas (H&E, original magnification ×40). (B) Zone 1 periportal steatosis with sparing of central vein region (H&E, original magnification ×100). (C) A patch of microvesicular steatosis in a case of NASH (H&E, original magnification ×600).

into hepatocyte plates. Microgranulomas are a common finding. Scattered apoptotic bodies/acidophil bodies are common but are not a conspicuous finding. Neutrophils may surround the ballooned hepatocytes, especially cells that have Mallory-Denk bodies (MDBs) in a pattern called satellitosis. Severe, confluent inflammation or bridging necrosis is not a feature of steatohepatitis and should prompt consideration of other diseases, such as autoimmune hepatitis or drug injury. Mild portal

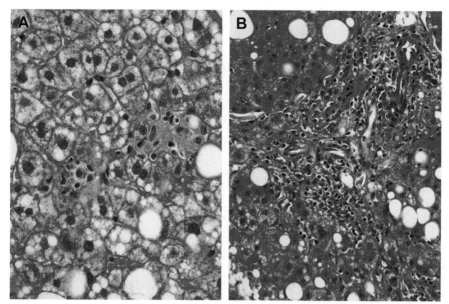

Fig. 2. Inflammatory infiltrates in NAFLD. (*A*) Lobular inflammation in NASH. A microgranuloma is seen to the right of the small lymphocytic infiltrate (H&E, original magnification ×600). (*B*) Portal inflammation is mild and may focally involve the limiting plate (H&E, original magnification ×400).

inflammation and mild ductular reaction are more common in NASH than in cases of steatosis alone.[18] Interface hepatitis, when present, is focal and mild, but, as with bridging necrosis, significant interface hepatitis should prompt consideration of other chronic inflammatory liver diseases. Although, portal inflammation is not a diagnostic criterion of NAFLD, it is reported to be associated with clinical and histologic features of advanced disease.[26,27] As the amount of fibrosis increases in steatohepatitis, more inflammation is observed in portal areas or within fibrous bands, so patients who are approaching cirrhosis have more inflammation in their fibrous tracts than patients who are early in their disease. However, when chronic portal inflammation is moderate or marked, clinicians should consider excluding other chronic liver diseases. The presence of lymphoid aggregates, as in hepatitis C; numerous plasma cells, as in autoimmune hepatitis; and bile duct injury, as in primary biliary cirrhosis is very unusual in NASH. Portal inflammation may persist or even increase after surgical or drug treatment of NASH, even as steatohepatitis resolves.[28–30]

The diagnostic feature of NASH is zone 3 hepatocellular injury. It takes the form of hepatocellular ballooning, with or without MDBs (**Fig. 3**). The ballooned hepatocytes are generally larger than the surrounding hepatocytes and have distinctive rarified cytoplasm that is irregularly stranded and clumped. There is some variation in this histologic appearance and cells with features that are between classic ballooned hepatocytes and normal cells may be identified. Some investigators have used the loss of staining for keratin 8 and 18 as a useful marker of ballooning.[31] Ballooning is not typically seen in young children, even those with fibrosis. The significance of ballooning was shown by the Cleveland Clinic study in which patients were subdivided into 4 types depending on histologic findings: types 1 and 2 had steatosis without or with inflammation, whereas types 3 and 4 also had ballooning and other features

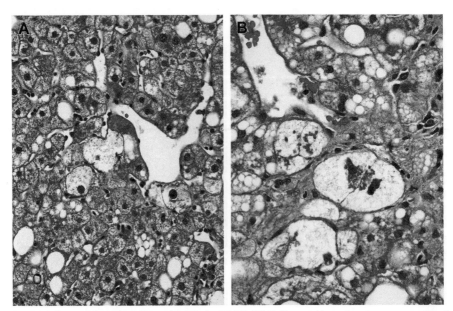

Fig. 3. Ballooned hepatocytes and MDBs in NASH. (*A*) Ballooned hepatocytes near a central vein (H&E, original magnification ×400). (*B*) Ballooned hepatocytes with large Mallory-Denk body cytoplasmic inclusions (H&E, original magnification ×600).

associated with the diagnosis of NASH.[14] Cirrhosis developed more frequently in types 3 and 4. A follow-up study using the same patient cohort showed that ballooning and MDBs were most closely associated with perivenular and perisinusoidal fibrosis in multivariable analysis of multiple histologic features.[32]

MDBs are a common finding in both ALD and NASH, although in NASH cases the MDBs are fewer and not as well formed as in typical cases of ALD. They may be seen in other diseases, particularly in severe cases of chronic cholestasis, in Wilson disease, and as a reaction to certain drugs. In NASH, the MDBs are associated with the ballooned hepatocytes in zone 3. MDBs have been noted to be a marker of severity or a progressive disease in alcoholic steatohepatitis and NASH. They result from active metabolic process and consist of aggregates of unfolded hyperphosphorylated keratins, heat shock proteins, ubiquitin, and an early response gene product known as p62.[33] MDBs can be highlighted using immunostains for ubiquitin or p62. When immunostaining is performed, they may also be seen in nonballooned hepatocytes.

Fibrosis in both ALD and NASH begins in the pericentral region or acinar zone 3; this fibrosis can become complex in the perisinusoidal spaces and eventually progresses to bridging fibrosis and cirrhosis (**Fig. 4**). This pattern of fibrosis is highly characteristic of steatohepatitis and is different from other chronic liver disease patterns in which the central veins are involved later in the disease process. Periportal fibrosis develops after the perisinusoidal fibrosis and is manifested as trapping of hepatocytes around the edge of the portal area and extension of short strands of collagen into the surrounding parenchyma. Fibrotic bridges may eventually form single bands between the portal areas and central veins without hepatocyte trapping or island formation. Masson trichrome or other connective tissue stains are essential to highlight the fibrosis and are particularly useful in early fibrosis of steatohepatitis. NASH cirrhosis may retain

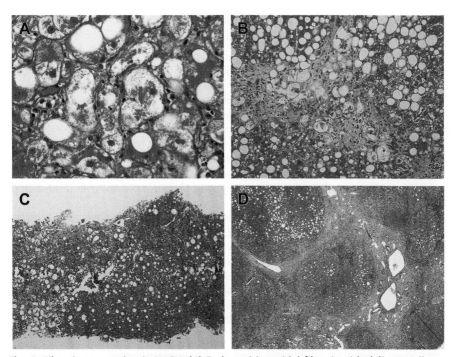

Fig. 4. Fibrosis progression in NASH. (*A*) Early perisinusoidal fibrosis with delicate collagen strands between ballooned hepatocytes (Masson, original magnification ×600). (*B*) Advanced perisinusoidal fibrosis (Masson, original magnification ×200). (*C*) Bridging fibrosis with extensive networks of perisinusoidal fibrosis nearly encircling a regenerative nodule (Masson, original magnification ×100). (*D*) Established cirrhosis (Masson, original magnification ×40).

all of the lesions of active steatohepatitis[34] but the steatosis may diminish below the 5% level. The active lesions of steatohepatitis may disappear in cirrhosis as well,[35,36] leading to a diagnosis of cryptogenic cirrhosis. It is likely that NASH is the underlying cause of most cases of cryptogenic cirrhosis.[37–39]

There are a variety of other findings in NAFLD and NASH that have less clinical and diagnostic significance. Megamitochondria or giant mitochondria have been described in ALD and NAFLD but they are more characteristic of alcohol-related steatohepatitis. Megamitochondria are small, intracytoplasmic, discrete, eosinophilic globules, 3 to 10 μm in diameter, sometimes rounded, and less often needle shaped. They are bright red on Masson trichrome stain and negative with periodic acid–Schiff stain, distinguishing them from alpha1-antitrypsin globules. On ultrastructural examination, they are dysmorphic and contain crystalline inclusions.[40] Lipogranulomas occur frequently in NASH, but are not helpful in the diagnosis. They may be associated with focal fibrosis and are frequently seen next to central veins or portal areas. However, this type of fibrosis should not be confused with the perisinusoidal fibrosis of steatohepatitis, and there is no evidence to suggest that this localized change contributes to progressive fibrosis. Glycogenated nuclei are also a common finding in NASH, but may be seen in other metabolic diseases. The hepatocyte nuclei appear empty and the change is seen more often in periportal hepatocytes.

NONALCOHOLIC FATTY LIVER DISEASE AND NONALCOHOLIC STEATOHEPATITIS IN CHILDREN AND ADOLESCENTS

With the increasing prevalence of obesity and diabetes in children and adolescents,[41] NAFLD and NASH have been identified in this population. Both teenagers and younger children may show the same patterns of NAFLD and NASH as adults, with zone 3–centered ballooning injury, inflammation, steatosis, and perisinusoidal fibrosis. The disease tends to be milder in children and biopsy surveys show only a few percent with cirrhosis. In a large study of children and adolescents enrolled by the NASH Clinical Research Network (NASH CRN) only 1 of 177 patients had cirrhosis on biopsy.[42] Another multicenter study in North America found no cases of cirrhosis among 108 children with NAFLD and NASH.[43] However, these same studies found that 14% and 20% of their respective cohort had bridging fibrosis, confirming that advanced liver disease can be found in children.

The typical adult pattern of NASH is seen mainly in adolescents, whereas preadolescent children tend to have an alternate pattern of progressive liver disease. This pattern is characterized by steatosis that is most prominent in zone 1, forming a collar around the portal areas (**Fig. 5**). The vacuoles of fat are largest in the hepatocytes nearest the portal areas and tend to decrease in diameter across the acinus to zone 3. Lobular and portal inflammation are present, but generally mild. Ballooned hepatocytes are difficult to identify, if present at all, and tend to be the same size as the surrounding nonballooned hepatocytes. MDBs are not seen in this pattern. The fibrosis

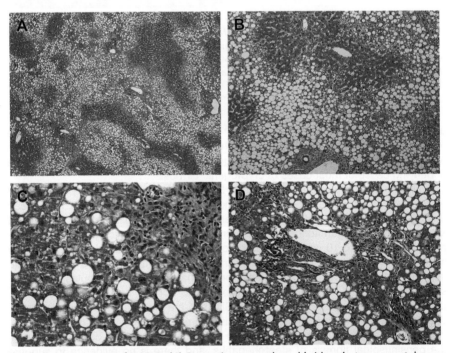

Fig. 5. Zone 1 pattern of NAFLD. (*A*) Steatosis surrounds and bridges between portal areas (H&E, original magnification ×40). (*B*) Steatosis spares the central vein (*top, center*) but surrounds the portal area (H&E, original magnification ×100). (*C*) Portal inflammation infiltrates adjacent parenchyma (H&E, original magnification ×200). (*D*) Periportal fibrosis is present (Masson, original magnification ×200).

pattern is also different, beginning around the portal areas, with hepatocyte trapping by collagen and extension of short septations into the surrounding parenchyma. When bridging fibrosis develops, the bridges connect the portal areas, leaving the central veins alone. Because of the zone 1–centric appearance of this pattern, the NASH CRN has termed this the zone 1 borderline pattern.[23,42] Because this pattern of NAFLD usually lacks the characteristic features of NASH (namely typical balloon cells and MDBs) there has been reluctance to use the diagnostic term steatohepatitis when describing this pattern. **Table 1** contrasts the features of classic NASH of adolescents and adults with the zone 1 borderline pattern.

GRADING, STAGING, AND SCORING IN NONALCOHOLIC FATTY LIVER DISEASE AND NONALCOHOLIC STEATOHEPATITIS

As NAFLD and NASH became subjects of serious clinical study, it became necessary for pathologists to develop systematic approaches for assessing the severity of the various lesions described earlier. However, unlike chronic hepatitis, in which inflammation and fibrosis are the only histologic features of importance, NAFLD and NASH have other characteristics that need to be tracked. Steatosis and ballooning injury are the main additions to inflammation and fibrosis in NAFLD scoring systems, but other features, including acidophil bodies, MDBs, and the zonal location of steatosis, are also important. Fibrosis staging is straightforward in chronic hepatitis, proceeding from none to portal/periportal to bridging to cirrhosis in a linear fashion. Although fibrosis in NAFLD and NASH proceeds generally from none to perisinusoidal to periportal and perisinusoidal to bridging to cirrhosis, the first manifestation of fibrosis may be periportal, particularly in children. The relative weight of perisinusoidal versus periportal fibrosis may vary and none of the current staging systems address this adequately. The risk is that efforts to simplify staging and grading for analysis may obscure key elements of pathophysiology. Pathologists and clinicians studying NAFLD and NASH should keep in mind that scoring systems are limited in their ability to capture the complexity of histological changes in this disease.

There are 3 scoring systems currently in regular use: the Brunt system,[44] the NASH CRN system,[45] and the SAF (steatosis, activity, and fibrosis) system.[46] A comparison of grading and staging of individual histologic features between these systems is shown in **Table 2**. The Brunt system was proposed primarily as a method for grading the severity of NASH and was not intended to be applied to cases that did not meet minimal criteria for steatohepatitis. The grading of steatohepatitis into mild, moderate, and

Table 1
Comparison of features of the pediatric zone 1 borderline pattern of NAFLD with typical steatohepatitis

Characteristic	Zone 1 Borderline Pattern	Typical NASH
Population	Mainly preadolescent children	Older adolescent children and adults
Steatosis	Zone 1 to panacinar distribution	Zone 3 to panacinar distribution
Inflammation	Portal inflammation equal to or greater than lobular inflammation in early disease	Lobular inflammation generally more prominent than portal inflammation in early disease
Ballooning	Indistinct or absent	Present, usually in zone 3
MDBs	Absent	Present
Fibrosis	Periportal fibrosis to portal-portal bridging fibrosis	Perisinusoidal fibrosis in zone 3 to portal-central bridging fibrosis

Table 2
Comparison of the essential elements of NAFLD/NASH grading and staging systems

Numerical Grade or Stage	Brunt System	NASH CRN System	SAF System
Fibrosis Stage			
0	None	None	None
1	Zone 3 perisinusoidal fibrosis only	Perisinusoidal or periportal fibrosis; 3 substages defined	Perisinusoidal or periportal fibrosis
2	Zone 3 perisinusoidal and periportal fibrosis	Perisinusoidal and periportal fibrosis	Perisinusoidal and periportal fibrosis
3	Bridging fibrosis	Bridging fibrosis	Bridging fibrosis
4	Cirrhosis	Cirrhosis	Cirrhosis
Ballooning Grade			
0	None	None	Only normal hepatocytes
1	Mild, zone 3	Few	Few: clusters of hepatocytes with rounded shape and reticulated cytoplasm
2	Prominent, zone 3	Many	Many: enlarged hepatocytes ($>2\times$ normal)
3	Marked, zone 3	—	—
Lobular Inflammation Grade			
0	No foci	No foci	No foci
1	1–2 foci per $20\times$ field	<2 foci per $20\times$ field	<2 foci per $20\times$ field
2	2–4 foci per $20\times$ field	2–4 foci per $20\times$ field	>2 foci per $20\times$ field
3	>4 foci per $20\times$ field	>4 foci per $20\times$ field	—
Portal Inflammation Grade			
0	None	None	—
1	Mild	Mild	—
2	Moderate	More than mild	—
3	Severe	—	—
Steatosis Grade (%)			
0	None	<5	<5
1	≤33	5–33	5–33
2	33–66	33–67	33–67
3	>66	>67	>67

severe was based on an overall impression of the severity of steatosis, inflammation, and ballooning, but most of the weight was given to ballooning. The NASH CRN system was developed specifically for use in clinical trials and natural history studies as a detailed method for tracking histologic change. It was designed with both pediatric and adult patterns in mind and in order to cover the spectrum of changes from the mildest forms of steatosis alone to the most severe forms of steatohepatitis. A composite grade, the NAFLD Activity Score (NAS), was developed as a summary of the overall severity of injury. It is defined as the unweighted sum of the steatosis, lobular inflammation, and ballooning scores and it varies from 0 to 8.[45] A diagnostic categorization of the changes as NAFLD but not NASH, zone 1 or zone 3 borderline patterns or definite steatohepatitis is made separately from the NAS. The SAF system is the most recent addition and has not yet been widely used in clinical trials. In this system, steatosis, activity, and fibrosis are separately assessed. Activity is defined as the sum of the lobular inflammation and ballooning scores and varies from 0 to 4. The SAF defines the presence or absence of NASH based directly on the scores, setting it apart from the other scoring systems (**Table 3**). Because it has no accommodation for the zone 1 pediatric pattern it should not be used to classify NAFLD and NASH in children. Cases with clear ballooning and inflammation but only minimal steatosis (<5%) are not classified as NASH in this system, which may cause interpretation problems in cases of cirrhosis or in evaluating a therapy that affects steatosis without changing the other features.

SAMPLE AND OBSERVER VARIABILITY

Although liver biopsy has remained as a core diagnostic tool and is regarded as the gold standard for evaluation of fatty liver diseases, there should be awareness of the sampling difficulties and problems of interobserver and intraobserver variation in grading and staging. The staging and grading systems described earlier were developed as semiquantitative scoring systems for assessing the severity of injury. Interobserver variability studies have been performed for the NASH CRN and SAF systems with adequate demonstration of reproducibility.[45–47]

In addition to issues of variation in interpretation, there are also potential pitfalls related to sampling.[48,49] A needle biopsy of liver represents at best 0.00002 of the liver and the severity of liver disease may not be evenly distributed throughout the liver. Bedossa and colleagues,[48] using computer modeling, showed that accurate grading and staging in chronic hepatitis requires a biopsy of at least 25 mm, which is an uncommon specimen in modern hepatological practice. Recent studies have shown

Table 3
The SAF diagnostic algorithm for defining NASH

Steatosis (S)	Lobular Inflammation	Ballooning	Total Activity Score (A)	Diagnosis
0	0, 1, or 2	0, 1, or 2	0–4	Not NAFLD
1, 2, or 3	0	0	0	NAFL
		1	1	NAFL
		2	2	NAFL
	1	0	1	NAFL
		1	2	NASH
		2	3	NASH
	2	0	2	NAFL
		1	3	NASH
		2	4	NASH

that this is also an important factor in evaluating NAFLD. In NAFLD, differences in findings, and thus in grade and stage, have been shown in recent studies.[50,51] Several studies have shown that experienced liver pathologists can have good or excellent agreement on the lesions of interest in NAFLD: steatosis, ballooning, lobular inflammation, and fibrosis.[45,47,52] Note that studies that attempt to define sample variation generally do not account for the noise contributed by observer variation and so overestimate the potential to miss lesions based on sampling.

HISTOLOGY-BASED NATURAL HISTORY STUDIES

The natural history of NAFLD has been studied for decades, even before NASH was characterized as a finding in NAFLD. Before 1980, there was significant debate in the medical and pathologic literature as to the significance of steatosis in nonalcoholic patients and its relationship to progressive fibrosis. Steatosis was a common finding, but evidence of chronic liver injury, namely advanced fibrosis and to a lesser extent inflammation, was often absent. Although alcohol-like steatohepatitic injury seemed to be present in specific cases, such as following intestinal bypass,[53] there was reluctance to extrapolate the association of steatosis and cirrhosis to the general population.[54,55]

The natural history of NAFLD has been explored in several types of studies. There have been large epidemiologic studies with populations defined by increases in the levels of liver enzymes coupled with risk factors like obesity and diabetes. On a smaller scale there have been retrospective studies of patients biopsied in the past and shown to have NAFLD or NASH who have then been followed to clinically determined end points. The third type of study involves paired biopsies. These studies are short term, with mean times between biopsies of 3 to 8 years. Information on disease progression can also be found in placebo arms of randomized clinical trials that use histology as an end point. **Table 4** highlights several paired biopsy studies in NAFLD and NASH, whereas **Table 5** shows studies with placebo groups that have paired biopsies.

Several general conclusions about fibrosis progression can be drawn from these studies. First, there is clear evidence of disease fluctuation in terms of fibrosis stage over the short term. Although some proportion of the apparent progression and regression is related to sample and observer variation, the percentage of the population that changes (20%–30%) is greater than observational noise would contribute. Note that placebo groups often show histologic improvement both in fibrosis and disease activity, possibly because of good medical care while patients are enrolled in a clinical trial. Second, although the percentages of progression and regression are similar in the short-term placebo-treated groups, in the longer term paired biopsies there is a clear bias toward progression. This finding was emphasized by 2 recent meta-analyses.[56,57] Singh and colleagues[57] found a mean fibrosis progression rate of 0.07 fibrosis stages per year in patients with fatty liver alone and 0.14 stages per year in patients with NASH. They identified an association between rapid progression and hypertension as well as a low aspartate aminotransferase/alanine aminotransferase ratio at baseline, but not with other clinical or histologic parameters. Argo and colleagues[56] found that fibrosis progression was associated with age and inflammation on the initial biopsy, but not with baseline obesity, diabetes, or hypertension. One of the most significant findings of the more recent meta-analysis as well as 2 of the most recent longitudinal studies[58,59] has been the observation that patients with NAFLD who do not have features of NASH are still at some risk of fibrosis progression and may develop NASH on subsequent biopsies. Because disease activity and stage apparently fluctuate over time, baseline risk factors for disease progression may be

Table 4
Longitudinal studies of NAFLD and NASH using paired biopsies

Author, Year	N	Follow-up (y)	Fibrosis Progressed (N)	Fibrosis Regressed (N)	Factors
Lee,[61] 1989	13	3.5	5	0	—
Powell et al,[36] 1990	13	3.5	4	1	—
Bacon et al,[62] 1994	2	5.5	1	0	—
Teli et al,[15] 1995	12		1	0	—
Ratziu et al,[63] 2000	14	5.2	2	4	—
Evans et al,[64] 2002	7	8.2	4	0	—
Harrison et al,[65] 2003	22	5.4	9	4	AST
Fassio et al,[66] 2004	22	5.3	7	4	Obesity, BMI
Adams et al,[67] 2005	103	3.2	38	30	DM, BMI, fibrosis stage
Hui et al,[68] 2005	17	6.1	9	0	None
Ekstedt et al,[69] 2006	68	13.8	29	11	None
Caldwell et al,[70] 2009	7	6	7	—	—
Feldstein et al,[71] 2009	5	3.4	4	0	—
Sorrentino et al,[72] 2010	132	6.4	45	11	Fibronectin, HTN, HOMA-IR
Wong et al,[73] 2010	52	3	14	13	Increased BMI and waist circumference
Hamaguchi et al,[74] 2010	39	2.4	11	12	Hemoglobin A1c
Pais et al,[75] 2011	6	5	6	—	—
Pais et al,[59] 2013	70	3.7	20	20	Age, DM
McPherson et al,[58] 2015	108	6.6	45	20	DM at follow-up
Total	712		37%	18%	—

Abbreviations: AST, aspartate aminotransferase; BMI, body mass index; DM, diabetes mellitus; HOMA-IR, Homeostatic model assessment of insulin resistance; HTN, hypertension.

difficult to identify. Although there is some suggestion that baseline obesity, diabetes, and other features of the metabolic syndrome play a role in disease progression, the size of the risk remains unclear. Nevertheless, long-term follow-up studies emphasize the importance of fibrosis stage in prognosis.[60] Because almost all cases of NASH have some degree of fibrosis it may be difficult to define the contribution of the severity of NASH (separate from stage) to long-term prognosis.

Although natural history studies of NAFLD and NASH have shed some light on disease progression over the short term, there remain unanswered questions:

- Is there a benign form of NAFLD or are all patients with NAFLD but not NASH at risk for progression?
- Can a reliable predictive model of progression be created, either from baseline clinical and histologic findings or from a combination of baseline data with some longitudinal data?

Table 5
Changes in fibrosis stage among placebo-treated patients in randomized trials

Author, Year	N	Treatment Time (wk)	Fibrosis Progressed (N)	Fibrosis Regressed (N)	Mean Fibrosis Change	Mean NAS Change
Harrison et al,[76] 2003	22	26	3	9	−0.27	−0.1
Lindor et al,[77] 2004	57	104	12	12	—	—
Belfort et al,[78] 2006	21	26	—	7	−0.15	−0.77
Dufour et al,[79] 2006	10	104	—	—	0.5	—
Aithal et al,[80] 2008	30	52	6	6	—	—
Ratziu et al,[81] 2008	31	52	6	5	−0.18	0
Abdelmalek et al,[82] 2009	28	52	—	—	0.4	−1
Haukeland et al,[83] 2009	24	26	—	4	0.08	−0.42
Nelson et al,[84] 2009	6	52	—	—	0	—
Leuschner et al,[85] 2010	91	78	—	—	−0.08	−1.03
Promrat et al,[86] 2010	10	48	—	—	−0.3	−1.4
Sanyal et al,[87] 2010	72	96	—	22	−0.1	−0.5
Lavine et al,[88] 2011	58	96	—	19	−0.2	−0.7
Van Wagner et al,[89] 2011	7	52	3	0	0.4	−0.3
Zein et al,[90] 2011	26	52	—	4	0.4	−0.1
Wong et al,[91] 2013	20	24	—	5	−0.1	−0.3
Sanyal et al,[92] 2014	55	52	—	—	0	−1
Takeshita et al,[93] 2014	12	24	—	—	0	−0.4
Neuschwander-Tetri et al,[94] 2015	109	72	31	19	0.1	−0.7
Summary	689	—	61 of 256 (24%)	112 of 477 (23%)	—	—

- How much is the natural history shifted by providing patients with a good standard of care for obesity and diabetes, without offering a specific pharmacologic intervention?
- How are changes in fibrosis tied to changes in other histologic and clinical parameters?

Longitudinal observational studies of NAFLD and NASH coupled with periodic bi-opsies have the potential to address these questions in ways that studies using only noninvasive methods cannot.

SUMMARY

NAFLD and its progressive subtype NASH are histologically complex diseases in which the pattern of changes drives the diagnostic classification. A liver biopsy re-mains the best method for characterizing the complexity of injury. Disease progression to cirrhosis occurs in patients with NASH, but some patients with steatosis alone may be at risk to develop NASH. The lesions of NAFLD and NASH can be graded and staged in a fashion similar to that used for other liver diseases and these methods can be used to study histologic change in patients enrolled in natural history studies and clinical trials.

REFERENCES

1. Sanyal AJ, Brunt EM, Kleiner DE, et al. Endpoints and clinical trial design for nonalcoholic steatohepatitis. Hepatology 2011;54(1):344–53.
2. Marrero JA, Fontana RJ, Su GL, et al. NAFLD may be a common underlying liver disease in patients with hepatocellular carcinoma in the United States. Hepatol-ogy 2002;36(6):1349–54.
3. Armstrong GL, Wasley A, Simard EP, et al. The prevalence of hepatitis C virus infec-tion in the United States, 1999 through 2002. Ann Intern Med 2006;144(10):705–14.
4. Williams CD, Stengel J, Asike MI, et al. Prevalence of nonalcoholic fatty liver dis-ease and nonalcoholic steatohepatitis among a largely middle-aged population utilizing ultrasound and liver biopsy: a prospective study. Gastroenterology 2011;140(1):124–31.
5. Lazo M, Clark JM. The epidemiology of nonalcoholic fatty liver disease: a global perspective. Semin Liver Dis 2008;28(4):339–50.
6. Wanless IR, Lentz JS. Fatty liver hepatitis (steatohepatitis) and obesity: an au-topsy study with analysis of risk factors. Hepatology 1990;12(5):1106–10.
7. Marchesini G, Bugianesi E, Forlani G, et al. Nonalcoholic fatty liver, steatohepa-titis, and the metabolic syndrome. Hepatology 2003;37(4):917–23.
8. Brunt EM, Ramrakhiani S, Cordes BG, et al. Concurrence of histologic features of steatohepatitis with other forms of chronic liver disease. Mod Pathol 2003;16(1): 49–56.
9. Vuppalanchi R, Gould RJ, Wilson LA, et al. Clinical significance of serum autoan-tibodies in patients with NAFLD: results from the nonalcoholic steatohepatitis clin-ical research network. Hepatol Int 2012;6:379–85.
10. Cotler SJ, Kanji K, Keshavarzian A, et al. Prevalence and significance of autoan-tibodies in patients with non-alcoholic steatohepatitis. J Clin Gastroenterol 2004; 38(9):801–4.
11. Adams LA, Angulo P. Role of liver biopsy and serum markers of liver fibrosis in non-alcoholic fatty liver disease. Clin Liver Dis 2007;11(1):25–35, viii.
12. Brunt EM. Histopathology of non-alcoholic fatty liver disease. Clin Liver Dis 2009; 13(4):533–44.
13. Nakano M, Fukusato T. Histological study on comparison between NASH and ALD. Hepatol Res 2005;33(2):110–5.
14. Matteoni CA, Younossi ZM, Gramlich T, et al. Nonalcoholic fatty liver disease: a spectrum of clinical and pathological severity. Gastroenterology 1999;116(6): 1413–9.

15. Teli MR, James OF, Burt AD, et al. The natural history of nonalcoholic fatty liver: a follow-up study. Hepatology 1995;22(6):1714–9.
16. Noureddin M, Lam J, Peterson MR, et al. Utility of magnetic resonance imaging versus histology for quantifying changes in liver fat in nonalcoholic fatty liver disease trials. Hepatology 2013;58(6):1930–40.
17. Cassidy FH, Yokoo T, Aganovic L, et al. Fatty liver disease: MR imaging techniques for the detection and quantification of liver steatosis. Radiographics 2009;29(1):231–60.
18. Neuschwander-Tetri BA, Clark JM, Bass NM, et al. Clinical, laboratory and histological associations in adults with nonalcoholic fatty liver disease. Hepatology 2010;52(3):913–24.
19. Wieckowska A, Zein NN, Yerian LM, et al. In vivo assessment of liver cell apoptosis as a novel biomarker of disease severity in nonalcoholic fatty liver disease. Hepatology 2006;44(1):27–33.
20. Sorbi D, McGill DB, Thistle JL, et al. An assessment of the role of liver biopsies in asymptomatic patients with chronic liver test abnormalities. Am J Gastroenterol 2000;95(11):3206–10.
21. Browning JD, Szczepaniak LS, Dobbins R, et al. Prevalence of hepatic steatosis in an urban population in the United States: impact of ethnicity. Hepatology 2004; 40(6):1387–95.
22. Kleiner DE, Berk PD, Hsu JY, et al. Hepatic pathology among patients without known liver disease undergoing bariatric surgery: observations and a perspective from the Longitudinal Assessment of Bariatric Surgery (LABS) study. Semin Liver Dis 2014;34(1):98–107.
23. Kleiner DE, Brunt EM. Nonalcoholic fatty liver disease: pathologic patterns and biopsy evaluation in clinical research. Semin Liver Dis 2012;32(1):3–13.
24. Chalasani N, Wilson L, Kleiner DE, et al. Relationship of steatosis grade and zonal location to histological features of steatohepatitis in adult patients with nonalcoholic fatty liver disease. J Hepatol 2008;48(5):829–34.
25. Seki S, Kitada T, Yamada T, et al. In situ detection of lipid peroxidation and oxidative DNA damage in non-alcoholic fatty liver diseases. J Hepatol 2002;37(1): 56–62.
26. Brunt EM, Kleiner DE, Wilson LA, et al. Portal chronic inflammation in nonalcoholic fatty liver disease (NAFLD): a histologic marker of advanced NAFLD-Clinicopathologic correlations from the Nonalcoholic Steatohepatitis Clinical Research Network. Hepatology 2009;49(3):809–20.
27. Gadd VL, Skoien R, Powell EE, et al. The portal inflammatory infiltrate and ductular reaction in human nonalcoholic fatty liver disease. Hepatology 2014;59(4): 1393–405.
28. Barker KB, Palekar NA, Bowers SP, et al. Non-alcoholic steatohepatitis: effect of Roux-en-Y gastric bypass surgery. Am J Gastroenterol 2006;101(2): 368–73.
29. Dixon JB, Bhathal PS, Hughes NR, et al. Nonalcoholic fatty liver disease: Improvement in liver histological analysis with weight loss. Hepatology 2004; 39(6):1647–54.
30. Neuschwander-Tetri BA, Brunt EM, Wehmeier KR, et al. Improved nonalcoholic steatohepatitis after 48 weeks of treatment with the PPAR-gamma ligand rosiglitazone. Hepatology 2003;38(4):1008–17.
31. Guy CD, Suzuki A, Burchette JL, et al. Costaining for keratins 8/18 plus ubiquitin improves detection of hepatocyte injury in nonalcoholic fatty liver disease. Hum Pathol 2012;43(6):790–800.

32. Gramlich T, Kleiner DE, McCullough AJ, et al. Pathologic features associated with fibrosis in nonalcoholic fatty liver disease. Hum Pathol 2004;35(2):196–9.
33. Zatloukal K, French SW, Stumptner C, et al. From Mallory to Mallory-Denk bodies: what, how and why? Exp Cell Res 2007;313(10):2033–49.
34. Charlton M, Kasparova P, Weston S, et al. Frequency of nonalcoholic steatohepatitis as a cause of advanced liver disease. Liver Transpl 2001;7(7):608–14.
35. Abdelmalek M, Ludwig J, Lindor KD. Two cases from the spectrum of nonalcoholic steatohepatitis. J Clin Gastroenterol 1995;20(2):127–30.
36. Powell EE, Cooksley WG, Hanson R, et al. The natural history of nonalcoholic steatohepatitis: a follow-up study of forty-two patients for up to 21 years. Hepatology 1990;11(1):74–80.
37. Caldwell SH, Oelsner DH, Iezzoni JC, et al. Cryptogenic cirrhosis: clinical characterization and risk factors for underlying disease. Hepatology 1999;29(3):664–9.
38. Poonawala A, Nair SP, Thuluvath PJ. Prevalence of obesity and diabetes in patients with cryptogenic cirrhosis: a case-control study. Hepatology 2000;32(4 Pt 1):689–92.
39. Struben VM, Hespenheide EE, Caldwell SH. Nonalcoholic steatohepatitis and cryptogenic cirrhosis within kindreds. Am J Med 2000;108(1):9–13.
40. Caldwell SH, Swerdlow RH, Khan EM, et al. Mitochondrial abnormalities in nonalcoholic steatohepatitis. J Hepatol 1999;31(3):430–4.
41. Ogden CL, Carroll MD, Curtin LR, et al. Prevalence of overweight and obesity in the United States, 1999-2004. JAMA 2006;295(13):1549–55.
42. Patton HM, Lavine JE, Van Natta ML, et al. Clinical correlates of histopathology in pediatric nonalcoholic steatohepatitis. Gastroenterology 2008;135(6): 1961–71.e1962.
43. Carter-Kent C, Yerian LM, Brunt EM, et al. Nonalcoholic steatohepatitis in children: a multicenter clinicopathological study. Hepatology 2009;50(4):1113–20.
44. Brunt EM, Janney CG, Di Bisceglie AM, et al. Nonalcoholic steatohepatitis: a proposal for grading and staging the histological lesions. Am J Gastroenterol 1999; 94(9):2467–74.
45. Kleiner DE, Brunt EM, Van Natta M, et al. Design and validation of a histological scoring system for nonalcoholic fatty liver disease. Hepatology 2005;41(6): 1313–21.
46. Bedossa P, Poitou C, Veyrie N, et al. Histopathological algorithm and scoring system for evaluation of liver lesions in morbidly obese patients. Hepatology 2012; 56(5):1751–9.
47. Bedossa P, Consortium FP. Utility and appropriateness of the fatty liver inhibition of progression (FLIP) algorithm and steatosis, activity, and fibrosis (SAF) score in the evaluation of biopsies of nonalcoholic fatty liver disease. Hepatology 2014; 60(2):565–75.
48. Bedossa P, Dargere D, Paradis V. Sampling variability of liver fibrosis in chronic hepatitis C. Hepatology 2003;38(6):1449–57.
49. Scheuer PJ. Liver biopsy size matters in chronic hepatitis: bigger is better. Hepatology 2003;38(6):1356–8.
50. Goldstein NS, Hastah F, Galan MV, et al. Fibrosis heterogeneity in nonalcoholic steatohepatitis and hepatitis C virus needle core biopsy specimens. Am J Clin Pathol 2005;123(3):382–7.
51. Ratziu V, Charlotte F, Heurtier A, et al. Sampling variability of liver biopsy in nonalcoholic fatty liver disease. Gastroenterology 2005;128(7):1898–906.
52. Younossi ZM, Gramlich T, Liu YC, et al. Nonalcoholic fatty liver disease: assessment of variability in pathologic interpretations. Mod Pathol 1998;11(6):560–5.

53. Drenick EJ, Simmons F, Murphy JF. Effect on hepatic morphology of treatment of obesity by fasting, reducing diets and small-bowel bypass. N Engl J Med 1970; 282(15):829–34.
54. Popper H, Schaffner F. Editorial: steatosis-Mallory's hyaline-cirrhosis: can their relationships be resolved by an experiment of nature? Gastroenterology 1974; 67(1):185–8.
55. Thaler H. Editorial: fatty liver-steatonecrosis-cirrhosis. Acta Hepatogastroenterol (Stuttg) 1975;22(5):271–3.
56. Argo CK, Northup PG, Al-Osaimi AM, et al. Systematic review of risk factors for fibrosis progression in non-alcoholic steatohepatitis. J Hepatol 2009;51(2): 371–9.
57. Singh S, Allen AM, Wang Z, et al. Fibrosis progression in nonalcoholic fatty liver vs nonalcoholic steatohepatitis: a systematic review and meta-analysis of paired-biopsy studies. Clin Gastroenterol Hepatol 2015;13(4):643–54.e1–9 [quiz: e639–40].
58. McPherson S, Hardy T, Henderson E, et al. Evidence of NAFLD progression from steatosis to fibrosing-steatohepatitis using paired biopsies: implications for prognosis and clinical management. J Hepatol 2015;62(5):1148–55.
59. Pais R, Charlotte F, Fedchuk L, et al. A systematic review of follow-up biopsies reveals disease progression in patients with non-alcoholic fatty liver. J Hepatol 2013;59(3):550–6.
60. Angulo P, Kleiner DE, Dam-Larsen S, et al. Liver fibrosis, but no other histologic features, associates with long-term outcomes of patients with nonalcoholic fatty liver disease. Gastroenterology 2015;149(2):389–97.e10.
61. Lee RG. Nonalcoholic steatohepatitis: a study of 49 patients. Hum Pathol 1989; 20(6):594–8.
62. Bacon BR, Farahvash MJ, Janney CG, et al. Nonalcoholic steatohepatitis: an expanded clinical entity. Gastroenterology 1994;107(4):1103–9.
63. Ratziu V, Giral P, Charlotte F, et al. Liver fibrosis in overweight patients. Gastroenterology 2000;118(6):1117–23.
64. Evans CD, Oien KA, MacSween RN, et al. Non-alcoholic steatohepatitis: a common cause of progressive chronic liver injury? J Clin Pathol 2002;55(9): 689–92.
65. Harrison SA, Torgerson S, Hayashi PH. The natural history of nonalcoholic fatty liver disease: a clinical histopathological study. Am J Gastroenterol 2003;98(9): 2042–7.
66. Fassio E, Alvarez E, Dominguez N, et al. Natural history of nonalcoholic steatohepatitis: a longitudinal study of repeat liver biopsies. Hepatology 2004;40(4): 820–6.
67. Adams LA, Sanderson S, Lindor KD, et al. The histological course of nonalcoholic fatty liver disease: a longitudinal study of 103 patients with sequential liver biopsies. J Hepatol 2005;42(1):132–8.
68. Hui AY, Wong VW, Chan HL, et al. Histological progression of non-alcoholic fatty liver disease in Chinese patients. Aliment Pharmacol Ther 2005;21(4):407–13.
69. Ekstedt M, Franzen LE, Mathiesen UL, et al. Long-term follow-up of patients with NAFLD and elevated liver enzymes. Hepatology 2006;44(4):865–73.
70. Caldwell SH, Lee VD, Kleiner DE, et al. NASH and cryptogenic cirrhosis: a histological analysis. Ann Hepatol 2009;8(4):346–52.
71. Feldstein AE, Charatcharoenwitthaya P, Treeprasertsuk S, et al. The natural history of non-alcoholic fatty liver disease in children: a follow-up study for up to 20 years. Gut 2009;58(11):1538–44.

72. Sorrentino P, Terracciano L, D'Angelo S, et al. Predicting fibrosis worsening in obese patients with NASH through parenchymal fibronectin, HOMA-IR, and hypertension. Am J Gastroenterol 2010;105(2):336–44.

73. Wong VW, Wong GL, Choi PC, et al. Disease progression of non-alcoholic fatty liver disease: a prospective study with paired liver biopsies at 3 years. Gut 2010;59(7):969–74.

74. Hamaguchi E, Takamura T, Sakurai M, et al. Histological course of nonalcoholic fatty liver disease in Japanese patients: tight glycemic control, rather than weight reduction, ameliorates liver fibrosis. Diabetes Care 2010;33(2):284–6.

75. Pais R, Pascale A, Fedchuck L, et al. Progression from isolated steatosis to steatohepatitis and fibrosis in nonalcoholic fatty liver disease. Clin Res Hepatol Gastroenterol 2011;35(1):23–8.

76. Harrison SA, Torgerson S, Hayashi P, et al. Vitamin E and vitamin C treatment improves fibrosis in patients with nonalcoholic steatohepatitis. Am J Gastroenterol 2003;98(11):2485–90.

77. Lindor KD, Kowdley KV, Heathcote EJ, et al. Ursodeoxycholic acid for treatment of nonalcoholic steatohepatitis: results of a randomized trial. Hepatology 2004; 39(3):770–8.

78. Belfort R, Harrison SA, Brown K, et al. A placebo-controlled trial of pioglitazone in subjects with nonalcoholic steatohepatitis. N Engl J Med 2006;355(22): 2297–307.

79. Dufour JF, Oneta CM, Gonvers JJ, et al. Randomized placebo-controlled trial of ursodeoxycholic acid with vitamin e in nonalcoholic steatohepatitis. Clin Gastroenterol Hepatol 2006;4(12):1537–43.

80. Aithal GP, Thomas JA, Kaye PV, et al. Randomized, placebo-controlled trial of pioglitazone in nondiabetic subjects with nonalcoholic steatohepatitis. Gastroenterology 2008;135(4):1176–84.

81. Ratziu V, Giral P, Jacqueminet S, et al. Rosiglitazone for nonalcoholic steatohepatitis: one-year results of the randomized placebo-controlled Fatty Liver Improvement with Rosiglitazone Therapy (FLIRT) Trial. Gastroenterology 2008;135(1): 100–10.

82. Abdelmalek MF, Sanderson SO, Angulo P, et al. Betaine for nonalcoholic fatty liver disease: results of a randomized placebo-controlled trial. Hepatology 2009;50(6): 1818–26.

83. Haukeland JW, Konopski Z, Eggesbo HB, et al. Metformin in patients with nonalcoholic fatty liver disease: a randomized, controlled trial. Scand J Gastroenterol 2009;44(7):853–60.

84. Nelson A, Torres DM, Morgan AE, et al. A pilot study using simvastatin in the treatment of nonalcoholic steatohepatitis: a randomized placebo-controlled trial. J Clin Gastroenterol 2009;43(10):990–4.

85. Leuschner UF, Lindenthal B, Herrmann G, et al. High-dose ursodeoxycholic acid therapy for nonalcoholic steatohepatitis: a double-blind, randomized, placebo-controlled trial. Hepatology 2010;52(2):472–9.

86. Promrat K, Kleiner DE, Niemeier HM, et al. Randomized controlled trial testing the effects of weight loss on nonalcoholic steatohepatitis. Hepatology 2010;51(1): 121–9.

87. Sanyal AJ, Chalasani N, Kowdley KV, et al. Pioglitazone, vitamin E, or placebo for nonalcoholic steatohepatitis. N Engl J Med 2010;362(18):1675–85.

88. Lavine JE, Schwimmer JB, Van Natta ML, et al. Effect of vitamin E or metformin for treatment of nonalcoholic fatty liver disease in children and adolescents: the TONIC randomized controlled trial. JAMA 2011;305(16):1659–68.

89. Van Wagner LB, Koppe SW, Brunt EM, et al. Pentoxifylline for the treatment of non-alcoholic steatohepatitis: a randomized controlled trial. Ann Hepatol 2011; 10(3):277–86.

90. Zein CO, Yerian LM, Gogate P, et al. Pentoxifylline improves nonalcoholic steatohepatitis: a randomized placebo-controlled trial. Hepatology 2011;54(5):1610–9.

91. Wong VW, Wong GL, Chan AW, et al. Treatment of non-alcoholic steatohepatitis with *Phyllanthus urinaria*: a randomized trial. J Gastroenterol Hepatol 2013; 28(1):57–62.

92. Sanyal AJ, Abdelmalek MF, Suzuki A, et al. No significant effects of ethyl-eicosapentanoic acid on histologic features of nonalcoholic steatohepatitis in a phase 2 trial. Gastroenterology 2014;147(2):377–84.e1.

93. Takeshita Y, Takamura T, Honda M, et al. The effects of ezetimibe on non-alcoholic fatty liver disease and glucose metabolism: a randomised controlled trial. Diabetologia 2014;57(5):878–90.

94. Neuschwander-Tetri BA, Loomba R, Sanyal AJ, et al. Farnesoid X nuclear receptor ligand obeticholic acid for non-cirrhotic, non-alcoholic steatohepatitis (FLINT): a multicentre, randomised, placebo-controlled trial. Lancet 2015;385(9972): 956–65.

Progression and Natural History of Nonalcoholic Fatty Liver Disease in Adults

Andrea Marengo, MD, Ramy Ibrahim Kamal Jouness, MD, Elisabetta Bugianesi, MD, PhD*

KEYWORDS

• Steatohepatitis • Hepatocellular carcinoma • Type 2 diabetes • Obesity • Cirrhosis

KEY POINTS

- Liver-related mortality is the third cause of death in patients with nonalcoholic fatty liver disease (NAFLD) and is significantly higher in patients with nonalcoholic steatohepatitis (NASH) compared with patients with simple steatosis (7.3% vs 0.9% respectively) within the first 15 years of follow-up.
- The presence and severity of fibrosis on liver biopsy is currently the best indicator of long-term liver outcomes in patients with NAFLD.
- The rate of fibrosis progression is at around 1 stage every 6 to 15 years in patients with NASH but is reduced by half in patients with simple steatosis; however some patients with NAFLD, also with simple steatosis, can progress rapidly to clinically significant fibrosis.
- Patients with NAFLD with cirrhosis have lower rates of liver-related complications but similar overall mortality as compared with patients with hepatitis C virus because of a higher incidence of cardiovascular events.
- Hepatocellular carcinoma incidence is growing in patients with NAFLD with or without cirrhosis, particularly among those with multiple metabolic risk factors.

INTRODUCTION

The three leading causes of death in patients with nonalcoholic fatty liver disease (NAFLD) in descending order are cardiovascular disease, cancer, and liver disease. Although the extrahepatic complications of NAFLD are described elsewhere, this section is focused on the potential liver-related morbidity and mortality that, along with the large prevalence and increasing incidence of this disease in the general population, clearly forecast the future impact of NAFLD on health care.

The authors have nothing to disclose.
Division of Gastroenterology and Hepatology, Department of Medical Sciences, A.O. Città della Salute e della Scienza di Torino, University of Turin, Corso Bramante 88, Turin I-10126, Italy
* Corresponding author.
E-mail address: elisabetta.bugianesi@unito.it

The burden of data on the liver-related complications of NAFLD comes from studies addressing both the clinical course and the progression of liver damage through paired liver biopsies, but tackling the natural history of NAFLD is one of the most difficult challenges for researchers. On one hand, the variety of criteria used to define NAFLD from the clinical point of view (abnormal liver enzymes, hepatic ultrasound, indices of liver fat, and liver biopsy), coupled with the lack of sensitivity and specificity of most of the tests used and the composite nature of NAFLD outcomes, has hampered most clinical studies. On the other hand, studies based on repeat biopsies are limited by sampling variability and by the lack of consensus on what is the best definition of nonalcoholic steatohepatitis (NASH). Several scoring systems have been described to classify liver histology in adults with NAFLD.[1–3] The NASH Clinical Research Network (CRN) classification is the most frequently used in recent studies; however, the NAFLD Activity Score (NAS) has often been used as a surrogate for the diagnosis of NASH, although it is not designed for it but rather for crude evaluation of disease severity, once the diagnosis has been established by the overall pathologic assessment. The prospectively designed Steatosis-Activity-Fibrosis score[2] has been recently introduced. Despite these caveats, the threat that NAFLD is going to replace chronic hepatitis C as major cause of liver morbidity and mortality should be no longer overlooked.

LIVER DISEASE PROGRESSION IN SIMPLE STEATOSIS AND NONALCOHOLIC STEATOHEPATITIS

Major prospective cohort studies have been derived from Western populations, whereas data in Asian, African, and Latin American populations are limited (**Table 1**). The overall long-term mortality of Western patients with the whole spectrum of NAFLD is 34% to 69% higher than the general population of the same age and sex within 15 years of follow-up and is mostly due to cardiovascular disease.[4] In a community-based study of 420 patients from the United States, liver disease was the third leading cause of death in patients with NAFLD, as compared with the 13th leading causes of death in the general Minnesota population.[5] However, only 21 (5%) patients were diagnosed with cirrhosis, and 3.1% developed liver-related complications, including one requiring liver transplantation (LT) and 2 developing hepatocellular carcinoma (HCC). Higher mortality was associated with age (hazard ratio [HR] per decade 2.2; 95% confidence interval [CI] 1.7–2.7), impaired fasting glucose (HR 2.6; 95% CI 1.3–5.2), and cirrhosis (HR 3.1; 95% CI 1.2–7.8).

Importantly, there is a prognostic association between the presence of NASH, the stage of liver disease (higher fibrosis stage), and the long-term prognosis of patients with NAFLD. In patients with NASH compared with patients with simple steatosis, both the prevalence of cirrhosis development (10.8% vs 0.7%, respectively) and the liver-related mortality are significantly higher (7.3% vs 0.9%) within the first 15 years of follow-up.[10] These findings have been repeatedly confirmed. In a landmark study,[9] although just 5% of the 129 patients with biopsy-proven NASH enrolled went on to develop end-stage liver disease, including 3 patients with HCC, liver-related mortality was increased 10-fold compared with the reference population. However, in patients with simple steatosis (or steatosis with mild inflammation/cellular injury), the overall and liver-related mortality risk was not different. In the long-term follow-up studies available thus far, only 1% of patients with simple steatosis developed cirrhosis and died a liver-related death after a mean 15.6 years of follow-up, compared with 11% of those with NASH having or developing cirrhosis, and 7.3% of those with NASH dying of a liver-related cause after a similar period of

Table 1
Prevalence of cirrhosis in patients with NAFLD diagnosed by liver biopsy

Author (Year)	Diagnosis	Number	Cirrhosis Prevalence (%)	Follow-up (y)	Main Findings
Teli et al,[6] 1995	Bland steatosis	40	0	9.6	There was no progression to NASH/cirrhosis.
Dam-Larsen et al,[7] 2004	Bland steatosis	109	1	16.7	Patients with NAFLD have a benign clinical course without excess mortality.
Matteoni et al,[8] 1999	NAFLD	98	20	8.3	Poor outcomes are more frequent in patients with NASH.
Adams et al,[5] 2005	NAFLD	420	5	7.6	Mortality among patients with NAFLD is higher than the general population.
Ekstedt et al,[9] 2006	NAFLD	129	7.8	13.7	NAFLD with elevated ALT/AST is associated with a significant risk of developing end-stage liver disease. Survival is lower in patients with NASH.
Söderberg et al,[10] 2010	NAFLD	143	9	28.0	Patients with NASH are at increased risk of death compared with the general population.
Lee,[11] 1989	NASH	39	16.3	3.8	NASH has the potential to progress into cirrhosis.
Powell et al,[12] 1990	NASH	42	7	4.5	NASH should be recognized as a further cause of CC.
Evans et al,[13] 2002	NASH	26	4	8.7	There is no evidence of progressive chronic liver injury in patients with NASH.
Hashimoto et al,[14] 2005	NASH septal fibrosis/cirrhosis	89	48	3.7	The most important consequence of patients with NAFLD with advanced fibrosis was HCC.
Sanyal et al,[15] 2006	Cirrhotic-stage NASH	152	100	10.0	NASH-cirrhosis has a lower mortality rate compared with HCV-cirrhosis but a greater CV mortality.
Ascha et al,[16] 2010	Cirrhotic-stage NASH	195	100	3.2	Patients with NASH-cirrhosis have an increased risk of HCC.
Bhala et al,[17] 2011	NASH septal fibrosis/cirrhosis	247	54	7.4	Patients with NAFLD-cirrhosis have lower rates of liver-related complications and HCC than patients with HCV infection but similar overall mortality.
Stepanova et al,[18] 2013	NASH	289	NA	12.5	Patients with NASH have a higher risk of liver-related mortality than non-NASH.

Abbreviations: ALT/AST, alanine/aspartate aminotransferase; CC, cryptogenic cirrhosis; CV, cardiovascular; HCC, hepatocellular carcinoma; NA, not available.

follow-up,[4] leading to the concept that simple steatosis is a relatively benign state, whereas NASH represents the form of NAFLD potentially progressive to cirrhosis and its complications (**Fig. 1**).

However, it is important to discriminate which of the histologic features of NASH are true determinants of long-term prognosis. In a cohort of 256 Swedish subjects, after a follow-up of up to 28 years, 40% of the 118 subjects with a histologic diagnosis of NAFLD died.[10] Compared with the total Swedish population, adjusted for sex, age, and calendar period, subjects with bland steatosis exhibited a 55% increased mortality and subjects with NASH 86%. Quite surprisingly, the study reported similar overall-related and liver-related mortality between the groups with and without definitive NASH (classified with the NASH CRN scoring system). However, 67% of patients classified as non-NASH in this study had liver fibrosis or even well-established cirrhosis, as fibrosis is not included in the NAS score. Thus, most likely the difference between the prognosis of NASH and simple steatosis is due to the greater likelihood of fibrosis being present in patients with NASH. This concept is supported by several studies. A more recent survey[19] conducted on 209 patients with NAFLD with a median 12 years of follow-up showed the presence of NASH correlated with liver mortality only when fibrosis was included in its definition, and the risk was highest with bridging fibrosis and cirrhosis (HR 5.68, 95% CI 1.5–21.5). Thus, it would seem likely that the presence and severity of fibrosis at liver biopsy would be the most important histologic determinant of long-term prognosis. Further evidence comes from recent studies demonstrating that noninvasive scoring systems correlating with the degree of fibrosis are capable of predicting liver-related events, LT, and death in patients with NAFLD.[20]

The rate of fibrosis progression in NAFLD is generally slow, and regression may also occur; but a subset of patients either with NASH or simple steatosis can develop severe liver damage quite rapidly (see **Fig. 1**). In a systematic review and meta-analysis[21] including 411 patients with biopsy-proven NAFLD (63% with NASH), over 2145.5 person-years of follow-up, 33.6% had fibrosis progression, 43.1% had stable fibrosis, and 22.3% had an improvement in fibrosis stage. The annual fibrosis progression rate in patients with NASH was doubled compared with that in patients with

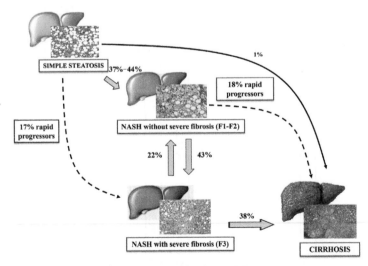

Fig. 1. Risk stratification for fibrosis progression in NAFLD.

simple steatosis; overall, one stage of fibrosis progression in patients with NASH occurred over 7.1 years in NASH versus 14.3 years in those with simple steatosis. However, the proportion of fibrosis progressors who moved from stage 0 to advanced (stage 3 or 4) fibrosis (rapid progressors) was identical in the 2 histologic subgroups (17% of patients with steatosis and 18% of patients with NASH). Similarly, a recent study has challenged the current concept that simple steatosis is a benign disease and cannot progress to significant liver damage. In a cohort of 108 patients from the United Kingdom with serial biopsies,[22] 81 had a baseline histologic diagnosis of NASH (75%) and 27 (25%) of NAFLD. The mean annual rate of fibrosis progression was 0.08 ± 0.25 stages. Remarkably, 44% of patients with baseline NAFLD developed NASH, including 10 patients in which fibrosis worsened over time (3 of 10 progressed by 1 stage, 5 by 2 stages, and 2 by 3 stages). No difference in the proportion exhibiting fibrosis progression was found between patients with steatosis or NASH at index biopsy (37% vs 43%), although all patients with steatosis developing fibrosis had also developed NASH on follow-up biopsy (see **Fig. 1**). Of note, 44% of the patients with steatosis developed NASH after a median 8 years of follow-up, suggesting that NASH usually develops after steatosis. Overall, these data suggest that the necro-inflammatory damage per se is not as important as fibrosis for the long-term prognosis of patients with NAFLD and accordingly the major focus of therapy should be in the resolution of fibrosis rather than of the other histologic features of NASH.

RISK FACTORS FOR DISEASE PROGRESSION IN SIMPLE STEATOSIS AND NONALCOHOLIC STEATOHEPATITIS

Provided that the presence and severity of fibrosis is the key factor determining long-term, liver-related mortality, the key question is which are the main determinants of NAFLD progression that can be identified without a liver biopsy. Age, body mass index (BMI), type 2 diabetes mellitus (T2DM) or metabolic syndrome (MetS), and insulin resistance assessed by homeostasis model assessment are well-recognized risk factors for advanced fibrosis in multiple cross-sectional studies; but few of them have also been examined in longitudinal studies and in relation to their ability to predict the progression of NAFLD. In the previously cited meta-analysis,[21] the presence of hypertension (odds ratio [OR] 1.94; 95% CI 1.00–3.74) and a low aspartate aminotransferase (AST)/alanine aminotransferase (ALT) ratio at the time of baseline biopsy was associated with the progression of fibrosis, whereas in a recent study,[22] most (80%) of the patients with NAFLD in which fibrosis worsened were diabetic and had a longer disease duration. Fibrosis progressors had also a significantly lower platelet count ($P = .04$) and higher AST/ALT ratio ($P = .04$) and Fibrosis 4 (FIB-4) score ($P = .02$) than nonprogressors. The same study identified the FIB-4 score as the only significant baseline factor able to predict fibrosis progression, whereas the presence of T2DM (OR 6.25; CI 1.88–20) and FIB-4 score (OR 3.1; CI 1.4–6.8, $P = .004$) at the time of follow-up liver biopsy were indicators of the presence of fibrosis.

Among genetic factors, homozygosity for the patatin-like phospholipase domain-containing protein (PNPLA3) 148M allele has been associated with a 3.3-fold increased risk of both NASH and liver fibrosis independent of BMI, T2DM, and steatosis (for NASH) and age, BMI, T2DM, steatosis, and NASH (for fibrosis).[23] The association between PNPLA3 I148M and the severity of fibrosis in NAFLD has been almost contemporarily replicated by independent groups in adults[24,25] and in the pediatric population[26] and confirmed by a recent meta-analysis.[27] Studies on the ability of genetic and other factors to predict the risk of disease progression are definitely needed, not only in the Western population but also in other developed and developing countries where the risk of NAFLD is paralleling the economic development.

LIVER DISEASE PROGRESSION IN NONALCOHOLIC STEATOHEPATITIS–RELATED CIRRHOSIS

It is well established that patients with severe liver damage are more likely to develop liver-related complications, and pooled data from long-term (~10 years) follow-up studies of patients with NAFLD with advanced fibrosis and cirrhosis demonstrate a 16% mortality with 60% of the deaths liver-related compared with only approximately 9% liver-related in long-term (~15 years) follow-up studies of patients with NAFLD without advanced fibrosis or cirrhosis.[4] However, the natural history of cirrhosis due to NASH has been addressed by only few studies.

In an Australian study of 23 patients with NASH cirrhosis identified from a hospital database, the 10-year survival rate was 84%. Comparing these patients to subjects affected by hepatitis C virus (HCV)–related cirrhosis, the study showed no difference between liver-related deaths or all-cause mortality between the two groups after adjustment for baseline differences, despite a trend toward improved survival in NASH.[28] In a larger study,[15] the 10-year survival in the NASH group was 80.9%, significantly better than in the HCV controls of similar age, sex, and Child-Pugh score, principally because of a lower risk of hepatic decompensation in the NASH cohort. In subjects with NASH-related cirrhosis, ascites was the first and most common clinical feature of decompensation but occurred at a slower rate than in patients with HCV. Once ascites developed, the rate of hepatorenal syndrome was similar in the two groups. Development of varices and the rates of variceal hemorrhage were similar in NASH-related and HCV-related cirrhosis, whereas the incidence of hepatic encephalopathy was intermediate between that for ascites and variceal hemorrhage. Remarkably, subjects with NASH-related cirrhosis had a significantly higher rate of cardiovascular mortality compared with HCV-related cirrhosis. These data have been corroborated in another independent cohort.[16] In a multicenter prospective study,[17] the long-term morbidity and mortality of 247 patients with NAFLD advanced fibrosis or cirrhosis was compared with 264 patients with HCV cirrhosis. Both cohorts were Child-Pugh class A and had cirrhosis confirmed by liver biopsy. In the NAFLD cohort, liver-related complications occurred in 19.4% of patients and deaths or LT in 13.4%, compared with 16.7% and 9.4%, respectively, in the HCV cohort. When adjusting for baseline differences in age and sex, the cumulative incidence of liver-related complications was lower in the NAFLD than the HCV cohort, including incident HCC; but cardiovascular events and overall mortality were similar in both groups. Thus, NAFLD seems to have lower rates of liver-related complications but a similar overall mortality compared with patients with HCV. Fibrosis stage and standard clinical and biochemical parameters are relevant in assessing the risk of future liver complications.

HEPATOCELLULAR CARCINOMA IN NONALCOHOLIC FATTY LIVER DISEASE

The exact burden of HCC related to NAFLD remains uncertain, but it is clear that NAFLD is going to be the most common underlying etiologic risk factor for HCC. In a population–based study in the United States, NAFLD accounted for 59% of HCC cases, with a cumulative incidence of 0.3% over a 6-year follow-up.[29] The mortality rates for HCC ranged from 0.25% to 2.3% over 8.3 and 13.7 years of follow-up in 2 further studies.[8,9] In the largest prospective community-based study performed so far,[30] after a mean follow-up of 7.6 years, only 0.5% patients developed HCC; but the rate among cirrhotic patients was 10%. As expected, the risk of HCC is more elevated when examining patients with advanced liver disease; but patients with NAFLD with HCC have a lower prevalence of cirrhosis than patients with HCC in HCV-related and other liver diseases. This prevalence is an important characteristic of HCC in NAFLD, which has been reported in multiple publications (**Table 2**).

Hepatocellular Carcinoma in Nonalcoholic Steatohepatitis–Related Cirrhosis

Two longitudinal studies on the natural history of NASH-related cirrhosis in the United States[15] and Japan[30] confirmed that HCC was the cause of 47% of deaths in patients with NASH, representing an independent risk factor for liver-related mortality (HR 7.96). Overall, the relative HCC risk and mortality rate in NASH-related cirrhosis seems to be lower in comparison with viral or alcohol-related cirrhosis. In a large cohort study, HCC was significantly more common in HCV than NAFLD (6.8% vs 2.4%, respectively)[17] and the HCV cohort had an approximate 0.15% risk per year of HCC development versus 0.05% in NAFLD. However, the perception that HCC is a rare and late complication of NAFLD has been denied by recent reports. In North East England, the overall incidence of HCC increased 1.8-fold from 2000 to 2010; but most shocking was a more than 10-fold increase in HCC associated with NAFLD, accounting for 34.8% of all the cases in 2010 and making it the single most common underlying cause.[39] Not surprisingly, this increasing incidence of HCC was associated with an increasing prevalence of overweight and obesity (61.0% in 2000 and 65.5% in 2010). This finding confirms that the apparently lower rates of HCC arising in NAFLD-cirrhosis compared with other causes of chronic liver disease are definitely outweighed by the much larger spread of NAFLD in the general population and open future scenarios in the approach to HCC.

Hepatocellular Carcinoma in Patients with Nonalcoholic Fatty Liver Disease Without Cirrhosis

The most worrisome issue consistently emerging in the last years is the onset of HCC in patients with NAFLD who do not have cirrhosis yet. A French study analyzed a cohort of 31 patients with HCC with MetS as the only risk factor for liver disease and found mild or no fibrosis in most cases, compared with those harboring HCC associated with an overt cause of liver disease (65% vs 26%, P<.0001).[38] The absence of cirrhosis was further confirmed in 38% of Japanese patients[41] and in one-third of patients from North East England with NAFLD-related HCC.[41] As patients without cirrhosis are not in surveillance programs, most (62.3%) presented symptomatically with larger tumors, and their median survival was just 7.2 months.[39]

In conclusion, HCC in NAFLD should not be underestimated for several reasons. First, once cirrhosis had developed, HCC represents a frequent complication, with an incidence of up to 10% over a 7-year follow-up. Secondly, HCC can also arise in the absence of cirrhosis in patients with NASH with multiple metabolic risk factors, mainly obesity and T2DM. These observations arouse an urgent need to better understand the risk factors linked to the development of HCC, especially in noncirrhotic livers, and to update screening programs.

Nonalcoholic Fatty Liver Disease in Lean Patients

A small but significant proportion of patients (7%–21%) develops NAFLD despite normal BMI, and they are defined as lean or normal weight NAFLD.[42–46] They are generally described in the Asian populations; but within the National Health and

Table 2
Principal studies on the association between NAFLD and HCC

Author (Year)	Diagnosis	Study Population	Main Findings
Bugianesi et al,[31] 2002	Cirrhosis	641 patients with cirrhosis-associated HCC	NAFLD-related features are more frequent in HCC arising in CC than viral or alcoholic cirrhosis.
Marrero et al,[32] 2002	Cirrhosis	105 patients with HCC	CC-related HCC was less likely to have undergone HCC surveillance and had larger tumors at diagnosis.
Regimbeau et al,[33] 2004	Cirrhosis	210 patients who underwent resection for HCC	Obesity and T2DM may be important risk factors for HCC, via NAFLD and CC.
Ascha et al,[16] 2010	Cirrhosis	510 patients with cirrhosis	Patients with NASH cirrhosis have an increased risk of HCC yearly cumulative incidence (2.6% vs 4.0% in HCV).
Yasui et al,[34] 2011	Cirrhosis and NAFLD/NASH	87 HCC cases; no cirrhosis in 43 patients	Most patients with NASH who develop HCC are men with features of MetS and at a less advanced stage of liver fibrosis.
Mittal et al,[35] 2015	Cirrhosis	1500 patients with HCC	NAFLD is the third most common risk factor for HCC. Cirrhosis was less common in NAFLD-related cases compared with alcoholic or HCV-related HCC.
Wong et al,[36] 2014	Cirrhosis	10,061 adult LT recipients for HCC	NAFLD is the most rapidly growing indication for LT in HCC cases in the United States.
Tateishi et al,[37] 2015	Cirrhosis	33,782 patients with HCC (596 NAFLD related)	Most cases of nonviral HCC are related to lifestyle factors, including obesity and T2DM.
Paradis et al,[38] 2009	NAFLD/NASH	31 patients with HCC with MetS as the only risk factor for liver disease	NAFLD contributes to noncirrhotic HCC.
Dyson et al,[39] 2014	Cirrhosis and NAFLD/NASH	623 patients with HCC	HCC cases without cirrhosis most commonly occurred in NAFLD. Patients without cirrhosis were not in surveillance programs, and most presented symptomatically with larger tumors.
Leung et al,[40] 2015	Cirrhosis and NAFLD/NASH	54 patients with NAFLD-associated HCC	HCC can develop in NAFLD without cirrhosis. At diagnosis, such tumors are larger than those in cirrhotic patients.

Abbreviation: CC, cryptogenic cirrhosis.

Nutrition Examination Survey III cohort, 7.4% of subjects had a normal BMI (<25 kg/m^2).[47] Lean individuals with NAFLD constitute a subgroup of patients relatively free from MetS, although insulin resistance can be increased anyway compared with healthy controls.[48] The common variant in the PNPLA3 gene (I148M) can partially explain the onset of NAFLD in lean patients; but in a recent study,[46] PNPLA3 polymorphism did not contribute to incident NAFLD.

The pivotal question is whether lean patients with NAFLD have a different disease progression compared with obese patients with NAFLD, but the answer is still unknown because of the paucity of clinical and histologic outcome data. In a biopsy series, leaner Asian patients with NASH were less likely to have advanced fibrosis and cirrhosis than Caucasians.[49] However, the preliminary report of an international study indicated a more severe prognosis in lean subjects with biopsy-proven NAFLD compared with overweight/obese subjects.[50] In a cohort of 1090 NAFLD patients, only 125 (11.5%) were classified as lean at first diagnosis. In accordance with previous studies, lean patients with NAFLD were characterized by a lower prevalence of T2DM, hypertension, hypertriglyceridemia, low high-density lipoproteins cholesterol, central obesity, and MetS as well as more frequently normal liver enzymes and a lower prevalence or severity of insulin resistance. Histology was characterized by milder degrees of steatosis and fibrosis but more severe lobular inflammation. In a subgroup of 483 patients, whereby the index liver biopsy had been performed before 2005, the difference in overall mortality between the lean and nonlean NAFLD group was analyzed. Over a follow-up of 11 years, 71 of the 483 (14.7%) patients died; surprisingly, the cumulative survival was significantly shorter in lean patients with NAFLD as compared with non–lean NAFLD (log-rank test = 5.6; P<.02). This difference remained significant when adjusted in a Cox regression model, with only lean NAFLD (HR 11.8; 95% CI 2.8–50.1; P = .001) and age (HR 1.05; 95% CI 1.008–1.1; P = .02) identified as prognostic factors. These provocative data point out that the definition of risk factors for the progression of NAFLD is still an open issue and that we should not quickly discharge lean patients with NAFLD from the gastroenterology outpatients clinic, overlooking their potential liver-related complications.

SUMMARY

Patients with NAFLD are at risk of liver-related complications and death; but fibrosis progression is generally slow, taking around 8 years to progress from stage 0 to stage 1 fibrosis, although there is a subgroup of rapid progressors who can progress 3 to 4 stages within 2 to 6 years. There is a prognostic association between the histologic stage of liver disease and the long-term prognosis of patients with NAFLD. Currently the presence and severity of fibrosis at index biopsy is the best indicator of the long-term liver outcome. Pooled data from long-term follow-up studies of NAFLD demonstrate only approximately 9% of liver-related deaths in patients without advanced fibrosis or cirrhosis, whereas patients with NAFLD with advanced fibrosis and cirrhosis demonstrate a 16% mortality with 60% of the deaths liver related. Among nonhistologic predictors, hypertension and T2DM at presentation are the factors most consistently associated with the risk of disease progression that is observed also in lean patients. HCC is a worrisome growing complication of NAFLD at any stage. Scientific advances in the understanding of mechanisms of fibrosis and carcinogenesis in NAFLD are awaited with interest in order to provide clinical indexes to predict and prevent the risk of liver-related deaths.

REFERENCES

1. Kleiner DE, Brunt EM, Van Natta M, et al. Design and validation of a histological scoring system for non-alcoholic fatty liver disease. Hepatology 2005;41: 1313–21.
2. Bedossa P, Flip Pathology Consortium. Utility and appropriateness of the fatty liver inhibition of progression (FLIP) algorithm and steatosis, activity, and fibrosis (SAF) score in the evaluation of biopsies of nonalcoholic fatty liver disease. Hepatology 2014;60:565–75.
3. Brunt EM, Kleiner DE, Wilson LA, et al. Nonalcoholic fatty liver disease (NAFLD) activity score and the histopathologic diagnosis in NAFLD: distinct clinicopathologic meanings. Hepatology 2011;53:810–20.
4. Angulo P. The natural history of NAFLD. In: Farrell GC, McCullough AJ, Day CP, editors. Non-alcoholic fatty liver disease: a practical guide. London: Wiley Blackwell Press; 2013. p. 37–45.
5. Adams LA, Lymp JF, St Sauver J, et al. The natural history of nonalcoholic fatty liver disease: a population-based cohort study. Gastroenterology 2005;129:113–21.
6. Teli MR, James OF, Burt AD, et al. The natural history of nonalcoholic fatty liver: a follow-up study. Hepatology 1995;22:1714–9.
7. Dam-Larsen S, Franzmann M, Andersen IB, et al. Long term prognosis of fatty liver: risk of chronic liver disease and death. Gut 2004;53:750–5.
8. Matteoni CA, Younossi ZM, Gramlich T, et al. Nonalcoholic fatty liver disease: a spectrum of clinical and pathological severity. Gastroenterology 1999;116:1413–9.
9. Ekstedt M, Franzen LE, Mathiesen UL, et al. Long-term follow-up of patients with NAFLD and elevated liver enzymes. Hepatology 2006;44:865–73.
10. Söderberg C, Stål P, Askling J, et al. Decreased survival of subjects with elevated liver function tests during a 28-year follow-up. Hepatology 2010;51:595–602.
11. Lee RG. Nonalcoholic steatohepatitis: a study of 49 patients. Hum Pathol 1989; 20:594–8.
12. Powell EE, Cooksley WG, Hanson R, et al. The natural history of nonalcoholic steatohepatitis: a follow-up study of forty-two patients for up to 21 years. Hepatology 1990;11:74–80.
13. Evans CD, Oien KA, MacSween RN, et al. Non-alcoholic steatohepatitis: a common cause of progressive chronic liver injury? J Clin Pathol 2002;55:689–92.
14. Hashimoto E, Yatsuji S, Kaneda H, et al. The characteristics and natural history of Japanese patients with nonalcoholic fatty liver disease. Hepatol Res 2005;33:72–6.
15. Sanyal AJ, Banas C, Sargeant C, et al. Similarities and differences in outcomes of cirrhosis due to nonalcoholic steatohepatitis and hepatitis C. Hepatology 2006; 43:682–9.
16. Ascha MS, Hanouneh IA, Lopez R, et al. The incidence and risk factors of hepatocellular carcinoma in patients with nonalcoholic steatohepatitis. Hepatology 2010;51:1972–8.
17. Bhala N, Angulo P, van der Poorten D, et al. The natural history of nonalcoholic fatty liver disease with advanced fibrosis or cirrhosis: an international collaborative study. Hepatology 2011;54:1208–16.
18. Stepanova M, Rafiq N, Makhlouf H, et al. Predictors of all-cause mortality and liver-related mortality in patients with non-alcoholic fatty liver disease (NAFLD). Dig Dis Sci 2013;58:3017–23.
19. Younossi ZM, Stepanova M, Rafiq N, et al. Pathologic criteria for nonalcoholic steatohepatitis: interprotocol agreement and ability to predict liver-related mortality. Hepatology 2011;53:1874–82.

20. Angulo P, Bugianesi E, Bjornsson ES, et al. Simple noninvasive systems predict long-term outcomes of patients with nonalcoholic fatty liver disease. Gastroenterology 2013;145:782–9.
21. Singh S, Allen AM, Wang Z, et al. Fibrosis progression in nonalcoholic fatty liver vs nonalcoholic steatohepatitis: a systematic review and meta-analysis of paired-biopsy studies. Clin Gastroenterol Hepatol 2015;13:643–54.
22. McPherson S, Hardy T, Henderson E, et al. Evidence of NAFLD progression from steatosis to fibrosing-steatohepatitis using paired biopsies: Implications for prognosis and clinical management. J Hepatol 2015;62:1148–55.
23. Valenti L, Al-Serri A, Daly AK, et al. Homozygosity for the patatin-like phospholipase-3/adiponutrin I148M polymorphism influences liver fibrosis in patients with nonalcoholic fatty liver disease. Hepatology 2010;51:1209–17.
24. Rotman Y, Koh C, Zmuda JM, et al. The association of genetic variability in patatin-like phospholipase domain-containing protein 3 (PNPLA3) with histological severity of nonalcoholic fatty liver disease. Hepatology 2010;52:894–903.
25. Speliotes EK, Butler JL, Palmer CD, et al. PNPLA3 variants specifically confer increased risk for histologic nonalcoholic fatty liver disease but not metabolic disease. Hepatology 2010;52:904–12.
26. Valenti L, Alisi A, Galmozzi E, et al. I148M patatinlike phospholipase domain-containing 3 gene variant and severity of pediatric nonalcoholic fatty liver disease. Hepatology 2010;52:1274–80.
27. Sookoian S, Pirola CJ. Meta-analysis of the influence of I148M variant of patatin-like phospholipase domain containing 3 gene (PNPLA3) on the susceptibility and histological severity of nonalcoholic fatty liver disease. Hepatology 2011;53:1883–94.
28. Hui JM, Kench JG, Chitturi S, et al. Long-term outcomes of cirrhosis in nonalcoholic steatohepatitis compared with hepatitis C. Hepatology 2003;38:420–7.
29. Sanyal A, Poklepovic A, Moyneur E, et al. Population-based risk factors and resource utilization for HCC: US perspective. Curr Med Res Opin 2010;26:2183–91.
30. Yatsuji S, Hashimoto E, Tobari M, et al. Clinical features and outcomes of cirrhosis due to non-alcoholic steatohepatitis compared with cirrhosis caused by chronic hepatitis C. J Gastroenterol Hepatol 2009;24:248–54.
31. Bugianesi E, Leone N, Vanni E, et al. Expanding the natural history of nonalcoholic steatohepatitis: from cryptogenic cirrhosis to hepatocellular carcinoma. Gastroenterology 2002;123:134–40.
32. Marrero JA, Fontana RJ, Su GL, et al. NAFLD may be a common underlying liver disease in patients with hepatocellular carcinoma in the United States. Hepatology 2002;36:1349–54.
33. Regimbeau JM, Colombat M, Mognol P, et al. Obesity and diabetes as a risk factor for hepatocellular carcinoma. Liver Transpl 2004;10:S69–73.
34. Yasui K, Hashimoto E, Komorizono Y, et al. Characteristics of patients with nonalcoholic steatohepatitis who develop hepatocellular carcinoma. Clin Gastroenterol Hepatol 2011;9:428–33.
35. Mittal S, Sada YH, El-Serag HB, et al. Temporal trends of nonalcoholic fatty liver disease-related hepatocellular carcinoma in the veteran affairs population. Clin Gastroenterol Hepatol 2015;13:594–601.
36. Wong RJ, Cheung R, Ahmed A. Nonalcoholic steatohepatitis is the most rapidly growing indication for liver transplantation in patient with hepatocellular carcinoma in the U.S. Hepatology 2014;59:2188–95.
37. Tateishi R, Okanoue T, Fujiwara N, et al. Clinical characteristics, treatment, and prognosis of non-B, non-C hepatocellular carcinoma: a large retrospective multicenter cohort study. J Gastroenterol 2015;50:350–60.

38. Paradis V, Zalinski S, Chelbi E, et al. Hepatocellular carcinomas in patients with metabolic syndrome often develop without significant liver fibrosis: a pathological analysis. Hepatology 2009;49:851–9.
39. Dyson J, Jaques B, Chattopadyhay D, et al. Hepatocellular cancer: the impact of obesity, type 2 diabetes and multidisciplinary team. J Hepatol 2014;60:110–7.
40. Leung C, Yeoh SW, Patrick D, et al. Characteristics of hepatocellular carcinoma in cirrhotic and non-cirrhotic non-alcoholic fatty liver disease. World J Gastroenterol 2015;21:1189–96.
41. Tokushige K, Hashimoto E, Horie Y, et al. Hepatocellular carcinoma in Japanese patients with nonalcoholic fatty liver disease, alcoholic liver disease, and chronic liver disease of unknown etiology: report of the nationwide survey. J Gastroenterol 2011;46:1230–7.
42. Wong VW, Chu WC, Wong GL, et al. Prevalence of non-alcoholic fatty liver disease and advanced fibrosis in Hong Kong Chinese: a population study using proton-magnetic resonance spectroscopy and transient elastography. Gut 2012;61: 409–15.
43. Das K, Das K, Mukherjee PS, et al. Nonobese population in a developing country has a high prevalence of nonalcoholic fatty liver and significant liver disease. Hepatology 2010;51:1593–602.
44. Kwon YM, Oh SW, Hwang SS, et al. Association of nonalcoholic fatty liver disease with components of metabolic syndrome according to body mass index in Korean adults. Am J Gastroenterol 2012;107:1852–8.
45. Liu CJ. Prevalence and risk factors for non-alcoholic fatty liver disease in Asian people who are not obese. J Gastroenterol Hepatol 2012;27:1555–60.
46. Wong VW, Wong GL, Yeung DK, et al. Incidence of non-alcoholic fatty liver disease in Hong Kong: a population study with paired proton-magnetic resonance spectroscopy. J Hepatol 2015;62:182–9.
47. Younossi ZM, Stepanova M, Negro F, et al. Nonalcoholic fatty liver disease in lean individuals in the United States. Medicine 2012;91:319–27.
48. Vos B, Moreno C, Nagy N, et al. Lean nonalcoholic fatty liver disease (Lean-NAFLD): a major cause of cryptogenic liver disease. Acta Gastroenterol Belg 2011;74: 389–94.
49. Wong VW, Vergniol J, Wong GL, et al. Diagnosis of fibrosis and cirrhosis using liver stiffness measurement in nonalcoholic fatty liver disease. Hepatology 2010;51:454–62.
50. Dela Cruz AC, Bugianesi E, George J, et al. Characteristics and long-term prognosis of lean patients with non-alcoholic fatty liver disease. Gastroenterology 2014;146: S-909.

The Progression and Natural History of Pediatric Nonalcoholic Fatty Liver Disease

CrossMark

Nidhi P. Goyal, MD, MPH[a,b], Jeffrey B. Schwimmer, MD[a,b],*

KEYWORDS

- Children • Adolescents • Nonalcoholic steatohepatitis • Obesity • Epidemiology
- Morbidity • Mortality • Outcomes

KEY POINTS

- Evidence suggests nonalcoholic fatty liver disease (NAFLD) may begin in the perinatal period in children of diabetic mothers.
- Pediatric NAFLD is typically diagnosed between 10 and 13 years of age.
- At diagnosis, among children with NAFLD, 25% to 50% of children have nonalcoholic steatohepatitis and 10% to 25% have advanced fibrosis.
- Cardiovascular derangement in the form of left ventricular dysfunction and increased left ventricular strain and mass is observed in adolescents with NAFLD, raising concern for premature cardiovascular morbidity and mortality.
- Obesity in childhood is a known risk factor for hepatocellular carcinoma in adulthood.

INTRODUCTION

The question of interest this review addresses is: What is the progression and natural history of nonalcoholic fatty liver disease (NAFLD) in children? The natural history of pediatric NAFLD is a complex topic, in that there is a paucity of longitudinal data in children with NAFLD. Understanding the natural history is also challenging because

Funding: This work was supported in part by R01DK088925, R01DK088831, R56DK090350, U01DK61734, and K12-HD000850. The funders did not participate in the design, preparation, review, or approval of the article. The contents of this work are solely the responsibility of the authors and do not necessarily represent the official views of the National Institutes of Health.
[a] Division of Gastroenterology, Hepatology, and Nutrition, Department of Pediatrics, University of California, San Diego, San Diego, CA, USA; [b] Department of Gastroenterology, Rady Children's Hospital, San Diego, CA, USA
* Corresponding author. Division of Gastroenterology, Hepatology, and Nutrition, Department of Pediatrics, University of California, San Diego, 3030 Children's Way, San Diego, CA 92123.
E-mail address: jschwimmer@ucsd.edu

it is difficult to properly date the onset of disease. Currently, there is insight about the range of disease severity at the time of biopsy diagnosis. With respect to progression over time, however, the data are lacking. One cannot assume that the time point of clinical diagnosis equals the starting point. In fact, for most children with NAFLD, disease onset is unknown. Thus, a better understanding of the severity range, variability, and associations of pediatric NAFLD is important, as children may represent different time points on a history continuum.

In order to answer the broad question of the natural history of NAFLD in children, this article is divided into the following series of subquestions to better address the comprehensive clinical phenotype:

1. When does NAFLD start in children?
2. What is the histologic starting point and severity?
3. What is the associated morbidity?
4. What is the longitudinal hepatic outcome?

When Does Nonalcoholic Fatty Liver Disease Start in Children?

Some data suggest that NAFLD begins in utero. Two studies have used neonatal magnetic resonance spectroscopy (MRS) to assess steatosis in infants born to mothers with gestational diabetes. Hepatic fat fraction (HFF) at 1 to 3 weeks of age was performed in neonates born to normal weight mothers (n = 13) and was compared with those born to obese mothers with gestational diabetes (n = 12). In this study, neonates born to obese mothers with gestational diabetes had a mean HFF that was 68% greater than infants born to normal weight mothers.[1] In a study by Modi and colleagues,[2] 105 mother/neonate dyads were studied to determine if maternal body mass index (BMI) influenced neonatal HFF. Their key finding was that maternal BMI at conception was associated with neonatal HFF. Similarly, the presence and severity of fetal hepatic steatosis were assessed in 33 stillborn babies of diabetic mothers compared with 48 stillborn babies of mothers without diabetes.[3] The diabetic mothers were more likely to be obese compared with controls (61% vs 33%). There was a substantially higher rate of hepatic steatosis in neonates born to mothers with diabetes (79%) versus controls (17%). It is not known, however, if the steatosis identified in the neonatal period progresses to the NAFLD that is typically diagnosed in adolescence.

There is evidence that postnatal factors may also have an effect in pediatric NAFLD. Breast-feeding, for example, has also been postulated to be protective for NAFLD. In a study of 191 Italian children with biopsy-proven NAFLD, hepatic steatosis, inflammation, hepatocyte ballooning, and fibrosis were worse in children who were not breast-fed compared with breast-fed children.[4]

If NAFLD begins in utero, at birth, or soon after, one would expect a meaningful prevalence of NAFLD in very young children. However, in the Study of Child and Adolescent Liver Epidemiology (SCALE), this was not the case in the younger age group, whereby the prevalence of NAFLD for a 10-year period 1993 to 2003 was 0.7% in children aged 2 to 4 years.[5] As opposed to a general population-based study, there may be unique populations of young children with higher rates of NAFLD. In a study of obese preschool-aged children in Chicago, elevated alanine aminotransferase (ALT) was reported in 26% of obese children aged 2 to 5 years.[6] In a study of Hispanic children in Houston with most of the children being obese, ALT greater than 35 U/L was reported in 15% of 4 to 5 year olds.[7] Several gaps remain. In the 2 studies of ALT in preschool children, it is not known how many actually had NAFLD. Also, this population does not typically have symptoms and is well below the age at which guidelines recommend screening for NAFLD. These studies were also conducted more recently than SCALE, and it is possible that the prevalence of NAFLD has increased. Notably, in NHANES (National Health and Nutrition Examination Survey), the rate of elevated ALT in children in the United States nearly tripled from 3.9% in 1988 to 1994 to 10.7% in 2007 to 2010.[8]

In the United States, NAFLD is typically diagnosed in children between age 12 and 13 years. Numerous large and multicenter studies consistently report mean ages within this range.[9–11] The largest clinical reports from outside the United States are from Italy, and it is notable that many such reports have a mean age of 10 to 11 years at diagnosis.[12,13] Whether there are differences in the age of onset by country or whether the difference in reported ages are due to differences in clinical practice are unknown. Moreover, whether the onset of NAFLD is truly between age 10 and 13 years or whether most of these children have NAFLD that is present earlier but clinically silent are also unknown. In order to answer this query, prepubertal children should be followed *before* the typical age at diagnosis, to determine if these younger patients may have undiagnosed NAFLD. This typical age at diagnosis was addressed in one study thus far in 123 prepubertal children ages 7 to 9, and those who were of normal weight had lower hepatic lipid load compared with obese children who were at risk for metabolic syndrome.[14] To track the progression of NAFLD that potentially begins during the perinatal period, infants with suspected steatosis born to diabetic mothers should be followed longitudinally for development or ongoing presence of NAFLD. This finding would be important clinically because, if NAFLD onset is in the perinatal period, it would have broader implications for preconception and pregnancy counseling as well as for earlier screening for NAFLD in infants born to diabetic mothers.[15]

When NAFLD begins may also be contingent on genetic risks. Recently, with the advancement of genetic technologies, emerging data have elucidated several genetic risk associations with complex and sporadic diseases such as NAFLD. Genetics is a potential disease modifier, and the natural history of NAFLD and progression of disease may depend on patient-specific genetic factors.

Although NAFLD pathogenesis and treatment options have been linked to environmental factors such as diet and physical activity, it is likely that NAFLD has a highly influential genetic component as well. There are 2 key observations that make a genetic link very plausible: (1) NAFLD has racial and ethnic differences, and (2) NAFLD clusters in families. The prevalence of NAFLD varies with respect to race and ethnicity with the highest prevalence in Hispanic children and lowest prevalence in black children. In the SCALE study, NAFLD was present in 1.5% of black children, 8.6% of white children, 10.2% of Asian children, and 11.8% of Hispanic children.[5] In a heritability study, 33 obese children with biopsy-proven NAFLD, 11 obese children without NAFLD, and 152 of their family members (parents, siblings, second- or third-degree relatives) were evaluated. In obese children without NAFLD, 17% of siblings and 37% of parents had MRI HFF of 5% or greater compared with 59% of siblings and 78% of parents of children with biopsy-proven NAFLD. The heritability estimates (with 0 being no heritability and 1 representing a trait that is completely heritable) were 0.85 for the unadjusted dichotomous variable for NAFLD.[16] When HFF was taken as a continuous measure, the heritability was 0.58. Thus, there is an intricate interplay of environment and genetics that requires further investigation.

A NAFLD genome-wide association study resulted in the discovery of a single-nucleotide polymorphism (SNP) common variant allele in *PNPLA3* that confers susceptibility to NAFLD.[17] This SNP is highly associated with hepatic fat content, as measured by MRS, independent of BMI, diabetes, or alcohol use.

In adults, the variant PNPLA3 allele is associated with increased hepatic fat as well as histologic severity, including fibrosis and cirrhosis.[18] Much remains to be understood in the pediatric population however, as pediatric histology studies have demonstrated conflicting results. In a study of 223 pediatric patients from the Nonalcoholic Steatohepatitis Clinical Research Network (NASH CRN), there was no association of the PNPLA3 locus with the histologic severity of NAFLD.[19] In contrast, in a study of 149 Italian children, the PNPLA3 variant allele was associated with histologic severity and presence of fibrosis.[13] Interestingly, there was an association with age in the NASH CRN cohort. Children carrying the G allele had a younger age at biopsy by 11 months. Hispanic ethnicity was also associated with younger age at biopsy,[19] suggesting a more severe phenotype presenting at a younger age in those with a genetic risk. Similarly, in a biopsy study of Italian children with NAFLD, age at first visit was an independent predictor of fibrosis.[13] These data suggest that patients carrying the risk allele of PNPLA3 may benefit from screening at a younger age to capture those with NAFLD. Given the emerging importance of this susceptibility gene and other genes in NAFLD pathophysiology along with the paucity of pediatric data, there is a great need for well-designed studies with biopsy-proven NAFLD in large pediatric cohorts. By understanding the genetics of NAFLD, it is possible this knowledge can aid diagnosis, guide treatment, and provide clinicians with tools to help with disease prognosis.

What Is the Histologic Starting Point and Severity?

Although the diagnosis of NAFLD is established at the time of biopsy, disease onset is unclear because this liver histology represents one time point of a chronic disease process. It is currently unknown if the disease begins with steatosis and progresses to NASH or if patients can start with NASH, because there is a lack of data for sequential biopsies over time. There is, however, an observed distribution of histologic severity at time of diagnosis. The authors performed a study of 347 overweight and obese children who were screened by their primary care providers per prevailing national guidelines and referred to Pediatric Gastroenterology in San Diego for suspected NAFLD based on elevated ALT. The combination of histology, clinical, and laboratory features yielded a diagnosis of NAFLD in only 55% of these children. Among the 193 children with NAFLD, 41% had steatohepatitis and 17% had advanced fibrosis.[20] The severity of liver disease depends on the study population, because the distribution of disease severity is shifted in a population selected to have the disease. In the SCALE study, a careful evaluation of liver histology from 742 children who had autopsies for rapid, unexpected deaths demonstrated that, of those children with NAFLD, 23% had NASH and 9% had advanced fibrosis.[5] Two types of histologic patterns have been described in pediatric NASH. Type 1, more common in adults, is characterized by steatosis, ballooning degeneration, and perisinusoidal fibrosis. Type 2, more common in non-Caucasian children, is characterized by steatosis, portal inflammation, and portal fibrosis. Type 1 NASH has an older age of onset, mean age 13.5, whereas type 2 NASH is more likely to be present in younger children, mean age 11.5,[21] suggesting these may be different diseases or a different disease process based on individual risk. Adolescents selected for extreme obesity may be biologically different that children with NAFLD who are seen in gastroenterology clinics. In the multicenter Teen LABS (Longitudinal Assessment of Bariatric Surgery) Study of adolescents undergoing bariatric surgery, 148 had intraoperative liver biopsies, and the prevalence of NAFLD in this cohort was 59%, with only 10% of those with NAFLD having definite NASH and 0.7% having advanced fibrosis.[22]

Many children with NAFLD have advanced disease at presentation. In a multicenter study from North America, of 108 children with NAFLD, 20% had advanced fibrosis at presentation.[10] In another US multicenter study in 2015 of biopsy-proven NAFLD, about 24% of children (mean age 13.3 years) had advanced fibrosis or cirrhosis at presentation.[23] When taken in aggregate, for children diagnosed with NAFLD through gastroenterology evaluation, a large number, 10% to 25%, have advanced fibrosis at initial presentation, and 25% to 50% have NASH. The data are limited regarding the evolution of NAFLD longitudinally after diagnosis and implications for prognosis in children with advanced stages of disease.

What Is the Associated Morbidity?

In addition to knowing the distribution of liver disease severity at diagnosis along with hepatic outcomes, it is crucial to also recognize the broader clinical phenotype, which is a key determinant not only of liver disease but also of clinical morbidity and mortality. This section focuses on the morbidity associated with NAFLD, including psychosocial, hepatic, cardiovascular, pulmonary, and metabolic.

Psychosocial

Although NAFLD can be asymptomatic, children with NAFLD report many symptoms that are only elicited through broad and detailed evaluation. In a study of 239 children with NAFLD enrolled in the NASH CRN, irritability was the most common individual symptom (reported by 73% of children), followed by fatigue (68%), headache (60%), trouble concentrating (55%), and muscle aches or cramps (53%).[24] Half of these children reported having 5 or more symptoms. Symptoms like pain and fatigue are more common in children with NAFLD; however, it is unclear if these symptoms arise from the disease itself or are associated symptoms.

In addition to the physical symptoms associated with NAFLD, NAFLD can also affect the quality of life in children. In an NASH CRN study, 39% of children with NAFLD had impaired quality of life. Fatigue, trouble sleeping, and sadness were the symptoms that accounted for nearly half of the variance in quality-of-life scores compared with controls.[24] In a study of psychosocial outcomes in children with NAFLD, children with NAFLD had higher levels of depression compared with obese controls.[25] Children with NAFLD may have a substantial psychological burden, and disease management should take potential psychosocial comorbidities into account to provide patient-centered care.

Hepatic

In adults, NAFLD is an increasingly common cause of hepatocellular carcinoma (HCC). The incidence of HCC in pediatric NAFLD is not known and is likely rare. There is one case report of HCC concurrent with NAFLD in a 7-year-old obese boy.[26] However, having NAFLD in childhood may be an important risk factor for HCC in adulthood. In a Dutch study of a cohort of more than 280,000 children followed for nearly 30 years, BMI at age 7 and 13 years was evaluated for longitudinal risk of HCC.[27] For every one point increase in BMI z-score at age 13, there was an increased risk of HCC of 33%. As opposed to BMI, there are no data specific to pediatric NAFLD. Although rare, HCC in the young adult is likely to increase given the percentage of children who have severe NAFLD (10%–25% with advanced fibrosis). This amount is a large pool of children who are at increased risk of developing HCC over the next few decades, thereby leading to increased amount of HCC in early adulthood stemming from pediatric NAFLD. This increased amount of HCC can have a devastating impact as the current estimated 5-year survival rate for HCC is only 15%.[28]

Cardiovascular

As more children with NAFLD are identified, more data are emerging about the associated cardiac and metabolic risks. NAFLD has been demonstrated to be more frequent in children with metabolic syndrome than in those without.[29] In a case-control study of 300 children, those with biopsy-proven NAFLD had a much higher cardiovascular risk profile, including higher total cholesterol, low-density lipoprotein (LDL), triglycerides, and systolic blood pressure than children with obesity alone. Similarly, in a cohort of 268 Italian children, obese children with ultrasound evidence of steatosis had a higher mean systolic blood pressure than those with obesity alone.[30] In a systematic, longitudinal study of blood pressure in 382 children with NAFLD, the prevalence of hypertension was 36% at the time of diagnosis. At 48-week follow-up, 21% of children with NAFLD had persistent hypertension. More severe steatosis was associated with odds of having hypertension. Of the children with severe steatosis, 45.2% had hypertension versus 35.1% in the normotensive group.[11] There were higher rates of hypertension in NAFLD cross-sectionally and longitudinally. Hypertension may cause structural and functional cardiac changes in children with NAFLD.

Dyslipidemia is also common in children with NAFLD. In a study of 120 Italian children with NAFLD, 63% had elevated triglycerides and 45% had low high-density lipoprotein (HDL). Cali and colleagues[31] evaluated serum lipids in 49 obese children and found that MRI HFF greater than 5.5% was associated with higher number of small, dense LDL and very LDL particles, which denote a more atherogenic lipid profile. Changes in lipids may also track with changes in liver histology. In a secondary analysis of TONIC (Treatment Of Nonalcoholic Fatty Liver Disease In Children), 173 children with NAFLD had a follow-up liver biopsy at 2 years, and histologic improvement was associated decreases in non-HDL cholesterol.[32]

Carotid intima-media thickness (CIMT) is a quantifiable cardiovascular phenotype for subclinical atherosclerosis and cardiovascular risk and has been evaluated in several studies of pediatric NAFLD. In 2 studies of obese children evaluated with liver ultrasonography, there was higher CIMT in those with suspected hepatic steatosis.[33,34] However, in a study of children with biopsy-proven NAFLD, there was no difference in CIMT compared with obese controls.[35] Because of small sample sizes and different methodology, the relationship between pediatric NAFLD and CIMT is unsettled. Data regarding alterations in left-ventricular mass (LVM) are most consistent. In a study of 117 Turkish children with ultrasound evidence of liver steatosis, those with liver steatosis and obesity had higher LVM compared with lean children or those with obesity alone.[36] In a study of 14 lean, 15 obese, and 15 obese children with MRS HFF greater than 5.6%, those with suspected NAFLD had significantly higher LV strain compared with children with obesity alone.[37] In a study of 136 Italian children by Pacifico and colleagues,[38] children with obesity and biopsy-proven NAFLD had significantly greater left ventricular dysfunction and higher LVM. Thus, children with NAFLD may be at increased risk of future heart failure and cardiovascular morbidity and mortality.

Pulmonary

Several recent studies have reported an association between NAFLD and obstructive sleep apnea (OSA). OSA results in a constellation of symptoms including daytime sleepiness, poor school performance, and snoring. Apnea can produce hypoxia and oxidative stress, which is speculated to contribute to the progression steatohepatitis and fibrosis due to ischemia-reperfusion injury.[39,40] There are a few studies of the association between NAFLD and OSA in children. In a study of 25 obese children with NAFLD, polysomnography demonstrated OSA in 60% of patients and those with OSA had more hepatic fibrosis.[41] In a study of 65 children with NAFLD, the prevalence of OSA was also 60%. OSA prevalence and severity were associated with NASH and fibrosis stage. In this study, the association with histologic severity was present even for children with NAFLD who were not obese.[42] In contrast, in a preliminary report of 53 children with NAFLD, OSA was again shown to be common, but was not associated with the severity of NAFLD.[43] In order to develop a thorough understanding of sleep and OSA in children with NAFLD, larger and longitudinal studies are needed. However, clinicians caring for children with NAFLD should be aware of the potential for undiagnosed OSA.

Metabolic

The metabolic comorbid conditions associated with pediatric NAFLD include metabolic syndrome, type 2 diabetes, low bone mineral density, and low vitamin D 25-OH levels.

In a study of obese adolescents, those with MRI HFF greater than 5.5% were 3 times as likely to have metabolic syndrome compared with those with HFF less than 5.5%.[44] In the series of 150 children with NAFLD compared with 150 children with obesity alone, children with NAFLD had higher fasting glucose and insulin.[29] Given that insulin resistance is important in the pathogenesis of NAFLD, the development of type 2 diabetes mellitus in children with NAFLD seems to be a logical progression. About 50% of children with type 2 diabetes have suspected NAFLD based on elevated ALT.[45] There are small studies in which the prevalence of type 2 diabetes is reported in children with NAFLD. Two studies looking at metabolic syndrome in biopsy-proven NAFLD have reported the prevalence of diabetes to be near 2%.[9,46] In a study of 43 children with biopsy-proven NAFLD, the prevalence of diabetes was 14%.[47] In a multicenter, retrospective study of patients with biopsy-proven NAFLD, the prevalence of diabetes was near 7% and did not correlate with the presence or absence of fibrosis on biopsy.[48] This finding is contrary to a study of adolescents undergoing bariatric surgery. In this study, 148 children underwent an intraoperative liver biopsy, and the detection of liver fibrosis was associated with pre-existing diabetes with an odds ratio of 3.56.[22] Based on these data, the frequency of type 2 diabetes in children lies somewhere between 2% and 14%, and whether diabetes is associated with the severity of NAFLD in children in unknown. Larger studies are needed to allow more stable estimates of prevalence and to clarify the relationship with disease progression.

Children with NAFLD may also be at increased risk for fractures. In a study of 38 children with NAFLD, obese children with NAFLD had significantly lower bone mineral density as measured by dual-energy X-ray absorptiometry compared with age-, sex-, and adiposity-matched obese children without NAFLD.[49] In addition, the bone mineral density for children with NASH was significantly lower compared with children with steatosis alone. In a cohort of 44 obese children with NAFLD, those with MRI HFF 5% or greater had significantly lower bone mineral density of the lumbar spine than those with MRI HFF less than 5%.[50] A subset of these patients had a liver biopsy, and children with NASH had a lower bone mineral density than those without NASH. When to evaluate children with NAFLD for fracture risk is unknown.

Vitamin D insufficiency and deficiency have been associated with obesity and may also have an association with NAFLD in children. Vitamin D deficiency, defined as vitamin D 25-OH levels less than 20 ng/mL, was present in 50% of 64 children with NAFLD.[51] In a follow-up study of 73 overweight and obese Italian children with NAFLD, vitamin D 25-OH levels were significantly lower in those children with NASH than those without NASH.[52] In contrast, in a study of 102 children in the NASH CRN, although low vitamin D 25-OH levels were common, there was no association with the histologic severity of disease.[53] Because of conflicting data, the role of vitamin D in pediatric NAFLD is unclear.

Pediatric NAFLD is a complex disease with potential for multiorgan complications and morbidity. Which of these complications arise directly as a result of liver disease and which are associated are challenging to determine. There are limited data regarding NAFLD and pediatric mortality. One retrospective study in Minnesota found children with NAFLD to be at higher risk for mortality compared with the general population, with a standardized mortality ratio of 13.6.[54] More studies are needed to assess the long-term outcomes in children with NAFLD in order to reduce the disease burden and associated morbidities that have the potential to significantly reduce life expectancy in these children.

What Is the Longitudinal Hepatic Outcome?

Longitudinal outcomes data are lacking in the pediatric NAFLD population. What is known, however, is that children can present with cirrhosis at diagnosis and that progression from NASH to cirrhosis can be rapid in a subset of patients. This rapid progression was first detailed in 2002 when Molleston and colleagues[55] reported a 12-year-old child with NASH and mild fibrosis at initial diagnosis who progressed to cirrhosis with variceal bleeding, ascites, and mild encephalopathy by age 14.

There are few longitudinal studies in pediatric NAFLD (**Table 1**). Several histology studies have a handful of patients with serial liver biopsies from their broader cohort, and some information can be gleaned from these studies. A study from 2008 included 18 patients between the ages of 7 and 19 years that had a follow-up biopsy at a mean interval of 28 months from initial diagnosis. In this study, 8 patients had no change in fibrosis, 7 patients had progression of fibrosis, and 3 patients had regression or disappearance of fibrosis after losing weight. Children who had resolution of fibrosis decreased their BMI by an average of 13%.[56] In another study from the Mayo Clinic in 2009, 5 children had repeat biopsies. The grade of steatosis and lobular inflammation either worsened or remained the same in all follow-up biopsies, and there was progression of fibrosis in 4 of 5 patients. One patient without fibrosis at initial biopsy developed cirrhosis by 57 months, and another without fibrosis at diagnosis progressed to stage 3 fibrosis by 82 months. Two patients with decompensated cirrhosis underwent liver transplant at follow-up. Both allografts had recurrence of NAFLD, and 1 of those 2 died after retransplantation.[54] Recently, a preliminary report described data from United Network for Organ Sharing/Organ Procurement and Transplantation Network (UNOS/OPTN) for liver transplants in patients less than the age of 40. There were 330 liver transplants performed for NASH in children and young adults.[57] Although most were not done before age 18, it is possible that many of these cases were the consequence of childhood NAFLD.

Longitudinal histology has been presented in 2 preliminary reports from the NASH CRN. In one study, there were 58 children, and in the other study, there were 102 children.[58,59] Over a time interval of 2 years, liver histology was stable in most children with NAFLD; however, about 25% demonstrated progression in this short time frame, and 20% of children had advanced fibrosis on follow-up liver histology.

Table 1
Longitudinal studies in pediatric nonalcoholic fatty liver disease

Study, y	Population	N	Age (y)	Follow-up (y)	Results
Peer-reviewed publications					
Molleston et al,[55] 2002	Single Site Pediatric Hepatology Clinic	2	10 and 14	N/A	• Patient 1: initial biopsy with cirrhosis • Patient 2: initial biopsy with NASH, within 2 y with portal hypertension, ascites, esophageal varices, and cirrhosis
A-Kader et al,[56] 2008		18	Range 7–19	2.3	• 8 patients: no change in fibrosis • 7 patients: progression of fibrosis • 3 patients: regression of fibrosis after losing weight • 2 patients with complete resolution of steatosis and fibrosis after decrease in BMI (23.9–19 kg/m² and 24.4–22.8 kg/m²)
Feldstein et al,[54] 2009		5	Mean 13.9	6.4	• Grade of steatosis and lobular inflammation either worsened or remained the same in all follow-up biopsies • Progression of fibrosis in 4/5 patients • 2 underwent liver transplant at follow-up; they presented with cirrhosis, one of those 2 died after retransplantation
Preliminary reports					
Lavine et al,[59] 2012	NASH CRN	58	Range 8–17	1.8	• Histologic improvement associated with improvement in ALT, insulin resistance, alkaline phosphatase, and BMI • 26% with progression of fibrosis on follow-up
Brunt et al,[58] 2014	NASH CRN	102	Range 11–17	2.2	• 20% of patients with advanced fibrosis on follow-up biopsy
Alkhouri et al,[57] 2015	UNOS/OPTN database for 1987–2010	330	Range 4–40	N/A	Transplants for NASH: • 14 children • 20 patients between ages 18 and 25 • 13 patients required retransplantation for NASH recurrence

With these data, it is clear that NAFLD in children can progress rapidly; it can present with severe cirrhosis and may ultimately require liver transplantation, which has additional implications for morbidity and mortality. Liver transplantation may not be uniformly curative, as data suggest recurrence of NASH and need for retransplantation in a meaningful subset. Given the lack of larger and more systematic studies, it is not known how frequently children with NAFLD should be monitored for progression of disease. What is clear, however, is severe fibrosis and cirrhosis are potential consequences of NAFLD and can occur within a few years of diagnosis in the most severe cases. Another unanswered question is determining which patients are at highest risk of rapid disease progression. Larger study populations are required to assess these outcomes data in pediatric NAFLD.

Table 2
Current understanding about the progression and natural history of pediatric nonalcoholic fatty liver disease

What Is Known	What Is Unknown
When does NAFLD start in children?	
Data support perinatal onset for some children of diabetic mothers	Does perinatal disease progress to adolescent NAFLD or is it a different disease?
Uncommon in children under 5 y	What is the disease process in younger children (perinatal and preadolescence)?
Average age at diagnosis in the United States between 12 and 13 y	Is the PNPLA3 gene associated with histologic severity in children?
PNPLA3 gene is associated with presence of NAFLD	Does PNPLA3 risk allele modify disease (ie, younger age of onset)?
What is the histologic starting point?	
25%–50% of children with NASH at time of diagnosis 10%–25% of children can present with advanced fibrosis and cirrhosis	Is there a linear progression from steatosis to NASH or can NASH be a starting point of disease?
What is the associated morbidity?	
NAFLD may be symptomatic: pain, fatigue, and lower quality of life	Are these symptoms associated with or caused by liver disease?
NAFLD can lead to HCC	Risk of HCC is unknown in pediatric NAFLD
Higher cardiovascular risk profiles, including hypertension, carotid intima media thickness, left ventricular dysfunction, and dyslipidemia	Need more data on pediatric mortality and NAFLD
Metabolic comorbid conditions include type 2 diabetes, low bone mineral density, and low vitamin D 25-OH levels	Is OSA associated with histologic severity or presence of NAFLD?
What is the longitudinal hepatic outcome?	
Progression from NASH to cirrhosis in a subset of patients can be rapid	Who is at risk for rapid disease progression?
Liver transplant is a potential outcome	How frequently should patients be biopsied to monitor disease progression?
Liver transplant is not uniformly curative; recurrence of NAFLD can occur	Very few longitudinal data exist with serial liver biopsies in the pediatric NAFLD population to make accurate conclusions about hepatic outcomes

SUMMARY

NAFLD is the leading cause of chronic liver disease in children; thus, more rigorous study of children with NAFLD over time is required in order to understand outcomes. Current observations and data can help elucidate portions of the natural history of NAFLD in children because there are data on the spectrum of histologic disease severity at diagnosis, evidence of multi-organ morbidity, and a few longitudinal studies, but much about the progression of disease remains unanswered (**Table 2**). NAFLD typically is a disease of peripuberty and adolescence because that is when children are diagnosed; however, disease onset is unknown. Does it start in utero for some and adolescence for others, and does genetics modify this age at presentation? Is it different diseases at different age groups?

With the present data, the field cannot accurately answer the question: What is the progression and natural history of pediatric NAFLD? In order to address this complicated question, studies with the following parameters would be needed: (1) very large sample size; (2) age, sex, racial, and geographic diversity; (3) per protocol follow-up histology; (4) standardized pathology evaluation; and (5) detailed phenotyping evaluation of BMI, liver transaminases, and NAFLD comorbidities at each biopsy time point.

NAFLD is not exclusively a liver disease; rather, it is a systemic disorder in which the liver acts with many other organ systems, and understanding those phenotypes and outcomes is critical to understanding NAFLD. Children with NAFLD need to be followed at regular and frequent intervals to watch for advancement of their liver and associated diseases, and to determine need for repeat biopsies depending on the clinical situation. However, the timing of this interval is unknown. Much remains to be uncovered about the natural history and progression of this disease spectrum as currently biopsy only provides one time point in the chronic disease process. It is with additional longitudinal pediatric data that the clinician can accurately anticipate prognosis, determine length of follow-up and need for repeat liver biopsies, and provide informed counseling to patients regarding their chronic disease.

REFERENCES

1. Brumbaugh DE, Tearse P, Cree-Green M, et al. Intrahepatic fat is increased in the neonatal offspring of obese women with gestational diabetes. J Pediatr 2013; 162(5):930–6.e1.
2. Modi N, Murgasova D, Ruager-Martin R, et al. The influence of maternal body mass index on infant adiposity and hepatic lipid content. Pediatr Res 2011; 70(3):287–91.
3. Patel KR, White FV, Deutsch GH. Hepatic steatosis is prevalent in stillborns delivered to women with diabetes mellitus. J Pediatr Gastroenterol Nutr 2015;60(2): 152–8.
4. Nobili V, Bedogni G, Alisi A, et al. A protective effect of breastfeeding on the progression of non-alcoholic fatty liver disease. Arch Dis Child 2009;94(10):801–5.
5. Schwimmer JB, Deutsch R, Kahen T, et al. Prevalence of fatty liver in children and adolescents. Pediatrics 2006;118(4):1388–93.
6. Beacher DA, Ariza AJ, Fishbein MH, et al. Screening for elevated risk of liver disease in preschool children (aged 2–5 years) being seen for obesity management. SAGE Open Med 2014;2.
7. Quiros-Tejeira RE, Rivera CA, Ziba TT, et al. Risk for nonalcoholic fatty liver disease in Hispanic youth with BMI > or =95th percentile. J Pediatr Gastroenterol Nutr 2007;44(2):228–36.

8. Welsh JA, Karpen S, Vos MB. Increasing prevalence of nonalcoholic fatty liver disease among United States adolescents, 1988-1994 to 2007-2010. J Pediatr 2013;162(3):496–500.e1.

9. Patton HM, Lavine JE, Van Natta ML, et al. Clinical correlates of histopathology in pediatric nonalcoholic steatohepatitis. Gastroenterology 2008;135(6): 1961–71.e2.

10. Carter-Kent C, Brunt EM, Yerian LM, et al. Relations of steatosis type, grade, and zonality to histological features in pediatric nonalcoholic fatty liver disease. J Pediatr Gastroenterol Nutr 2011;52(2):190–7.

11. Schwimmer JB, Zepeda A, Newton KP, et al. Longitudinal assessment of high blood pressure in children with nonalcoholic fatty liver disease. PLoS One 2014; 9(11):e112569.

12. Nobili V, Marcellini M, Devito R, et al. NAFLD in children: a prospective clinical-pathological study and effect of lifestyle advice. Hepatology 2006; 44(2):458–65.

13. Valenti L, Alisi A, Galmozzi E, et al. I148M patatin-like phospholipase domain-containing 3 gene variant and severity of pediatric nonalcoholic fatty liver disease. Hepatology 2010;52(4):1274–80.

14. Bennett B, Larson-Meyer DE, Ravussin E, et al. Impaired insulin sensitivity and elevated ectopic fat in healthy obese vs. nonobese prepubertal children. Obesity (Silver Spring) 2012;20(2):371–5.

15. Ugalde-Nicalo PA, Schwimmer JB. On the origin of pediatric nonalcoholic fatty liver disease. J Pediatr Gastroenterol Nutr 2015;60(2):147–8.

16. Schwimmer JB, Celedon MA, Lavine JE, et al. Heritability of nonalcoholic fatty liver disease. Gastroenterology 2009;136(5):1585–92.

17. Romeo S, Kozlitina J, Xing C, et al. Genetic variation in PNPLA3 confers susceptibility to nonalcoholic fatty liver disease. Nat Genet 2008;40(12):1461–5.

18. Valenti L, Al-Serri A, Daly AK, et al. Homozygosity for the patatin-like phospholipase-3/adiponutrin I148M polymorphism influences liver fibrosis in patients with nonalcoholic fatty liver disease. Hepatology 2010;51(4):1209–17.

19. Rotman Y, Koh C, Zmuda JM, et al. The association of genetic variability in patatin-like phospholipase domain-containing protein 3 (PNPLA3) with histological severity of nonalcoholic fatty liver disease. Hepatology 2010;52(3): 894–903.

20. Schwimmer JB, Newton KP, Awai HI, et al. Paediatric gastroenterology evaluation of overweight and obese children referred from primary care for suspected nonalcoholic fatty liver disease. Aliment Pharmacol Ther 2013;38(10):1267–77.

21. Schwimmer JB, Behling C, Newbury R, et al. Histopathology of pediatric nonalcoholic fatty liver disease. Hepatology 2005;42(3):641–9.

22. Xanthakos SA, Jenkins TM, Kleiner DE, et al. High prevalence of nonalcoholic fatty liver disease in adolescents undergoing bariatric surgery. Gastroenterology 2015;149(3):623–34.e8.

23. Mansoor S, Yerian L, Kohli R, et al. The evaluation of hepatic fibrosis scores in children with nonalcoholic fatty liver disease. Dig Dis Sci 2015;60(5):1440–7.

24. Kistler KD, Molleston J, Unalp A, et al. Symptoms and quality of life in obese children and adolescents with non-alcoholic fatty liver disease. Aliment Pharmacol Ther 2010;31(3):396–406.

25. Kerkar N, D'Urso C, Van Nostrand K, et al. Psychosocial outcomes for children with nonalcoholic fatty liver disease over time and compared to obese controls. J Pediatr Gastroenterol Nutr 2012;56(1):77–82.

26. Nobili V, Alisi A, Grimaldi C, et al. Non-alcoholic fatty liver disease and hepatocellular carcinoma in a 7-year-old obese boy: coincidence or comorbidity? Pediatr Obes 2014;9(5):e99–102.
27. Berentzen TL, Gamborg M, Holst C, et al. Body mass index in childhood and adult risk of primary liver cancer. J Hepatol 2014;60(2):325–30.
28. Jemal A, Bray F, Center MM, et al. Global cancer statistics. CA Cancer J Clin 2011;61(2):69–90.
29. Schwimmer JB, Pardee PE, Lavine JE, et al. Cardiovascular risk factors and the metabolic syndrome in pediatric nonalcoholic fatty liver disease. Circulation 2008;118(3):277–83.
30. Sartorio A, Del Col A, Agosti F, et al. Predictors of non-alcoholic fatty liver disease in obese children. Eur J Clin Nutr 2007;61(7):877–83.
31. Cali AM, Zern TL, Taksali SE, et al. Intrahepatic fat accumulation and alterations in lipoprotein composition in obese adolescents: a perfect proatherogenic state. Diabetes Care 2007;30(12):3093–8.
32. Corey KE, Vuppalanchi R, Vos M, et al. Improvement in liver histology is associated with reduction in dyslipidemia in children with nonalcoholic fatty liver disease. J Pediatr Gastroenterol Nutr 2015;60(3):360–7.
33. Demircioglu F, Koçyiğit A, Arslan N, et al. Intima-media thickness of carotid artery and susceptibility to atherosclerosis in obese children with nonalcoholic fatty liver disease. J Pediatr Gastroenterol Nutr 2008;47(1):68–75.
34. Pacifico L, Cantisani V, Ricci P, et al. Nonalcoholic fatty liver disease and carotid atherosclerosis in children. Pediatr Res 2008;63(4):423–7.
35. Manco M, Bedogni G, Monti L, et al. Intima-media thickness and liver histology in obese children and adolescents with non-alcoholic fatty liver disease. Atherosclerosis 2010;209(2):463–8.
36. Sert A, Pirgon O, Aypar E, et al. Relationship between left ventricular mass and carotid intima media thickness in obese adolescents with non-alcoholic fatty liver disease. J Pediatr Endocrinol Metab 2012;25(9–10):927–34.
37. Singh GK, Vitola BE, Holland MR, et al. Alterations in ventricular structure and function in obese adolescents with nonalcoholic fatty liver disease. J Pediatr 2013;162(6):1160–8, 1168.e1.
38. Pacifico L, Di Martino M, De Merulis A, et al. Left ventricular dysfunction in obese children and adolescents with nonalcoholic fatty liver disease. Hepatology 2014; 59(2):461–70.
39. Mathurin P, Durand F, Ganne N, et al. Ischemic hepatitis due to obstructive sleep apnea. Gastroenterology 1995;109(5):1682–4.
40. Henrion J, Colin L, Schapira M, et al. Hypoxic hepatitis caused by severe hypoxemia from obstructive sleep apnea. J Clin Gastroenterol 1997;24(4): 245–9.
41. Sundaram SS, Sokol RJ, Capocelli KE, et al. Obstructive sleep apnea and hypoxemia are associated with advanced liver histology in pediatric nonalcoholic fatty liver disease. J Pediatr 2014;164(4):699–706.e1.
42. Nobili V, Cutrera R, Liccardo D, et al. Obstructive sleep apnea syndrome affects liver histology and inflammatory cell activation in pediatric nonalcoholic fatty liver disease, regardless of obesity/insulin resistance. Am J Respir Crit Care Med 2014;189(1):66–76.
43. Daniel JL, Behling C, Proudfoot J, et al. Is sleep disordered breathing associated with non-alcoholic fatty liver disease in pediatric patients? Am J Respir Crit Care Med 2015;191:A5054.

44. Burgert TS, Taksali SE, Dziura J, et al. Alanine aminotransferase levels and fatty liver in childhood obesity: associations with insulin resistance, adiponectin, and visceral fat. J Clin Endocrinol Metab 2006;91(11):4287–94.

45. Nadeau KJ, Klingensmith G, Zeitler P. Type 2 diabetes in children is frequently associated with elevated alanine aminotransferase. J Pediatr Gastroenterol Nutr 2005;41(1):94–8.

46. Manco M, Marcellini M, Devito R, et al. Metabolic syndrome and liver histology in paediatric non-alcoholic steatohepatitis. Int J Obes (Lond) 2008;32(2):381–7.

47. Schwimmer JB, Deutsch R, Rauch JB, et al. Obesity, insulin resistance, and other clinicopathological correlates of pediatric nonalcoholic fatty liver disease. J Pediatr 2003;143(4):500–5.

48. Carter-Kent C, Yerian LM, Brunt EM, et al. Nonalcoholic steatohepatitis in children: a multicenter clinicopathological study. Hepatology 2009;50(4):1113–20.

49. Pardee PE, Dunn W, Schwimmer JB. Non-alcoholic fatty liver disease is associated with low bone mineral density in obese children. Aliment Pharmacol Ther 2012;35(2):248–54.

50. Pacifico L, Bezzi M, Lombardo CV, et al. Adipokines and C-reactive protein in relation to bone mineralization in pediatric nonalcoholic fatty liver disease. World J Gastroenterol 2013;19(25):4007–14.

51. Manco M, Ciampalini P, Nobili V. Low levels of 25-hydroxyvitamin D(3) in children with biopsy-proven nonalcoholic fatty liver disease. Hepatology 2010;51(6):2229 [author reply: 2230].

52. Nobili V, Giorgio V, Liccardo D, et al. Vitamin D levels and liver histological alterations in children with nonalcoholic fatty liver disease. Eur J Endocrinol 2014; 170(4):547–53.

53. Hourigan SK, Abrams S, Yates K, et al. Relation between vitamin D status and nonalcoholic fatty liver disease in children. J Pediatr Gastroenterol Nutr 2015; 60(3):396–404.

54. Feldstein AE, Charatcharoenwitthaya P, Treeprasertsuk S, et al. The natural history of non-alcoholic fatty liver disease in children: a follow-up study for up to 20 years. Gut 2009;58(11):1538–44.

55. Molleston JP, White F, Teckman J, et al. Obese children with steatohepatitis can develop cirrhosis in childhood. Am J Gastroenterol 2002;97(9):2460–2.

56. A-Kader HH, Henderson J, Vanhoesen K, et al. Nonalcoholic fatty liver disease in children: a single center experience. Clin Gastroenterol Hepatol 2008;6(7): 799–802.

57. Alkhouri N, Hanouneh IA, Zein NN, et al. Su1038 Liver Transplantation for Nonalcoholic Steatohepatitis (NASH) in children and young adults: the true burden of pediatric nonalcoholic fatty liver disease. Gastroenterology 2015;148(4):S-1046.

58. Brunt EM, Kleiner DE, Belt PH, et al. Pediatric Nonalcoholic Fatty Liver Disease (NAFLD): histological feature changes over time in paired biopsies from the NASH CRN. Hepatology 2014;60:290a.

59. Lavine JE, Yates KP, Brunt EM, et al. The natural history of nonalcoholic fatty liver disease in children and adolescents assessed in placebo recipients in the TONIC trial. Hepatology 2012;56:905a.

Effect of Weight Loss, Diet, Exercise, and Bariatric Surgery on Nonalcoholic Fatty Liver Disease

William N. Hannah Jr, MD[a], Stephen A. Harrison, MD[b],*

KEYWORDS

- Nonalcoholic fatty liver disease • Weight loss • Diet • Exercise • Bariatric surgery

KEY POINTS

- Lifestyle modifications to include diet, exercise, and weight loss remain the most effective therapy for nonalcoholic fatty liver disease (NAFLD).
- Weight loss of 3% to 5% is associated with decreased steatosis; however, a 7% to 10% decrease is necessary to achieve NAFLD/nonalcoholic steatohepatitis remission and fibrosis regression.
- Independent of weight loss, exercise reduces hepatic steatosis and improves metabolic indices.
- No specific dietary intervention or exercise regimen has proven beneficial beyond calorie restriction coupled with energy reduction.
- Bariatric surgery in morbidly obese individuals who have failed to lose weight through lifestyle modifications can improve steatosis, inflammation, and fibrosis.

INTRODUCTION

Nonalcoholic fatty liver disease (NAFLD) now represents the most common form of liver disease in developed countries with an estimated prevalence of 20% to 30% and increasing to 50% in diabetics and 70% in obese individuals.[1] Worldwide, obesity

Disclosure Statement: The views expressed are those of the authors and should not be construed as official views of the United States Air Force, United States Army, or Department of Defense. Dr W.N. Hannah has nothing to disclose. Dr S.A. Harrison is an advisor for Fibrogen, Chronic Liver Disease Foundation, NGM Biopharmaceuticals, Nimbus Discovery, and Gilead.
 a Department of Medicine, San Antonio Military Medical Center, JBSA, 3551 Roger Brooke Drive, Fort Sam Houston, TX 78234-4504, USA; b Division of Gastroenterology, Department of Medicine, San Antonio Military Medical Center, JBSA, 3551 Roger Brooke Drive, Fort Sam Houston, TX 78234-4504, USA
* Corresponding author.
E-mail address: stephen.a.harrison.mil@mail.mil

has become a major global health care concern, with the number of obese and overweight individuals reaching 2.1 billion in 2013.[2] The United States alone accounts for 13% of obese people globally.[2] With NAFLD representing the hepatic manifestation of the metabolic syndrome, the rates of NAFLD continue to increase as obesity reaches pandemic proportions. Of those with NAFLD, the prevalence of biopsy-proven nonalcoholic steatohepatitis (NASH) has been estimated at 12.2% in a prospective community cohort.[3] Importantly, individuals with NASH and fibrosis have a substantial risk of progression to advanced disease, and increased body mass index has been associated with advanced fibrosis in NASH.[4] Because of the established role of obesity in the pathophysiology of NAFLD, efforts targeted at obesity reduction remain the primary therapeutic intervention. In this review, the authors summarize the effects of weight loss, diet, exercise, and bariatric surgery on NAFLD.

WEIGHT LOSS

Because obesity plays such a central role in the underlying pathophysiology of NAFLD, efforts at weight reduction represent the mainstay of management and first line therapy for NAFLD. The beneficial effects of weight loss on NAFLD have been demonstrated in numerous clinical trials.[5–9] In 2012, Musso and colleagues[10] evaluated the effects of weight loss in NAFLD from 8 randomized controlled trials, 4 of which included posttreatment histology. From their metaanalysis, a 5% or greater weight loss improved hepatic steatosis, and a 7% or greater weight loss also showed improvement in the NAFLD Activity Score (NAS). Unfortunately, only 50% of subjects were able to attain a weight loss of 7% or greater even with significant intervention. Overall fibrosis was unchanged. Most recently, Patel and colleagues[11] demonstrated a reduction in body mass index of at least 5% was associated with significant decreases in liver fat and volume in patients with biopsy-proven NASH. In a study by Promrat and colleagues,[7] 8 participants achieved a 10% or greater weight reduction with a trend toward reduced NAS for those who lost more weight. Similarly, Harrison and colleagues[5] showed improvement in steatosis, ballooning, inflammation, and NAS in those subjects who lost 9% or more of body weight compared with those who did not. In a recent seminal paper by Vilar-Gomez et al,[12] the effects of weight loss through lifestyle modifications from 261 patients with paired liver biopsies were evaluated. Their results demonstrate the degree of weight loss is associated independently with improvements in all NASH-related histology. Further, for those individuals who lost 10% or more of body weight, 45% had regression of fibrosis, 90% had resolution of steatohepatitis, and 100% demonstrated improvements in NAS. Finally, Wong and colleagues[13] demonstrated through proton-magnetic resonance spectroscopy that weight loss of 3% to 4.9% was associated with remission of NAFLD in 41% of patients, whereas those with more than 10% weight loss had 97% remission of NAFLD. Although the exact upper limit for weight loss in the treatment of NAFLD has not been established, current evidence suggests that weight loss of at least 7% is essential to improved histologic disease activity. Current practice guidelines from the American Association for the Study of Liver Diseases recommends that loss of at least 3% to 5% of body weight seems to be necessary to improve steatosis, but a greater weight loss (up to 10%) may be needed to improve necroinflammation[14] and fibrosis[12] (**Fig. 1**).

DIETARY INTERVENTIONS

Current guidelines suggest that individuals at metabolic risk should follow a low calorie diet with a 30% energy deficit.[15,16] Although strategies to obtain significant weight loss

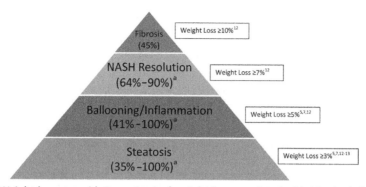

Fig. 1. Weight loss pyramid. Percentage of weight loss associated with histologic improvement in nonalcoholic fatty liver disease. [a] Depending on the degree of weight loss. NASH, nonalcoholic steatohepatitis. (*Data from* Refs.[5,7,12,13])

are critical in NAFLD management, only about 50% of patients are able to achieve the necessary weight loss goal of 7% to 10% in clinical trials.[10,12] As such, any dietary intervention should promote long-term sustainability and have demonstrated improvement in NAFLD. Prior studies have demonstrated the benefits of caloric restriction on hepatic steatosis; however, the most effective dietary interventions have yet to be elucidated.[6,17]

LOW CARBOHYDRATE AND LOW FAT DIETS

In a small pilot study of only 5 patients, Tendler and colleagues[8] evaluated the effects of a low carbohydrate, ketogenic diet on NAFLD. After 6 months of therapy, significant improvements were noted in steatosis, inflammatory grade, and fibrosis on liver biopsy specimens. Haufe and colleagues[18] compared the effects of reduced fat and reduced carbohydrate diets on intrahepatic fat by liver spectroscopy. Of the 102 patients who completed the study, both hypocaloric diets decreased intrahepatic lipid content with the largest response in those with elevated fat content at baseline. Similarly, de Luis and colleagues[19] evaluated the effect of hypocaloric low fat and low carbohydrate diets on transaminases and insulin resistance in patients with NAFLD. In the 28 patients with NAFLD, weight reduction owing to both the hypocaloric diets was associated with an improvement in ALT and improved insulin resistance as measured by the homeostasis model assessment for insulin sensitivity. Based on these studies, the benefits obtained seem to be related to calorie restriction rather than the specific dietary restriction. No rigorous longitudinal prospective trials have linked specific dietary compositions with histologic improvements in NAFLD, and it remains unclear whether low carbohydrate or low fat diets produce benefits in the absence of significant weight reduction.

FRUCTOSE

Fructose intake has now become a major component of the modern diet.[20] The main sources of fructose include sucrose (table sugar), corn syrup, fruits, and honey. To an increasing degree, consumption of sweetened beverages is contributing to the overall intake of fructose and is associated with high energy intake, increased body weight, and metabolic and cardiovascular disease.[20] In fact, Vos and colleagues[21] determined that as much as 10% of daily calories for American children and adults results from consumption of fructose with the largest source being sugar-sweetened beverages.

Ingestion of fructose stimulates de novo lipogenesis, increased visceral fat and may contribute to the pathogenesis of NAFLD.[22]

Abdelmalek and colleagues[23] performed a cross-sectional analysis of 427 adults to investigate the impact of increased fructose consumption on the metabolic syndrome and histologic features of NAFLD. The authors found that intake of 7 or more sweetened beverages per week was associated with higher fibrosis and lobular inflammation. After controlling for confounders, daily fructose consumption was associated with higher fibrosis stage in all age groups. For those age greater than 48 years, daily consumption demonstrated increased hepatic inflammation and hepatocyte ballooning. Jin and colleagues[24] recently completed a 4-week trial to assess the effects of reduced dietary fructose on 24 obese Hispanic-American adolescents. These individuals in the reduced fructose arm were given glucose-only beverages but were calorie matched to the control arm. At the conclusion of the study, those in the reduced fructose cohort experienced improvements in cardiovascular profile, but no changes were seen in hepatic steatosis.

Kanerva and colleagues[25] assessed the effects of high fructose intake with the risk of NAFLD in older Finnish adults. In this cross-sectional study of 2003 Finnish men and women, those individuals in the highest fructose quartile had a lower risk of NAFLD and NAFLD liver fat score after adjusting for age, sex, and energy intake. These conflicting results raise the question as to whether the effects of fructose are mediated directly or through excess calories via fructose overconsumption. In fact, few studies have distinguished between the effects of energy excess and body weight from high intake of fructose. To address this "fructose hypothesis," Chung and colleagues[26] completed a systemic review to evaluate fructose intake on liver disease. Overall the metaanalysis included 21 interventional studies. The authors concluded that there was low evidence that hypercaloric fructose diet increases liver fat and aspartate aminotransferase in healthy men and insufficient evidence to draw conclusions on the effects of high fructose corn syrup or sucrose on NAFLD. Some authors have recommended that it is prudent to recommend restriction in fructose-rich food and beverage until further studies are available[1]; however, current evidence is lacking to draw any firm conclusions with respect to NAFLD.

POLYUNSATURATED FATTY ACIDS

Hepatic tissue has been shown to have a depletion of long chain *n*-3 polyunsaturated fatty acids (PUFAs), accumulation of triglycerides, and increased lipogenesis in patients with NAFLD compared with control subjects.[27] PUFAs coordinate the upregulation of lipid oxygenation and downregulation of lipid synthesis. Fatty acid oxidative effects are mediated through binding of PUFAs to proliferator activated receptor-α and the resultant transcription of several genes associated with fatty acid oxidation.[28] PUFAs also suppress lipid synthesis by reducing the expression of sterol regulatory element-binding protein-1, which regulates the synthesis and storage of triglycerides in the liver.[28] Furthermore, PUFAs have shown to reduce inflammation through the generation of eicosanoids.[29] Because of these effects, PUFAs may be an effective treatment option for NAFLD.

In 2007, Spadaro and colleagues[30] assessed the effects of PUFAs in subjects with NAFLD. Twenty patients with NAFLD were given an American Heart Association diet and 2 g per day of polyunsaturated acids for 6 months. These patients were compared with a control group who only received the American Heart Association diet. At the conclusion of the study in the diet plus PUFA cohort, a significant improvement was noted in serum alanine aminotransferase (ALT), gamma-glutamyl transferase, triglyceride levels, and an increase in high-density lipoprotein levels. The authors also noted a significant decrease in the homeostasis model assessment for insulin sensitivity as well as a notable improvement in echogenicity score. In a similar study by Zhu and colleagues,[31] 144 patients with NAFLD were given either PUFAs from seal oils and a standard diet or diet alone. After 24 weeks of treatment, significant improvements were noted in total symptom scores, ALT, and triglycerides in the PUFA and diet group compared with the diet alone group. Twenty percent of patients in the PUFA group experienced a complete fatty liver regression as measured by ultrasonography.

In a small study by Cussons and colleagues,[32] 25 women with the polycystic ovary syndrome were randomized to 4 g of omega-3 fatty acids compared with placebo. At the end of 8 weeks, hepatic fat content was measured using proton magnetic resonance spectroscopy. Overall there was a significant reduction in hepatic fat in the omega-3 fatty acid treatment group with the most improvement noted in women with liver fat greater than 5%. Statistically significant reductions were also noted in triglycerides, systolic blood pressure, and diastolic blood pressure. In 2012, Parker and colleagues[33] performed a systematic review and metaanalysis of omega-3 supplementation and NAFLD. Of the 9 studies that were reviewed, PUFA treatment was associated with decreases in hepatic fat and aspartate aminotransferase. When only randomized controlled trials were included in a subanalysis, a significant reduction in liver fat remained but not for ALT.

More recently completed studies have evaluated the effects of PUFAs on liver histology. Argo and colleagues[34] completed a double-blind, randomized, placebo-controlled trial comparing fish oil with placebo for 1 year with typical counseling on caloric intake and physical activity. Of the 17 patients given 3 g of n-3 fish oil per day, there was no difference in NAS reduction, although a significant reduction in fat reduction was seen by abdominal MRI. In a similar study performed by Dasarathy and colleagues,[35] 37 patients with NASH and diabetes were randomized to PUFAs containing eicosapentaenoic acid and docosahexaenoic acid or an identical, isocaloric, corn oil placebo for 48 weeks. At the completion of the study, patients in the PUFA treatment group showed no changes in NAS. Interestingly, the placebo group demonstrated a significant improvement in NAS, although lobular inflammation worsened. Finally, Nogueira and colleagues[36] compared the effects of PUFAs with a placebo group given mineral oil in patients with biopsy-proven NASH. Similar to the Argo and Dasarathy studies, histologic scores as measured by NAS failed to show significant changes between the PUFA and placebo groups. The authors did report an improvement in NAS in the subset of patients who experienced an increase in alpha-linolenic and eicosapentaenoic plasma levels. It remains to be seen whether higher doses or longer treatment durations with PUFAs may prove beneficial. At present, however, there is insufficient evidence to support routine use of PUFA in dietary supplementation with NAFLD.

EXERCISE

Likely as a result of cultural and socioeconomic changes in Western societies, individuals are much more sedentary compared with our ancestors. Risk factors associated with NAFLD include advancing age, increasing weight, and the metabolic syndrome and insulin resistance.[37] Physical inactivity has also been associated with increased body weight, central adiposity and insulin resistance,[38] increased risk of the metabolic syndrome,[39] NAFLD,[40] and severity of NASH.[37] Therefore, lifestyle modifications targeted specifically at physical activity that do not require significant weight loss are attractive therapeutic options.

Johnson and colleagues[41] studied the effects of aerobic exercise training on hepatic and visceral lipids in obese individuals in the absence of weight loss. The authors placed 12 sedentary obese individuals on a progressive aerobic exercise program for 4 weeks. At the end of the exercise program, there were significant reductions in visceral adiposity and hepatic triglyceride concentration. St. George and colleagues[42] evaluated 141 patients with NAFLD and randomized them to low or moderate intensity lifestyle interventions or a control group. Activity levels as low as 60 to 149 minutes per week showed significant improvement in liver enzymes, and the greatest improvement in liver enzymes were in those who maintained physical activity more than 150 minutes per week or those who increased their activity by more than 60 minutes per week. Subjects in the sedentary group had no changes in liver enzymes. Hallsworth and colleagues[43] compared sedentary adults with NAFLD who completed 8 weeks of resistance exercise with continued normal treatment. At the completion of the study, significant reductions were noted in hepatic steatosis, lipid oxidation, glucose control, and the homeostasis model assessment for insulin sensitivity. In all of these studies, the effects were independent of weight loss. A more recent metaanalysis of exercise and NAFLD by Keating and colleagues[44] reviewed 12 randomized controlled trails, and the Johnson and Hallsworth studies were included. When comparing a control arm versus exercise alone, there was a significant reduction in hepatic fat, but there was no significant difference in ALT. The only study to evaluate the effects of exercise with posttreatment histology was performed by Eckard and colleagues.[45] Fifty-six participants were randomized to standard care; a low-fat diet and moderate exercise; a moderate-fat, low-carbohydrate diet and moderate exercise; or moderate exercise alone for 6 months. At the end of the study, there was a significant reduction in before to after intervention NAS for the subgroups as a whole when compared with standard therapy. The moderate exercise group alone failed to demonstrate any change in NAS.

The current literature on exercise for NAFLD remains limited by low sample sizes and statistical power as well as lack of prospective trials evaluating changes in liver histology. Independent of weight loss, exercise does seem to reduce hepatic fat as well as other metabolic indices. The most rigorous systematic review completed to date did show a reduction in hepatic steatosis, but failed to observe an exercise benefit on ALT.[44] Therefore, current clinical recommendations seem to favor physical activity for reduction of hepatic fat and cardiovascular risk reduction, but no formal guidelines regarding the specific exercise, duration, or frequency are available at this time.

DIET AND EXERCISE

Recommendations for lifestyle modification as the treatment for NAFLD are generally meant to include both diet and exercise. Research that has examined the combined effects of diet and exercise on weight loss makes it clear that both energy expenditure and caloric restriction lead to weight loss.[46] In a metaanalysis of 18 trials, Wu and colleagues[47] evaluated the effectiveness of both diet and exercise compared with diet interventions on long-term weight loss. In their pooled analysis, interventions that included a diet plus exercise produced a 1.14-kg greater long-term weight loss than diet alone.

To assess the effects of exercise and diet combined on NALFD, Thoma and colleagues performed a systematic review.[48] Only 5 studies with 306 participants combined diets with specific aerobic exercise programs for 3 to 6 months. All of these studies demonstrated reductions on measures of liver fat and/or liver enzymes as well as weight reductions of 4.2% to 10.6%. Two studies reported histologic end-points.[9,49] Vilar-Gomez et al[49] reported significant reductions in inflammation, ballooning, and fibrosis relative to baseline, whereas Ueno and colleagues[9] only noted significant reductions in steatosis. To our knowledge, there are no large, prospective, randomized clinical trials directly comparing the effects of diet alone, exercise alone, or combined diet and exercise on NAFLD. Thus, although combined interventions of diet restriction and physical activity are more beneficial in the general public, limitations with study designs and reporting of patient adherence make it difficult to make firm recommendations on the combined effects of diet and exercise as compared with diet or physical activity alone for patients with NAFLD.

BARIATRIC SURGERY

Although the mainstay of therapy for NAFLD remains weight loss through exercise and lifestyle modification, only a small minority of individuals are able to achieve sustained weight reduction. Similarly, pharmacologic strategies for weight loss have limited efficacy. Bariatric surgery, on the other hand, can provide long-term weight loss and improvement in diseases associated with obesity. Bariatric surgery has proven to have an important and beneficial role in managing obesity.[50] Similarly, bariatric surgery can achieve significant weight loss, improved insulin sensitivity, and reduction of diabetes mellitus type 2.[51–54] In addition, bariatric surgery has also shown reduced cardiovascular death and improved overall mortality.[55,56] Because the metabolic syndrome and diabetes are critically linked to NAFLD, bariatric surgery has the potential to have lasting and meaningful improvements in liver related metabolic disease. In fact, 25% of those patients presenting for bariatric surgery had NASH, and of those, 42% had advanced fibrosis.[57]

Bower and colleagues[58] completed a systematic review of 29 studies to assess liver biochemistry and histology in obese patients undergoing bariatric surgery. Statistically significant improvements were noted in steatosis, hepatocyte ballooning, lobular inflammation, fibrosis, ALT, aspartate aminotransferase, and gamma-glutamyl transferase. Importantly, hepatocyte ballooning was significantly reduced by as much as 67.7%. Prior studies have correlated hepatocyte ballooning with progression to fibrosis; thus, improvements in this histologic feature are associated with improved clinical outcomes.[59] Although these studies suggest that bariatric surgery is associated with significant improvements in NAFLD, the relative small size of most studies and presence of significant heterogeneity limit firm conclusions. Large, prospective, randomized controlled trials are still needed.

In the largest prospective trial to evaluate the effects of bariatric surgery on NAFLD, Mathurin and colleagues[60] performed bariatric surgery on 381 patients, which included gastric banding, biliointestinal bypass, and gastric bypass procedures. The researchers performed liver biopsies at the time of surgery and again at 1 and 5 years. Although major reductions in steatosis and ballooning degeneration were seen, no differences were observed between the 3 groups, suggesting that no specific procedure was superior. There was a small but significant increase in fibrosis seen at 1 and 5 years, although there was remarkable stability seen in all aspects of liver histology suggesting the improvements in steatosis and ballooning and increase in fibrosis were associated with rapid weight loss after surgery. Unfortunately, there have been no head-to-head trials investigating the most effective procedure for NAFLD. Bariatric procedures vary in their complexity, risk–benefit profile, and extent of gastrointestinal interruption. Coupled with patient specific factors, the choice of which procedure to perform in NAFLD has not been elucidated.

Recently, Alizai and colleagues[61] evaluated liver recovery after bariatric surgery using the LiMAx test. This test is a validated bedside test for the determination of liver functional capacity based on the kinetics of C-methacetin used mainly in liver surgery and liver transplantation.[62] In the study by Alizai and associates, the mean liver function capacity increased significantly at both 6 and 12 months postoperatively from baseline. Although further studies are needed to validate the use of the LiMAx test in post bariatric surgery patients, results from this initial study are further evidence of overall improved hepatic function after bariatric surgery.

SUMMARY

NAFLD represents the hepatic manifestation of the metabolic syndrome. In parallel with the obesity pandemic, NAFLD has become the most common form of liver disease. As obesity rates continue to soar in Western societies, so too can we expect the prevalence of NAFLD to increase. To date, no single pharmacologic agent has proven consistently effective at treating NAFLD. Therefore, lifestyle modifications targeted at weight loss, dietary modifications, and exercise remain first-line therapy (**Table 1**).

Weight reduction is the primary goal for the management of NAFLD given that obesity plays such a central role in the pathophysiology of NAFLD. Current evidence suggests that a weight loss of at least 3% to 5% improves hepatic steatosis and that weight reduction of 5% to 7% is necessary for reductions in inflammatory activity. Furthermore, weight loss in excess of 10% has demonstrated regression of fibrosis. Physical activity in the absence of weight loss does seem to reduce hepatic steatosis and other metabolic indices. Despite this apparent benefit, there is insufficient

Table 1 Recommendations for lifestyle interventions for the treatment of nonalcoholic fatty liver disease	
Lifestyle Modification	**Recommendation**
Weight loss	Loss of 3%–5% of body weight to improve hepatic steatosis Loss of 7% to improve NAFLD activity score Loss of ≥10% to promote regression of fibrosis
Diet	Calorie restriction with 30% energy reduction
Fructose	Restriction of foods and beverages high in fructose may be beneficial
Polyunsaturated fatty acids	Insufficient evidence to support routine dietary supplementation
Exercise	Physical activity to improve hepatic steatosis and cardiovascular risk reduction Insufficient evidence for specific activities, duration, frequency, or intensity Consider American College of Sports Medicine guidelines for exercise/activity
Diet and exercise	Insufficient evidence to recommend specific combined diet and activity for NAFLD patients Combined diet and exercise programs produce greater long-term weight loss in general public
Bariatric surgery	In morbidly obese individuals improves hepatic steatosis, inflammation and fibrosis Insufficient evidence to recommend bariatric procedure of choice

Abbreviations: NAFLD, nonalcoholic fatty liver disease; NASH, nonalcoholic steatohepatitis.

evidence to recommend an individual activity, duration, or intensity of exercise. Current lifestyle modification recommendations promote both weight loss and physical activity for NAFLD, although rigorous data supporting the combination of diet and exercise in NAFLD are lacking.

Many different dietary strategies designed to promote weight loss and improve NAFLD have been evaluated. At this time, no specific dietary composition has been linked to histologic improvements in NAFLD nor is there sufficient evidence that any diet produces benefits in the absence of significant weight loss. PUFAs have effects on the regulation of lipid oxygenation and lipid synthesis and antiinflammatory activity. Despite this role in lipid regulation, routine dietary supplementation with PUFAs for the treatment of NAFLD is not currently supported in the literature. Similarly, fructose intake stimulates de novo lipogenesis, increased visceral fat, and is likely linked to the pathophysiology of NAFLD. Although limiting fructose intake may be prudent, current evidence for limiting fructose-rich foods and beverages in NAFLD management is lacking.

Unfortunately, only about one-half of patients in monitored settings such as clinical trials are able to achieve appropriate weight loss targets despite diet and physical activity. For morbidly obese individuals who are unable to achieve and sustain weight loss, bariatric surgery should be considered. Bariatric surgery results in reduced cardiovascular death and improved overall mortality, but also lasting improvements in the metabolic syndrome and NAFLD disease activity to include steatosis, fibrosis, and inflammation. Patient-specific factors, surgical complexity, and other risks and benefits should dictate the procedure of choice.

REFERENCES

1. Barrera F, George J. The role of diet and nutritional intervention for the management of patients with NAFLD. Clin Liver Dis 2014;18(1):91–112.
2. Ng M, Fleming T, Robinson M, et al. Global, regional, and national prevalence of overweight and obesity in children and adults during 1980-2013: a systematic analysis for the Global Burden of Disease Study 2013. Lancet 2014;384(9945): 766–81.
3. Williams CD, Stengel J, Asike MI, et al. Prevalence of nonalcoholic fatty liver disease and nonalcoholic steatohepatitis among a largely middle-aged population utilizing ultrasound and liver biopsy: a prospective study. Gastroenterology 2011;140(1):124–31.
4. Angulo P, Keach JC, Batts KP, et al. Independent predictors of liver fibrosis in patients with nonalcoholic steatohepatitis. Hepatology 1999;30(6):1356–62.
5. Harrison SA, Fecht W, Brunt EM, et al. Orlistat for overweight subjects with nonalcoholic steatohepatitis: a randomized, prospective trial. Hepatology 2009;49(1): 80–6.
6. Huang MA, Greenson JK, Chao C, et al. One-year intense nutritional counseling results in histological improvement in patients with non-alcoholic steatohepatitis: a pilot study. Am J Gastroenterol 2005;100(5):1072–81.
7. Promrat K, Kleiner DE, Niemeier HM, et al. Randomized controlled trial testing the effects of weight loss on nonalcoholic steatohepatitis. Hepatology 2010;51(1): 121–9.
8. Tendler D, Lin S, Yancy WS Jr, et al. The effect of a low-carbohydrate, ketogenic diet on nonalcoholic fatty liver disease: a pilot study. Dig Dis Sci 2007;52(2): 589–93.
9. Ueno T, Sugawara H, Sujaku K, et al. Therapeutic effects of restricted diet and exercise in obese patients with fatty liver. J Hepatol 1997;27(1):103–7.

10. Musso G, Cassader M, Rosina F, et al. Impact of current treatments on liver disease, glucose metabolism and cardiovascular risk in non-alcoholic fatty liver disease (NAFLD): a systematic review and meta-analysis of randomised trials. Diabetologia 2012;55(4):885–904.

11. Patel NS, Doycheva I, Peterson MR, et al. Effect of weight loss on magnetic resonance imaging estimation of liver fat and volume in patients with nonalcoholic steatohepatitis. Clin Gastroenterol Hepatol 2015;13(3):561–8.e1.

12. Vilar-Gomez E, Martinez-Perez Y, Calzadilla-Bertot L, et al. Weight loss via lifestyle modification significantly reduces features of nonalcoholic steatohepatitis. Gastroenterology 2015;149(2):367–78.e5.

13. Wong VW, Chan RS, Wong GL, et al. Community-based lifestyle modification programme for non-alcoholic fatty liver disease: a randomized controlled trial. J Hepatol 2013;59(3):536–42.

14. Chalasani N, Younossi Z, Lavine JE, et al. The diagnosis and management of non-alcoholic fatty liver disease: practice guideline by the American Gastroenterological Association, American Association for the Study of Liver Diseases, and American College of Gastroenterology. Gastroenterology 2012;142(7): 1592–609.

15. Rosenzweig JL, Ferrannini E, Grundy SM, et al. Primary prevention of cardiovascular disease and type 2 diabetes in patients at metabolic risk: an endocrine society clinical practice guideline. J Clin Endocrinol Metab 2008;93(10):3671–89.

16. Jensen MD, Ryan DH, Apovian CM, et al. 2013 AHA/ACC/TOS guideline for the management of overweight and obesity in adults: a report of the American College of Cardiology/American Heart Association Task Force on Practice Guidelines and the Obesity Society. Circulation 2014;129(25 Suppl 2):S102–38.

17. Drenick EJ, Simmons F, Murphy JF. Effect on hepatic morphology of treatment of obesity by fasting, reducing diets and small-bowel bypass. N Engl J Med 1970; 282(15):829–34.

18. Haufe S, Engeli S, Kast P, et al. Randomized comparison of reduced fat and reduced carbohydrate hypocaloric diets on intrahepatic fat in overweight and obese human subjects. Hepatology 2011;53(5):1504–14.

19. de Luis DA, Aller R, Izaola O, et al. Effect of two different hypocaloric diets in transaminases and insulin resistance in nonalcoholic fatty liver disease and obese patients. Nutr Hosp 2010;25(5):730–5.

20. Tappy L, Le KA. Metabolic effects of fructose and the worldwide increase in obesity. Physiol Rev 2010;90(1):23–46.

21. Vos MB, Kimmons JE, Gillespie C, et al. Dietary fructose consumption among US children and adults: the Third National Health and Nutrition Examination Survey. Medscape J Med 2008;10(7):160.

22. Basaranoglu M, Basaranoglu G, Bugianesi E. Carbohydrate intake and nonalcoholic fatty liver disease: fructose as a weapon of mass destruction. Hepatobiliary Surg Nutr 2015;4(2):109–16.

23. Abdelmalek MF, Suzuki A, Guy C, et al. Increased fructose consumption is associated with fibrosis severity in patients with nonalcoholic fatty liver disease. Hepatology 2010;51(6):1961–71.

24. Jin R, Welsh JA, Le NA, et al. Dietary fructose reduction improves markers of cardiovascular disease risk in Hispanic-American adolescents with NAFLD. Nutrients 2014;6(8):3187–201.

25. Kanerva N, Sandboge S, Kaartinen NE, et al. Higher fructose intake is inversely associated with risk of nonalcoholic fatty liver disease in older Finnish adults. Am J Clin Nutr 2014;100(4):1133–8.

26. Chung M, Ma J, Patel K, et al. Fructose, high-fructose corn syrup, sucrose, and nonalcoholic fatty liver disease or indexes of liver health: a systematic review and meta-analysis. Am J Clin Nutr 2014;100(3):833–49.
27. Araya J, Rodrigo R, Videla LA, et al. Increase in long-chain polyunsaturated fatty acid n - 6/n - 3 ratio in relation to hepatic steatosis in patients with non-alcoholic fatty liver disease. Clin Sci 2004;106(6):635–43.
28. Clarke SD. Nonalcoholic steatosis and steatohepatitis. I. Molecular mechanism for polyunsaturated fatty acid regulation of gene transcription. Am J Physiol Gastrointest Liver Physiol 2001;281(4):G865–9.
29. Calder PC. n-3 polyunsaturated fatty acids, inflammation, and inflammatory diseases. Am J Clin Nutr 2006;83(6 Suppl):1505S–19S.
30. Spadaro L, Magliocco O, Spampinato D, et al. Effects of n-3 polyunsaturated fatty acids in subjects with nonalcoholic fatty liver disease. Dig Liver Dis 2008;40(3): 194–9.
31. Zhu FS, Liu S, Chen XM, et al. Effects of n-3 polyunsaturated fatty acids from seal oils on nonalcoholic fatty liver disease associated with hyperlipidemia. World J Gastroenterol 2008;14(41):6395–400.
32. Cussons AJ, Watts GF, Mori TA, et al. Omega-3 fatty acid supplementation decreases liver fat content in polycystic ovary syndrome: a randomized controlled trial employing proton magnetic resonance spectroscopy. J Clin Endocrinol Metab 2009;94(10):3842–8.
33. Parker HM, Johnson NA, Burdon CA, et al. Omega-3 supplementation and non-alcoholic fatty liver disease: a systematic review and meta-analysis. J Hepatol 2012;56(4):944–51.
34. Argo CK, Patrie JT, Lackner C, et al. Effects of n-3 fish oil on metabolic and histological parameters in NASH: a double-blind, randomized, placebo-controlled trial. J Hepatol 2015;62(1):190–7.
35. Dasarathy S, Dasarathy J, Khiyami A, et al. Double-blind randomized placebo-controlled clinical trial of omega 3 fatty acids for the treatment of diabetic patients with nonalcoholic steatohepatitis. J Clin Gastroenterol 2015;49(2):137–44.
36. Nogueira MA, Oliveira CP, Ferreira Alves VA, et al. Omega-3 polyunsaturated fatty acids in treating non-alcoholic steatohepatitis: a randomized, double-blind, placebo-controlled trial. Clin Nutr 2015. [Epub ahead of print].
37. Kang H, Greenson JK, Omo JT, et al. Metabolic syndrome is associated with greater histologic severity, higher carbohydrate, and lower fat diet in patients with NAFLD. Am J Gastroenterol 2006;101(10):2247–53.
38. McGavock JM, Anderson TJ, Lewanczuk RZ. Sedentary lifestyle and antecedents of cardiovascular disease in young adults. Am J Hypertens 2006;19(7):701–7.
39. Zhu S, St-Onge MP, Heshka S, et al. Lifestyle behaviors associated with lower risk of having the metabolic syndrome. Metabolism 2004;53(11):1503–11.
40. Church TS, Kuk JL, Ross R, et al. Association of cardiorespiratory fitness, body mass index, and waist circumference to nonalcoholic fatty liver disease. Gastroenterology 2006;130(7):2023–30.
41. Johnson NA, Sachinwalla T, Walton DW, et al. Aerobic exercise training reduces hepatic and visceral lipids in obese individuals without weight loss. Hepatology 2009;50(4):1105–12.
42. St George A, Bauman A, Johnston A, et al. Independent effects of physical activity in patients with nonalcoholic fatty liver disease. Hepatology 2009;50(1):68–76.
43. Hallsworth K, Fattakhova G, Hollingsworth KG, et al. Resistance exercise reduces liver fat and its mediators in non-alcoholic fatty liver disease independent of weight loss. Gut 2011;60(9):1278–83.

44. Keating SE, Hackett DA, George J, et al. Exercise and non-alcoholic fatty liver disease: a systematic review and meta-analysis. J Hepatol 2012;57(1):157–66.
45. Eckard C, Cole R, Lockwood J, et al. Prospective histopathologic evaluation of lifestyle modification in nonalcoholic fatty liver disease: a randomized trial. Therap Adv Gastroenterol 2013;6(4):249–59.
46. Gerber LH, Weinstein A, Pawloski L. Role of exercise in optimizing the functional status of patients with nonalcoholic fatty liver disease. Clin Liver Dis 2014;18(1):113–27.
47. Wu T, Gao X, Chen M, et al. Long-term effectiveness of diet-plus-exercise interventions vs. diet-only interventions for weight loss: a meta-analysis. Obes Rev 2009;10(3):313–23.
48. Thoma C, Day CP, Trenell MI. Lifestyle interventions for the treatment of non-alcoholic fatty liver disease in adults: a systematic review. Journal of Hepatology 2012;56(1):255–66.
49. Vilar Gomez E, Rodriguez De Miranda A, Gra Oramas B, et al. Clinical trial: a nutritional supplement Viusid, in combination with diet and exercise, in patients with nonalcoholic fatty liver disease. Aliment Pharmacol Ther 2009;30(10):999–1009.
50. Buchwald H, Oien DM. Metabolic/bariatric surgery worldwide 2011. Obes Surg 2013;23(4):427–36.
51. Castagneto-Gissey L, Mingrone G. Insulin sensitivity and secretion modifications after bariatric surgery. J Endocrinol Invest 2012;35(7):692–8.
52. Mingrone G, Panunzi S, De Gaetano A, et al. Bariatric surgery versus conventional medical therapy for type 2 diabetes. N Engl J Med 2012;366(17):1577–85.
53. Schauer PR, Kashyap SR, Wolski K, et al. Bariatric surgery versus intensive medical therapy in obese patients with diabetes. N Engl J Med 2012;366(17):1567–76.
54. Ikramuddin S, Korner J, Lee WJ, et al. Roux-en-Y gastric bypass vs intensive medical management for the control of type 2 diabetes, hypertension, and hyperlipidemia: the Diabetes Surgery Study randomized clinical trial. JAMA 2013; 309(21):2240–9.
55. Pontiroli AE, Morabito A. Long-term prevention of mortality in morbid obesity through bariatric surgery. a systematic review and meta-analysis of trials performed with gastric banding and gastric bypass. Ann Surg 2011;253(3):484–7.
56. Adams TD, Gress RE, Smith SC, et al. Long-term mortality after gastric bypass surgery. N Engl J Med 2007;357(8):753–61.
57. Dixon JB, Bhathal PS, O'Brien PE. Nonalcoholic fatty liver disease: predictors of nonalcoholic steatohepatitis and liver fibrosis in the severely obese. Gastroenterology 2001;121(1):91–100.
58. Bower G, Toma T, Harling L, et al. Bariatric surgery and non-alcoholic fatty liver disease: a systematic review of liver biochemistry and histology. Obes Surg 2015. [Epub ahead of print].
59. Matteoni CA, Younossi ZM, Gramlich T, et al. Nonalcoholic fatty liver disease: a spectrum of clinical and pathological severity. Gastroenterology 1999;116(6): 1413–9.
60. Mathurin P, Hollebecque A, Arnalsteen L, et al. Prospective study of the long-term effects of bariatric surgery on liver injury in patients without advanced disease. Gastroenterology 2009;137(2):532–40.
61. Alizai PH, Wendl J, Roeth AA, et al. Functional liver recovery after bariatric surgery-a prospective cohort study with the LiMAx test. Obes Surg 2015;25(11): 2047–53.
62. Stockmann M, Lock JF, Riecke B, et al. Prediction of postoperative outcome after hepatectomy with a new bedside test for maximal liver function capacity. Ann Surg 2009;250(1):119–25.

Current Pharmacologic Therapy for Nonalcoholic Fatty Liver Disease

Swaytha Ganesh, MD[a],*, Vinod K. Rustgi, MD, MBA[b]

KEYWORDS

- NASH • Pharmacologic therapy • Weight loss • Lifestyle modification
- Insulin sensitizers • Fatty acids • Antioxidants

KEY POINTS

- Modest but sustained weight loss, regular exercise, and diet composition modification seem to improve biochemical and histologic abnormalities.
- Other therapies directed at insulin resistance, oxidative stress, cytoprotection, and fibrosis may also offer benefits, but further studies are required.
- A multifaceted approach of lifestyle modifications, weight loss, and pharmacotherapy can be used in combination, but no single treatment approach has proved universally applicable to the general population with nonalcoholic steatohepatitis (NASH).
- Continuous clinical and preclinical studies on existing and potential drugs are needed to improve treatment of nonalcoholic fatty liver disease/NASH, which is a burgeoning health care problem.

INTRODUCTION

Nonalcoholic fatty liver disease (NAFLD) is now the most frequent chronic liver disease in Western countries, affecting more than 30% of the general population, and has emerged as a serious public health burden. The prevalence of this syndrome is increasing worldwide in parallel with the increase in obesity (**Table 1**).[1] Recent surveys indicate that NAFLD may account for approximately 80% of cases, and that 1 in 4 or 5 American adults has NAFLD.[2,3]

Disclosure: The authors have nothing to disclose.
[a] Division of Gastroenterology, Hepatology and Nutrition, University of Pittsburgh Medical Center, Presbyterian, M2, C-Wing, 200 Lothrop Street, Pittsburgh, PA 15213, USA; [b] Liver Transplantation, The Thomas Starzl Transplant Institute, UPMC Montefiore, Room N758.1, 3459 Fifth Avenue, Pittsburgh, PA 15213, USA
* Corresponding author.
E-mail address: ganesx@upmc.edu

Table 1
Summary: pharmacologic therapies in the treatment of Non Alcoholic Steatohepatitis (NASH)

Treatment	Mechanism	Biochemical Effects	Histologic Effects	Comments
Orlistat	Weight loss	↓ LFTs and insulin resistance	↓ Steatosis, inflammation, NAS score	Improvement in inflammation and NAS seen if weight loss ≥9%
Rimonabant	Weight loss, possible peripheral effects	↓ Insulin resistance, triglyceride levels, LFTs; ↑ HDL and adiponectin levels	↓ Steatosis	Animal data, psychiatric side effects
Incretin analogues (exendin-4)	Weight loss	↓ LFTs, insulin resistance, hemoglobin A_1C levels	↓ Steatosis	Animal and pilot studies in NAFLD; extensively studied in type 2 diabetes mellitus
TZDs	PPAR-γ agonists	↓ LFTs, insulin resistance, and TNF-α levels; ↑ Adiponectin levels	↓ Steatosis, inflammation and fibrosis	Side effects: weight gain, peripheral edema, cardiac, fractures, need for maintenance therapy
Metformin	↑ AMP kinase	↓ LFTs and insulin resistance; No effect on adiponectin levels	+/− improvement in steatosis, inflammation, and fibrosis	Data conflicting; no RCTs
Vitamin E	↓ Oxidative stress	↓ LFTs	Uncertain	Large trials with histologic follow-up evaluation required
Betaine	↓ Oxidative stress	↓ LFTs	↓ Steatosis, inflammation, fibrosis	Pilot study only
UDCA	Hepatoprotective	No change	No change	Not beneficial in large RCT
Pentoxifylline	Hepatoprotective	↓ LFTs, TNF-α levels	↓ Steatosis, inflammation	Pilot study only
HMG CoA-reductase inhibitors	Improve lipid panel	? LFTs	Uncertain	Conflicting studies
Ezetimibe	Blocks cholesterol absorption in intestine	? LFTs	↓ Steatosis and fibrosis	Animal data
Angiotensin receptor blockers	? Inhibits stellate cells	↓ LFTs	↓ Fibrosis	Animal and pilot studies

The symbol "↓" indicates a decrease, "↑" indicates an increase, and "?" indicates that the effect is uncertain.
Abbreviations: AMP, adenosine 5′-monophosphate; HMG CoA, 3-hydroxy-3-methylglutaryl-coenzyme A; LFTs, liver function tests; PPAR, peroxisome proliferator-activated receptor; TNF, tumor necrosis factor, TZDs, thiazolidinediones.
From Torres DM, Harrison SA. Diagnosis and therapy of nonalcoholic steatohepatitis. Gastroenterology 2008;134:1689; with permission.

CURRENT TREATMENT OPTIONS

At present, there is no approved treatment (medical or surgical) for NAFLD. Several studies have concluded that body weight loss is the only proven effective therapy for NAFLD. However, many agents have shown promising results.[4,5] A prior meta-analysis of randomized controlled trials (RCTs) showed that 5% weight loss improved steatosis and associate metabolic parameters but higher degrees of weight loss were required to ameliorate necroinflammation and overall disease activity.[5] There are also no US Food and Drug Administration (FDA)–approved therapies for nonalcoholic stea-tohepatitis (NASH). There is therefore a need to develop better diagnostic and thera-peutic strategies for patients with NASH, targeting both those with early stage disease as well as those with advanced liver fibrosis.[6] Treatment of NAFLD includes lifestyle modifications and pharmacotherapy aiming at increasing insulin sensitivity, and atten-uating inflammation and hepatic fibrosis. Weight reduction has consistently been shown to reduce levels of liver enzymes and insulin resistance. Although dietary inter-vention and exercise remain the first-line therapy, because of low patient compliance with these measures, pharmacotherapy or surgical approaches are often required.[7–9] Despite several trials of pharmacologic agents, no highly effective treatment yet ex-ists[8–10] for NASH. The ideal diet composition for patients with NASH has not been established, although the general consensus has been that excessive intake of either fat or carbohydrate is harmful. An RCT of low-fat versus low-carbohydrate diets showed greater weight loss and improved lipid panels in the low-carbohydrate group.[11] A small pilot trial of 5 patients with NAFLD who followed a low-carbohydrate (<20 g/d) diet for 6 months showed histologic improvements in 4 of the 5 patients, who had a mean weight loss of 12.8 kg (**Fig. 1**).[12]

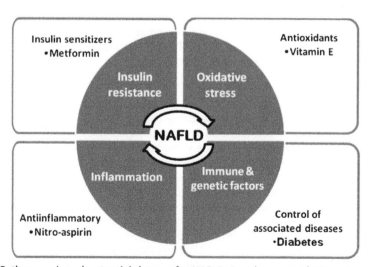

Fig. 1. Pathogenesis and potential therapy for NAFLD. Development of NAFLD is caused by interaction between multiple factors, mainly insulin resistance, oxidative stress, inflamma-tion, and genetic predisposition. The potential therapies of NAFLD target one or more of these factors. (*From* Ibrahim MA, Kelleni M, Geddawy A. Nonalcoholic fatty liver disease: current and potential therapies. Life Sci 2013;92(2):115; with permission.)

POTENTIAL THERAPIES FOR NONALCOHOLIC FATTY LIVER DISEASE
Medical Therapies That Improve Metabolic Profiles

Omega-3 fatty acids

A large multicenter study of omega-3 fatty acid (eicosapentaenoic acid) to treat NASH is ongoing in the United States. It might be considered as a first-line agent in treating hypertriglyceridemia in patients with NAFLD. Another prospective, randomized, double-blind, placebo-controlled study was performed in patients with NASH with diabetes. A total of 37 patients with well-controlled diabetes (hemoglobin A_1C <8.5%) were randomized to receive either polyunsaturated fatty acid (PUFA) containing eicosapentaenoic acid (2160 mg) and docosahexaenoic acid (1440 mg) daily or an isocaloric, identical placebo containing corn oil for 48 weeks. PUFA provided no benefit compared with placebo in patients with NASH with diabetes. The effects of PUFA on histology and insulin resistance were inferior to placebo. These data provide no support for PUFA supplements in NASH.[13] PUFAs have been used in the treatment of hyperlipidemia and cardiovascular disease (CVD), and more recently in the treatment of NAFLD. Studies have highlighted the correlation between insulin resistance and changes in fatty acids, specifically a deficiency in n-3 PUFA. Capanni and colleagues investigated the effects of n-3 PUFA supplementation (1 g/d for 12 months) in 56 patients with NAFLD. The results indicated that PUFA improves biochemical aspects of NAFLD as well as liver steatosis. Similarly, a literature review conducted by Masterton and colleagues[14] found that in animal studies n-3 PUFA reduced hepatic steatosis, and improved insulin sensitivity and biochemical markers of inflammation; human studies yielded similar results. Masterton and colleagues[14] and Capanni and colleagues[15] concluded that PUFA is a promising therapeutic approach to the treatment of NAFLD.[16] Prior systematic search of the literature was conducted for studies pertaining to the effect of omega-3 PUFA supplementation on NAFLD in humans. Nine eligible studies, involving 355 individuals given either omega-3 PUFA or control treatment, were included. Primary outcome measures were liver fat levels and liver function tests. The pooled data suggest that omega-3 PUFA supplementation may decrease liver fat levels. The optimal dose required has not been determined, but benefits are seen with greater than or equal to 0.83 g/d of omega-3. There was significant heterogeneity between studies. Well-designed RCTs that quantify the magnitude of effect of omega-3 PUFA supplementation on liver fat are needed.[17]

Insulin sensitizers

In previous studies for the treatment of NASH, use of thiazolidinediones (TZDs; especially pioglitazone) has been most extensively evaluated. Glitazones are those with the best evidence-based data and also with the strongest pathogenesis-based rationale for treatment of NASH. Pioglitazone is the best studied pharmacologic agent in NASH. The largest trial so far, the PIVENS trial (Pioglitazone, Vitamin E, or Placebo for Nonalcoholic Steatohepatitis), compared pioglitazone at a low dose of 30 mg/d versus vitamin E (800 IU/d) versus placebo for 2 years in 247 patients without full-blown diabetes.[18] Pioglitazone improved all individual histologic features (except for fibrosis) and achieved resolution of steatohepatitis. It showed a significant improvement in alanine aminotransferase (ALT) levels, aspartate aminotransferase (AST) levels (P<.001), hepatic steatosis (P<.001), and lobular inflammation after treatment with pioglitazone 30 mg/d (n = 80) for 96 weeks. Hajiaghamohammadi and colleagues[20] compared the effects of metformin 500 mg/d (n = 22), pioglitazone 15 mg/d (n = 22), and silymarin 140 mg/d (n = 22). After 8 weeks, pioglitazone led to a significant improvement in AST and ALT levels and, of the 3 therapies, was associated with the most significant reduction in average fasting blood sugar, triglycerides, and serum insulin levels, and Homeostasis Model Assessment index.[19,20] Lomonaco and colleagues[21] showed a significant reduction in adipose tissue insulin resistance (Adipo-IR) score (fasting nonesterified fatty acid level times fasting insulin level) in nondiabetic patients with biopsy-proven NASH after 16 weeks of treatment with pioglitazone. The NAFLD activity score (NAS) improved in 73% of patients treated with pioglitazone compared with 24% in the placebo group.[21]

The reduction in this score was associated with an improvement in steatosis and necroinflammation.[21] The Adipo-IR score reduction did not persist at 96 weeks, which was thought to be secondary to a significant amount of weight gain observed in the pioglitazone group.[22] It has been suggested, but not confirmed, that glitazones strongly improve adipose tissue insulin resistance, which correlates with the reduction in steatosis and necroinflammation.[23,24]

Studies have shown that metformin and TZDs may improve insulin sensitivity, serum aminotransferase concentrations, and liver histology. These results indicate that treatment with an insulin-sensitizing agent can lead to improvement in biochemical and histologic features of NASH and support the role of insulin resistance in the pathogenesis of this disease.[25] TZDs improved steatosis and inflammation, but yielded significant weight gain. Little evidence exists regarding the sustained effects after drug discontinuation, which, together with their side effects, limits the widespread use of these agents in clinical practice.[7–9] However insulin-sensitizing agents are promising drugs in NAFLD management in patients with insulin resistance. There is evidence that both biguanides (eg, metformin) and TZDs (eg, pioglitazone and rosiglitazone) produce positive effects on biochemical parameters with variable effects on liver histology. Although these studies provided some evidence that the TZDs may be beneficial in the short term, the long-term benefits remain to be seen. Moreover, a recent meta-analysis of diabetic male patients taking rosiglitazone has suggested an increased risk of cardiovascular events.[26] There has been an adverse side effect profile described as well. Modest weight gain has been shown routinely and seems to be caused by increased peripheral fat deposition. Some retrospective studies also suggest that TZDs promote bone loss and may contribute to osteoporosis and increased incidence of fractures, particularly in postmenopausal women.[27] The risk of congestive heart failure exacerbation with the use of TZDs also has been reported. The long-term safety of TZDs (heart failure, bone loss, and bladder cancer) has been under much debate. Regarding bladder cancer, the FDA currently recommends avoidance of pioglitazone if active bladder cancer is present, and caution if there is prior history of the disease.[21] In contrast, pioglitazone has been shown to reduce CVD in patients with type 2 diabetes mellitus.[28]

The guidelines from the American Association for the Study of Liver Diseases, American College of Gastroenterology, and the American Gastroenterological Association recommend the use of pioglitazone in patients with biopsy-proven NASH, but more studies are needed to assess efficacy and safety of the drug in the long term.[29]

Pioglitazone 30 mg/d may be considered in patients with biopsy-proven NASH with type 2 diabetes who do not have congestive heart failure or increased risk of fracture, although long-term effects have not yet been established.[19]

Metformin acts through the activation of adenosine monophosphate activated protein kinase, a master regulator of glucose and lipid metabolism. This agent could be therapeutically advantageous in people with type 2 diabetes, in whom NAFLD occurs frequently.[4]

One of the other studies has shown that metformin leads to improvements in liver histology and ALT levels in 30% of patients with NASH, probably by its effects in causing weight loss, but not for nonobese patients who develop NAFLD. Twenty-eight adult patients with biopsy-proven NASH were enrolled in the study and completed the 48 weeks of therapy with metformin at 2 g/d. This treatment was associated with improvements in liver histology and insulin sensitivity in more than half of patients with NASH. There was an improvement in serum aminotransferase levels. Histologic improvements were found predominantly in hepatocellular injury and parenchymal inflammation, with fewer effects on steatosis and little measurable effect on portal inflammation or fibrosis. Importantly, metformin also caused weight loss. Twenty-one of the 26 patients (81%) lost weight during the 48 weeks of treatment and in 5 (19%) the weight loss was marked (>10 kg). The patients with the most weight loss tended to have the greatest improvement in liver histology and those with no weight loss tended to have no improvement in histology. Thirty percent achieved a histologic response. Most patients lost weight, the average being 6 kg. There was a marked association between weight loss and improvements in NASH activity index and ALT levels (both $P<.01$). Insulin sensitivity also improved, but the degree of change did not correlate with histologic improvement.[30] Several smaller studies have reported reductions in plasma aminotransferase levels with metformin; however, improvement of liver steatosis, inflammation, and fibrosis has been reported in only a few small studies, with more recent studies, including 3 RCTs, finding no benefit.[31–38] Metformin still has clinical value in patients with NASH because it controls hyperglycemia (common in these patients) and may reduce CVD in patients with type 2 diabetes mellitus.[39,40]

Antioxidants

Vitamin E
Lower levels of serum antioxidants are present in patients with NASH. Depletion of antioxidants via lipid peroxidation and free oxygen radical species renders the liver more susceptible to oxidative damage. The use of vitamin E, a lipophilic antioxidant, counteracts these lower levels of antioxidant enzymes and slows the progression of NAFLD to NASH. The depletion of antioxidants within hepatocytes resulting in impaired reactive oxygen species inactivation is the basis for antioxidant supplementation as a potential treatment of NASH. The lipid-soluble antioxidant, alpha-tocopherol (vitamin E), has been shown to inhibit lipid peroxidation and suppress inflammatory cytokines such as tumor necrosis factor (TNF) alpha, and its use in the treatment of NASH has been studied.[41] Vitamin E is associated with a decrease in levels of aminotransferases; can cause improvement in steatosis and inflammation, and ballooning and resolution of steatohepatitis; and has no effect on hepatic fibrosis.[18,42]

A more recent 2-year RCT in nondiabetic patients with biopsy-proven NASH reported a significant difference in the response to the primary histologic end point for patients receiving vitamin E compared with placebo-treated patients (43% vs 19%; $P = .001$). The primary histologic end point was an improvement of greater than or equal to 2 grades in the NAS, with at least 1 point improvement in hepatocellular ballooning and 1 point in either the lobular inflammation or steatosis score, with no worsening of fibrosis. Using this end point, only 34% of patients on pioglitazone improved. However, more patients in the pioglitazone group lacked hepatocellular ballooning at study entry (a component of the primary end point and thus classified as nonresponders) and did not have a posttreatment liver biopsy (therefore considered by default as nonresponders), both negatively affecting the efficacy comparisons of pioglitazone. Moreover, there were no statistical differences between the treatments when patients receiving vitamin E and pioglitazone were matched for baseline histology (ie, ballooning) or when histologic outcomes were examined under a variety of sensitivity analysis scenarios.[18]

In recent years, the therapeutic effects of vitamin E for NAFLD have been widely studied. With the aim of evaluating the therapeutic efficacy, a meta-analysis was conducted to study the effects of vitamin E supplement in lowering the aspartate transaminase (AST) and alanine transaminase (ALT) levels in patients with NAFLD and NASH. A total of 8 articles were reviewed and evidence currently available supports the theory that vitamin E supplementation can optimize aminotransferase levels for patients with NAFLD and NASH, and more well-designed, large-scale clinical trials are encouraged to examine the therapeutic effect of vitamin E for these disorders.[43] The major concern with vitamin E is the increase in all-cause mortality with high doses, which was showed in a few meta-analyses, but others failed to show such an association.[44,45] Another RCT showed that vitamin E administered at a dose of 400 IU/d increased the risk of prostate cancer in relatively healthy men.[46] However, given the adequate evidence on vitamin E, the current guidelines recommend the use vitamin E at the dose of 800 IU/d in nondiabetic patients with biopsy-proven NASH. Because vitamin E improves the liver histology, this should be considered as the first-line pharmacotherapy in this patient population.

Betaine

Adipose tissue dysfunction, characterized by insulin resistance and/or dysregulated adipokine production, plays a central role not only in disease initiation but also in the progression to NASH and cirrhosis. Promising beneficial effects of betaine supplementation on NAFLD have been reported in both clinical investigations and experimental studies; however, data related to betaine therapy in NAFLD are still limited. Betaine is a natural component of many foods and is safe in dosages ranging from 3 to 30 g/d; therefore, unlike other insulin sensitizers with potential side effects, betaine may represent an ideal therapeutic agent for NAFLD. The potential therapeutic role of betaine needs to be further evaluated.[47]

Medical Therapies That Augment Weight Loss

Orlistat

Orlistat is a drug that inhibits enteric lipid absorption and has been promoted as a weight-loss aid. Orlistat blocks approximately 30% of dietary triglycerides. It has shown promising effects in treatment of NAFLD, by reducing 10% of body weight, and reduction in hemoglobin A_1C and AST/ALT levels, along with improved steatosis and fibrosis.[48] Orlistat, in addition to lifestyle modification, was evaluated as a potential therapy for NASH in a double-blind randomized placebo-controlled trial on 52 patients with NAFLD diagnosed by ultrasonography, of whom 40 were confirmed by liver biopsy. Subjects were randomized to receive either orlistat (120 mg 3 times daily for 6 months) or placebo. Orlistat improves serum ALT level and features of steatosis on ultrasonography in patients with NAFLD beyond its effect on weight reduction. Although ALT levels were significantly decreased in both groups, the orlistat group showed a larger reduction. There was also a reduction in fatty liver by ultrasonography in the orlistat group. However, this finding could not be confirmed by biopsy because of a lack of follow-up.[49,50] In another trial, calorie-restricted patients were asked to take vitamin E and then were randomly assigned to either a placebo group or a group that was administered orlistat. Patients taking orlistat did not benefit from significant weight loss or histologic improvement compared with the placebo group. Weight loss is the common pathway through which orlistat may exert a beneficial effect. Other weight loss medications are under investigation. These data, combined with diet and exercise studies, suggest that modest amounts of weight loss, on the order of 5% to 10%, lead to improvement in both biochemical and histopathologic abnormalities seen in NASH.[49] In conclusion, ingestion of orlistat does not add any further cardiometabolic or histologic changes compared with lifestyle modification alone. Based on these data, the evidence supporting the efficacy of orlistat in patients with NASH is lacking, hence this treatment is not recommended in patients with NASH.[51]

Cytoprotective Agents

Ursodeoxycholic acid

Cytoprotective agents are thought to work by preventing apoptosis and downregulating the inflammatory cascade that has been shown to occur in patients with NAFLD. Ursodeoxycholic acid (UDCA) is the most studied and initial pilot trials proved promising as a NASH-specific therapy. However, a well-conducted, multicenter, double-blind, placebo-controlled trial of UDCA for 2 years failed to show significant change in biochemical or histologic parameters in patients with NAFLD.[48,52] In this study, 166 patients with liver biopsy–proven NASH were randomized to receive between 13 and 15 mg/kg/d of UDCA or placebo for 2 years. End points included changes in liver test results and liver histology at 2 years of therapy. The treatment groups were comparable at entry with regard to age, gender, risk factors for NASH, serum liver biochemistries, and baseline liver histology. A total of 126 patients completed 2 years of therapy. UDCA was well tolerated and serum liver biochemistries were stable in both the UDCA and placebo groups. Changes in the degree of steatosis, necroinflammation, or fibrosis that occurred with therapy were not significantly different between the UDCA and placebo groups.[52] This agent currently is not recommended in treatment of NASH.

Pentoxifylline

TNF-α, which is implicated in NASH, is inhibited by pentoxifylline. As an anti-TNF agent that targets the inflammatory process directly, pentoxifylline has been investigated for the treatment of NASH in individual studies and in pilot trials for years.[53] In a systematic review of 6 studies on the treatment of pentoxifylline in patients with NAFLD (2 randomized, double-blind, placebo-controlled trials; 4 prospective cohort studies) extracted from 11,604 references, the pentoxifylline-treated patients showed significantly decreased AST (n = 37; P = .01) and ALT (n = 50; P = .03) levels, but no significant effect on interleukin-6 (n = 36; P = .33) and TNF-α (n = 68; P = .26) levels compared with placebo. Pentoxifylline reduces AST and ALT levels and may improve liver histologic scores in patients with NALFD/NASH, but does not seem to affect cytokine levels.[53]

Another small study showed that pentoxifylline reduces TNF-α and ALT levels in patients with histologically proven NASH.[54] A recent study showed that pentoxifylline improved histologic features of NASH and liver fibrosis in patients with NASH. Fifty-five adults with biopsy-confirmed NASH were randomized to receive pentoxifylline at a dose of 400 mg 3 times a day (n = 26) or placebo (n = 29) over 1 year. After 1 year, intention-to-treat analysis showed a decrease of greater than or equal to 2 points in the NAS in 38.5% of patients on pentoxifylline versus 13.8% of those on placebo (P = .036). Per protocol analysis, a decrease of greater than or equal to 2 points in the NAS from baseline was observed in 50% of the patients on pentoxifylline versus 15.4% of those on placebo (P = .01).[55]

Previous studies have also shown that pentoxifylline improved biochemical parameters, steatosis, and necroinflammation in patients with NASH. One such study with 48 patients (25 men/23 women, aged 55 ± 7.54 years) with histologically confirmed NASH were enrolled between 2001 and 2005. Thirteen nonhypertensive/nondyslipidemic patients received pentoxifylline 400 mg twice a day. Mean duration of treatment was 37.8 ± 5.4 weeks. Patients treated with pentoxifylline showed a reduction of mean ALT and GGT (Gamma-Glutamyl Transferase) levels and necroinflammatory score.[56]

Pentoxifylline treatment in combination with diet and exercise results in significantly greater reduction in AST levels in patients with NASH compared with controls. Patients with biopsy-proven NASH and persistently increased ALT levels greater than 1.5 times the upper limit of normal were randomized to 3 months of treatment with a step 1 American Heart Association diet and daily exercise with pentoxifylline or placebo. Three months of pentoxifylline treatment in combination with diet and exercise resulted in significantly greater reduction in AST levels in patients with NASH compared with controls.[57] Twelve months of pentoxifylline 400 mg 3 times daily given in 2 recent pilot trials improved serum aminotransferase levels as well as steatosis and lobular inflammation.[54,58]

Pentoxifylline is safe, well tolerated, and improves transaminase levels and histology in patients with NASH compared with baseline. However, in many studies, pentoxifylline failed to reduce transaminase levels compared with placebo and did not positively affect any of the metabolic markers postulated to contribute to NASH.[59] Novel evidence supports that the beneficial effects of pentoxifylline in patients with NASH are likely partly mediated through decreasing lipid oxidation, largely free radical–mediated lipid oxidation.[60] Larger RCTs are needed to validate the effects of pentoxifylline on NAFLD/NASH. Administration of pentoxifylline requires caution because it can be associated with adverse effects such as nausea and vomiting.[23]

Lipid Level–lowering Agents

Statins
The most studied of this family of lipid level–lowering medicines are the statins, which work through inhibition of 3-hydroxy-3-methylglutaryl-coenzyme A reductase. Initially statins were noted to cause increases in hepatic transaminase levels in patients when used to treat hyperlipidemia and were thought to be harmful to liver function; however, studies have shown statins to be safe when given to patients with NAFLD. Several studies have suggested that statins may improve liver biochemistries and histology in patients with NASH, 70% of whom have dyslipidemia. Controlling dyslipidemia with diet, exercise, and lipid level–lowering agents may help stabilize or reverse NAFLD.[61] These studies consisted of small numbers of patients and have not been rigorously designed.[48,62–64]

Until RCTs with histologic end points prove their efficacy, statins should not be used specifically to treat NASH. Given the lack of evidence to show that patients with NAFLD and NASH are at increased risk for serious drug-induced liver injury from statins, statins can be used to treat dyslipidemia in patients with NAFLD and NASH.

Ezetimibe
Zetia is another lipid level–lowering medication that may have hepatic benefits in the treatment of NASH. This medication selectively inhibits intestinal cholesterol absorption and in controlled studies with statins seems to lower serum low-density lipoprotein cholesterol levels by 24% as well as triglyceride levels by 16%. Prior studies showed improved insulin resistance and decreased lipid deposition and fibrosis in obese rats treated with ezetimibe. No clinical trials with this therapy have been published.[65,66]

Others

Probiotics and synbiotics
Probiotics, such as a multistrain cocktail composed of *Streptococcus thermophilus* and several species of *Lactobacillus* and bifidobacteria, have been used to prevent and treat inflammatory conditions of the gastrointestinal tract. Gut microorganisms

play a role in the development of insulin resistance, hepatic steatosis, necroinflammation, and fibrosis; therefore, the potential benefits of probiotics and synbiotics on NAFLD/NASH have been suggested.[23] Preliminary data show a protective effect of VSL3# on the major key pathogenetic events of liver damage, suggesting the potential clinical utility of probiotics in limiting oxidative and inflammatory liver damage in patients with NAFLD. In one of the pilot studies, 52 patients with NAFLD were supplemented twice daily for 28 weeks with either a synbiotic or a placebo capsule. Both groups were advised to follow an energy-balanced diet and physical activity recommendations. At the end of the study, the ALT concentration decreased in both groups; this reduction was significantly greater in the synbiotic group.[67,68] Although promising results have been obtained in most of the previous experimental and clinical studies, the effects of probiotics and synbiotics on NAFLD/NASH need to be confirmed in larger RCTs. Also, the most effective preparations and dosages need to be established.

Angiotensin receptor blockers
The renin-angiotensin-aldosterone system modulates insulin sensitivity and is associated with pathogenesis of NAFLD/NASH. Thus, the effects of angiotensin II type 1 blockers (eg, telmisartan, valsartan, and losartan) on NAFLD have been investigated.[23] In a clinical trial, losartan improved serum aminotransferase levels and liver histology (necroinflammation and fibrosis).[69] However, in an open-label trial, combination therapy with rosiglitazone and losartan conferred no greater benefit than rosiglitazone alone with respect to histopathology. Well-designed RCTs are needed to confirm the effects of angiotensin receptor blockers on NASH. In addition, the use of angiotensin receptor blockers for normotensive patients requires caution because of their hypotensive effects.

Rimonabant
Increasing evidence suggests that the endocannabinoid system is enhanced in the setting of overweight or obesity. Activation of cannabinoid (CB-1) receptors located both centrally and peripherally (to include organs involved in energy homeostasis, such as the liver, adipocytes, and possibly skeletal muscle and pancreas), lead to enhanced weight gain and altered energy metabolism. Inhibition of these receptors has been the subject of recent intense investigation.[48] The recent association of this medication with psychiatric issues, including depression, may limit its future use, and it is currently not available in the United States outside of clinical research trials. No studies have been conducted in NAFLD.

Glucagonlike protein-1–receptor agonist (incretin analogues)
Peptides that are derived from glucagonlike protein-1–receptor agonists such as exenatide also may prove to be potential therapeutic agents in the treatment of NASH. These agents have been studied in patients with type 2 diabetes mellitus and have been found to produce weight loss. They promote insulin secretion, suppress inappropriate glucagon secretion, slow gastric emptying, and induce satiety. There are only animal studies at this time. There are studies that have supported the glycemic benefits of exenatide (exendin-4) with further well-designed studies specific to NASH populations required.[4,48]

SUMMARY

Statins seem to be safe agents for the treatment of hyperlipidemia and have shown a decrease in aminotransferase values in patients with NAFLD; however, further conclusions cannot be drawn.[56,61] Based on recent clinical trials, weight loss medications like orlistat, UDCA, and antioxidant agents could potentially be used as adjunctive therapy, but consistent evidence suggesting their use as a primary treatment of NASH across multiple trials remains to be seen.[49,51]

Modest but sustained weight loss, regular exercise, and diet composition modification also seem to improve biochemical and histologic abnormalities. Other therapies directed at insulin resistance, oxidative stress, cytoprotection, and fibrosis also may offer benefit but further studies are required. At present, insulin sensitizers (TZDs) and vitamin E seem to be the most promising. However, they cause side effects such as weight gain and may increase all-cause mortality, respectively. A multifaceted approach of lifestyle modifications, weight loss, and pharmacotherapy can be used in combination, but no single treatment approach has proved universally applicable to the general population with NASH. Continuous clinical and preclinical studies on existing and potential drugs are needed to improve treatment of NAFLD/NASH, which is a burgeoning health care problem.

REFERENCES

1. Asrih M, Jornayvaz FR. Metabolic syndrome and nonalcoholic fatty liver disease: is insulin resistance the link? Mol Cell Endocrinol 2015. [Epub ahead of print].
2. Falck-Ytter Y, Younossi ZM, Marchesini G, et al. Clinical features and natural history of nonalcoholic steatosis syndromes. Semin Liver Dis 2001;21:17–26.
3. Clark JM, Brancati FL, Diehl AM. Nonalcoholic fatty liver disease. Gastroenterology 2002;122:1649–57.
4. Ibrahim MA, Kelleni M, Geddawy A. Nonalcoholic fatty liver disease: current and potential therapies. Life Sci 2013;92:114–8.
5. Musso G, Gambino R, Cassader M, et al. A meta-analysis of randomized trials for the treatment of nonalcoholic fatty liver disease. Hepatology 2010;52:79–104.
6. Sanyal AJ, Friedman SL, McCullough AJ, et al. Challenges and opportunities in drug and biomarker development for nonalcoholic steatohepatitis: findings and recommendations from an American Association for the Study of Liver Diseases (AASLD) - Food and Drug Administration (FDA) joint workshop. Hepatology 2015; 61(4):1392–405.
7. Duvnjak M, Tomasic V, Gomercic M, et al. Therapy of nonalcoholic fatty liver disease: current status. J Physiol Pharmacol 2009;60(Suppl 7):57–66.
8. Dowman JK, Armstrong MJ, Tomlinson JW, et al. Current therapeutic strategies in non-alcoholic fatty liver disease. Diabetes Obes Metab 2011;13:692–702.
9. Caldwell SH, Oelsner DH, Iezzoni JC, et al. Cryptogenic cirrhosis: clinical characterization and risk factors for underlying disease. Hepatology 1999;29:664–9.
10. Preiss D, Sattar N. Non-alcoholic fatty liver disease: an overview of prevalence, diagnosis, pathogenesis and treatment considerations. Clin Sci (Lond) 2008; 115:141–50.
11. Yancy WS Jr, Olsen MK, Guyton JR, et al. A low-carbohydrate, ketogenic diet versus a low-fat diet to treat obesity and hyperlipidemia: a randomized, controlled trial. Ann Intern Med 2004;140:769–77.
12. Tendler D, Lin S, Yancy WS Jr, et al. The effect of a low-carbohydrate, ketogenic diet on nonalcoholic fatty liver disease: a pilot study. Dig Dis Sci 2007;52: 589–93.
13. Dasarathy S, Dasarathy J, Khiyami A, et al. Double-blind randomized placebo-controlled clinical trial of omega 3 fatty acids for the treatment of diabetic patients with nonalcoholic steatohepatitis. J Clin Gastroenterol 2015;49:137–44.

14. Masterton GS, Plevris JN, Hayes PC. Review article: omega-3 fatty acids - a promising novel therapy for non-alcoholic fatty liver disease. Aliment Pharmacol Ther 2010;31:679–92.
15. Capanni M, Calella F, Biagini MR, et al. Prolonged n-3 polyunsaturated fatty acid supplementation ameliorates hepatic steatosis in patients with non-alcoholic fatty liver disease: a pilot study. Aliment Pharmacol Ther 2006;23:1143–51.
16. Schwenger KJ, Allard JP. Clinical approaches to non-alcoholic fatty liver disease. World J Gastroenterol 2014;20:1712–23.
17. Parker HM, Johnson NA, Burdon CA, et al. Omega-3 supplementation and non-alcoholic fatty liver disease: a systematic review and meta-analysis. J Hepatol 2012;56:944–51.
18. Sanyal AJ, Chalasani N, Kowdley KV, et al. Pioglitazone, vitamin E, or placebo for nonalcoholic steatohepatitis. N Engl J Med 2010;362:1675–85.
19. Pearlman M, Loomba R. State of the art: treatment of nonalcoholic steatohepatitis. Curr Opin Gastroenterol 2014;30:223–37.
20. Hajiaghamohammadi AA, Ziaee A, Oveisi S, et al. Effects of metformin, pioglitazone, and silymarin treatment on non-alcoholic fatty liver disease: a randomized controlled pilot study. Hepat Mon 2012;12:e6099.
21. Lomonaco R, Ortiz-Lopez C, Orsak B, et al. Effect of adipose tissue insulin resistance on metabolic parameters and liver histology in obese patients with nonalcoholic fatty liver disease. Hepatology 2012;55:1389–97.
22. Bell LN, Wang J, Muralidharan S, et al. Relationship between adipose tissue insulin resistance and liver histology in nonalcoholic steatohepatitis: a pioglitazone versus vitamin E versus placebo for the treatment of nondiabetic patients with nonalcoholic steatohepatitis trial follow-up study. Hepatology 2012;56:1311–8.
23. Takahashi Y, Sugimoto K, Inui H, et al. Current pharmacological therapies for nonalcoholic fatty liver disease/nonalcoholic steatohepatitis. World J Gastroenterol 2015;21:3777–85.
24. Gastaldelli A, Harrison SA, Belfort-Aguilar R, et al. Importance of changes in adipose tissue insulin resistance to histological response during thiazolidinedione treatment of patients with nonalcoholic steatohepatitis. Hepatology 2009;50:1087–93.
25. Promrat K, Lutchman G, Uwaifo GI, et al. A pilot study of pioglitazone treatment for nonalcoholic steatohepatitis. Hepatology 2004;39:188–96.
26. Nissen SE, Wolski K. Effect of rosiglitazone on the risk of myocardial infarction and death from cardiovascular causes. N Engl J Med 2007;356:2457–71.
27. Murphy CE, Rodgers PT. Effects of thiazolidinediones on bone loss and fracture. Ann Pharmacother 2007;41:2014–8.
28. Cusi K. Role of obesity and lipotoxicity in the development of nonalcoholic steatohepatitis: pathophysiology and clinical implications. Gastroenterology 2012; 142:711–25.e6.
29. Chalasani N, Younossi Z, Lavine JE, et al. The diagnosis and management of non-alcoholic fatty liver disease: practice guideline by the American Gastroenterological Association, American Association for the Study of Liver Diseases, and American College of Gastroenterology. Gastroenterology 2012;142:1592–609.
30. Loomba R, Lutchman G, Kleiner DE, et al. Clinical trial: pilot study of metformin for the treatment of non-alcoholic steatohepatitis. Aliment Pharmacol Ther 2009;29: 172–82.
31. Fabbrini E, Mohammed BS, Magkos F, et al. Alterations in adipose tissue and hepatic lipid kinetics in obese men and women with nonalcoholic fatty liver disease. Gastroenterology 2008;134:424–31.

32. Browning JD, Horton JD. Molecular mediators of hepatic steatosis and liver injury. J Clin Invest 2004;114:147–52.
33. Cusi K, Consoli A, DeFronzo RA. Metabolic effects of metformin on glucose and lactate metabolism in noninsulin-dependent diabetes mellitus. J Clin Endocrinol Metab 1996;81:4059–67.
34. Uygun A, Kadayifci A, Isik AT, et al. Metformin in the treatment of patients with non-alcoholic steatohepatitis. Aliment Pharmacol Ther 2004;19:537–44.
35. Bugianesi E, Gentilcore E, Manini R, et al. A randomized controlled trial of metformin versus vitamin E or prescriptive diet in nonalcoholic fatty liver disease. Am J Gastroenterol 2005;100:1082–90.
36. Choi SH, Ginsberg HN. Increased very low density lipoprotein (VLDL) secretion, hepatic steatosis, and insulin resistance. Trends Endocrinol Metab 2011;22: 353–63.
37. Caldwell SH, de Freitas LA, Park SH, et al. Intramitochondrial crystalline inclusions in nonalcoholic steatohepatitis. Hepatology 2009;49:1888–95.
38. Haukeland JW, Konopski Z, Eggesbo HB, et al. Metformin in patients with non-alcoholic fatty liver disease: a randomized, controlled trial. Scand J Gastroenterol 2009;44:853–60.
39. Holman RR, Paul SK, Bethel MA, et al. Long-term follow-up after tight control of blood pressure in type 2 diabetes. N Engl J Med 2008;359:1565–76.
40. Holman RR, Paul SK, Bethel MA, et al. 10-year follow-up of intensive glucose control in type 2 diabetes. N Engl J Med 2008;359:1577–89.
41. Sanyal AJ. ACP Journal Club: vitamin E, but not pioglitazone, improved nonalcoholic steatohepatitis in nondiabetic patients. Ann Intern Med 2010;153:JC3–12.
42. Lavine JE, Schwimmer JB, Van Natta ML, et al. Effect of vitamin E or metformin for treatment of nonalcoholic fatty liver disease in children and adolescents: the TONIC randomized controlled trial. JAMA 2011;305:1659–68.
43. Ji HF. Vitamin E therapy on aminotransferase levels in NAFLD/NASH patients. Nutrition 2015;31:899.
44. Miller ER 3rd, Pastor-Barriuso R, Dalal D, et al. Meta-analysis: high-dosage vitamin E supplementation may increase all-cause mortality. Ann Intern Med 2005;142:37–46.
45. Bjelakovic G, Nikolova D, Gluud LL, et al. Mortality in randomized trials of antioxidant supplements for primary and secondary prevention: systematic review and meta-analysis. JAMA 2007;297:842–57.
46. Klein EA, Thompson IM Jr, Tangen CM, et al. Vitamin E and the risk of prostate cancer: the Selenium and Vitamin E Cancer Prevention Trial (SELECT). JAMA 2011;306:1549–56.
47. Wang Z, Yao T, Pini M, et al. Betaine improved adipose tissue function in mice fed a high-fat diet: a mechanism for hepatoprotective effect of betaine in nonalcoholic fatty liver disease. Am J Physiol Gastrointest Liver Physiol 2010;298:G634–42.
48. Torres DM, Harrison SA. Diagnosis and therapy of nonalcoholic steatohepatitis. Gastroenterology 2008;134:1682–98.
49. Zelber-Sagi S, Kessler A, Brazowsky E, et al. A double-blind randomized placebo-controlled trial of orlistat for the treatment of nonalcoholic fatty liver disease. Clin Gastroenterol Hepatol 2006;4:639–44.
50. Younossi ZM, Reyes MJ, Mishra A, et al. Systematic review with meta-analysis: non-alcoholic steatohepatitis - a case for personalised treatment based on pathogenic targets. Aliment Pharmacol Ther 2014;39:3–14.
51. Harrison SA, Fecht W, Brunt EM, et al. Orlistat for overweight subjects with nonalcoholic steatohepatitis: a randomized, prospective trial. Hepatology 2009;49:80–6.

52. Lindor KD, Kowdley KV, Heathcote EJ, et al. Ursodeoxycholic acid for treatment of nonalcoholic steatohepatitis: results of a randomized trial. Hepatology 2004;39: 770–8.

53. Li W, Zheng L, Sheng C, et al. Systematic review on the treatment of pentoxifylline in patients with non-alcoholic fatty liver disease. Lipids Health Dis 2011;10:49.

54. Satapathy SK, Sakhuja P, Malhotra V, et al. Beneficial effects of pentoxifylline on hepatic steatosis, fibrosis and necroinflammation in patients with non-alcoholic steatohepatitis. J Gastroenterol Hepatol 2007;22:634–8.

55. Zein CO, Yerian LM, Gogate P, et al. Pentoxifylline improves nonalcoholic steato-hepatitis: a randomized placebo-controlled trial. Hepatology 2011;54:1610–9.

56. Georgescu EF, Georgescu M. Therapeutic options in non-alcoholic steatohepati-tis (NASH). Are all agents alike? Results of a preliminary study. J Gastrointest Liver Dis 2007;16:39–46.

57. Lee YM, Sutedja DS, Wai CT, et al. A randomized controlled pilot study of Pentox-ifylline in patients with non-alcoholic steatohepatitis (NASH). Hepatol Int 2008;2: 196–201.

58. Adams LA, Zein CO, Angulo P, et al. A pilot trial of pentoxifylline in nonalcoholic steatohepatitis. Am J Gastroenterol 2004;99:2365–8.

59. Van Wagner LB, Koppe SW, Brunt EM, et al. Pentoxifylline for the treatment of non-alcoholic steatohepatitis: a randomized controlled trial. Ann Hepatol 2011; 10:277–86.

60. Zein CO, Lopez R, Fu X, et al. Pentoxifylline decreases oxidized lipid products in nonalcoholic steatohepatitis: new evidence on the potential therapeutic mecha-nism. Hepatology 2012;56:1291–9.

61. Hyogo H, Tazuma S, Arihiro K, et al. Efficacy of atorvastatin for the treatment of nonalcoholic steatohepatitis with dyslipidemia. Metabolism 2008;57:1711–8.

62. Browning JD. Statins and hepatic steatosis: perspectives from the Dallas Heart Study. Hepatology 2006;44:466–71.

63. Ekstedt M, Franzen LE, Mathiesen UL, et al. Statins in non-alcoholic fatty liver dis-ease and chronically elevated liver enzymes: a histopathological follow-up study. J Hepatol 2007;47:135–41.

64. Gomez-Dominguez E, Gisbert JP, Moreno-Monteagudo JA, et al. A pilot study of atorvastatin treatment in dyslipemid, non-alcoholic fatty liver patients. Aliment Pharmacol Ther 2006;23:1643–7.

65. Mikhailidis DP, Sibbring GC, Ballantyne CM, et al. Meta-analysis of the cholesterol-lowering effect of ezetimibe added to ongoing statin therapy. Curr Med Res Opin 2007;23:2009–26.

66. Deushi M, Nomura M, Kawakami A, et al. Ezetimibe improves liver steatosis and insulin resistance in obese rat model of metabolic syndrome. FEBS Lett 2007; 581:5664–70.

67. Esposito E, Iacono A, Bianco G, et al. Probiotics reduce the inflammatory response induced by a high-fat diet in the liver of young rats. J Nutr 2009;139: 905–11.

68. Eslamparast T, Poustchi H, Zamani F, et al. Synbiotic supplementation in nonalco-holic fatty liver disease: a randomized, double-blind, placebo-controlled pilot study. Am J Clin Nutr 2014;99:535–42.

69. Yokohama S, Yoneda M, Haneda M, et al. Therapeutic efficacy of an angiotensin II receptor antagonist in patients with nonalcoholic steatohepatitis. Hepatology 2004;40:1222–5.

Emerging Therapies for Nonalcoholic Fatty Liver Disease

Bilal Hameed, MD*, Norah Terrault, MD, MPH

KEYWORDS

- Nonalcoholic fatty liver disease • FXR agonists • Insulin sensitizers • PPAR agonists
- Antifibrotic agents

KEY POINTS

- There is a large unmet need for new therapeutics for patients with nonalcoholic steatohepatitis (NASH). No treatment to date has shown efficacy in greater than 50% of patients.
- The ideal treatment of NASH should improve liver histology and cardiovascular outcomes and have good tolerability and an excellent safety profile.
- Because insulin resistance is central to the pathogenesis of NASH, many new NASH drugs have insulin sensitization as one of their primary modes of action; however, other drug classes are emerging.
- There has been an increased effort to develop antifibrotic agents to treat patients with NASH complicated by significant fibrosis to reduce progression to end-stage disease.

INTRODUCTION

Nonalcoholic fatty liver disease (NAFLD) is the most common liver disease in the developed world, with prevalence estimates varying from 25% to 40% across different countries.[1,2] In the United States, the estimated prevalence is about 20% to 30%.[3] At present there are no drug therapies that have been approved for the treatment of nonalcoholic steatohepatitis (NASH) by the US Food and Drug Administration. Among drugs studied to date, few have achieved an efficacy of greater than 50%, highlighting the great need for new therapeutics for patients with NASH.

Current clinical practice guidelines recommend that only patients with biopsy-confirmed NASH, those with any degree of fibrosis, or those with both should be considered for liver-directed therapy.[2] This group is at greatest risk of liver-related

Disclosure: The authors have nothing to disclose.
Division of Gastroenterology, University of California San Francisco S357, 513 Parnassus Avenue, San Francisco, CA 94143-0538, USA
* Corresponding author. 350 Parnassus Avenue, Suite 300, San Francisco, CA 94143.
E-mail address: Bilal.Hameed@ucsf.edu

Clin Liver Dis 20 (2016) 365–385
http://dx.doi.org/10.1016/j.cld.2015.10.015
liver.theclinics.com

complications with progressive disease and likely to benefit most from effective therapy. An added complexity in treatment of NASH is the recognition that it represents a multifaceted condition with variable coexisting metabolic complications. The ideal therapy would effectively reverse the liver injury and fibrosis and improve, or at least have no negative impact on, other metabolic parameters or cardiovascular comorbidities. In addition, the ideal therapy should have good tolerability and an excellent safety profile with longer-term use, because many drugs may need to be used for years to obtain the desired clinical benefits.

Although changes on liver biopsy are used to define NASH and identify patients who are candidates for therapy, these histologic manifestations of disease represent the result of multiple different but interrelated pathogenetic pathways (**Fig. 1**), which are likely of variable importance in each individual. Looking to the future, it can be envisioned that therapy will be individualized, with specific metabolic and liver disease profiles treated with specific types of medications. Combinations of drugs working in complimentary or synergistic ways are likely to be the future of effective NASH therapy.

CHALLENGES IN DRUG DEVELOPMENT FOR NONALCOHOLIC STEATOHEPATITIS
Multiplicity of Pathways to Liver Injury

There are multiple different pathways described for the pathogenesis of NAFLD and each of them can be a potential target of the therapy (**Table 1**). It is also likely that more than 1 target is involved in the disease development and progression (**Fig. 2**). There is not a perfect animal model to study NAFLD. Many of the pharmacologic agents showing promise in animal models fail to show benefits in humans with NASH.[4] Clinical trials currently underway in patients with NASH are summarized in **Table 2**.

Defining Study End Points

The common primary outcomes used in NASH studies are either resolution of steatohepatitis with no worsening of fibrosis or a minimum of 2-point improvement in NASH activity score (NAS), with at least a 1-point improvement in more than 1 category and no worsening of fibrosis. Primary outcomes used in current randomized controlled trials in NASH are shown in **Table 3**.

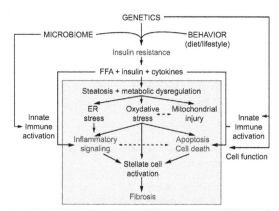

Fig. 1. Pathogenetic pathways for NASH highlighting potential targets for NASH. ER, endoplasmic reticulum; FFA, free fatty acid. (*From* Ratziu V, Goodman Z, Sanyal A. Current efforts and trends in the treatment of NASH. J Hepatol 2015;62(1 Suppl):S66; with permission.)

Table 1
New drugs for NASH by primary mechanism of action

Drug Class	Primary Proposed Mechanism of Action	Examples
FXR agonist	Carbohydrate, lipid metabolism, and regulation of insulin sensitivity	OCA
Insulin sensitizers	PPAR alpha/delta agonists SGLT2 Inhibitors GLP-1 receptor agonists Angiotensin-converting enzyme inhibitors and angiotensin-II receptor blockers	Elafibranor (GFT505) Remogliflozin etabonate Liraglutide (GLP-1 analogue) Telmisartan, losartan
Modulators of lipogenesis	n-3 PUFAs Fatty acid–bile acid conjugates LXR-α inhibitor	Ethyl-eicosapentanoic acid (EPA-E) Aramchol Oltipraz
Antioxidants	GSH repletion	Cysteamine
Antiinflammatory/ apoptotic	Caspase inhibitor Chemokine receptor type 2 and 5 antagonists	Emricasan and GS-9450 Cenicriviroc
Antifibrotic agents	Monoclonal antibody (IgG4) against LOXL2 Galectin-3 inhibitor	Simtuzumab GR-MD-02

Abbreviations: EPA-E, ethyl-eicosapentaenoic acid; FXR, farnesoid X receptor; GLP-1; glucagonlike peptide-1; GR-MD-02, galactoarabino-rhamnogalacturnate; GSH, glutathione; IgG4, immunoglobulin G4; LOXL2, lysyl oxidaselike-2; LXR-α, liver X receptor alpha; n-3 PUFAs, n-3 polyunsaturated fatty acids; OCA, obeticholic acid; PPAR, peroxisome proliferator–activated receptor; SGLT2, sodium glucose-dependent renal transporter 2.

NAS was developed by the NASH CRN to evaluate disease activity.[5] The NAS has not been validated as a marker for likelihood of progression to cirrhosis or mortality. It is unclear whether improvement of this score is a reflection of clinically significant end points, including liver-related mortality. Therefore, if NAS is used as a primary end point, a minimum of 2-point improvement with contribution from more than 1 parameter and no worsening of fibrosis should be used.[6]

Trials involving the cirrhotic population need to include different end points. Key end points of interest in this population include the development of portal hypertension (measurement of hepatic venous pressure gradient [HVPG], imaging or endoscopic findings); worsening Model for End-stage Liver Disease or Child-Pugh-Turcotte scores; and development of clinical complications of cirrhosis, such as variceal hemorrhage, ascites, encephalopathy, and hepatocellular carcinoma, as well as liver and all-cause mortality. If an agent with the promise of reversal of cirrhosis is studied, then the end point of fibrosis reduction is used, but ideally is accompanied by markers of reduced portal hypertension, such as improvement in the HVPG.[6]

The primary end point should be easy to measure, quantified consistently, and clinically meaningful. Current histologic end points are not ideal, because they are invasive and subject to measurement error. A noninvasive study end point that reflects liver-related and metabolic complications is highly desirable.[4]

Short-term Versus Long-term Efficacy

The optimum duration for therapy when evaluating new drug therapies for NASH is unclear. With a histologic end point, duration must be sufficient to allow changes to be

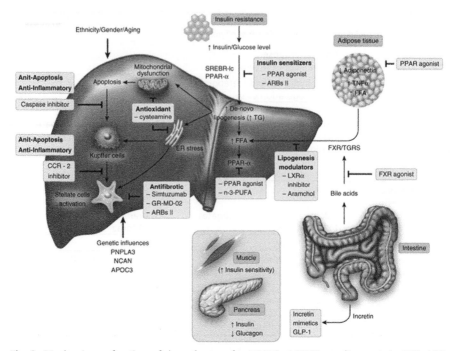

Fig. 2. Mechanisms of action of drug therapy for NAFLD. APOC3, apolipoprotein C-III; ARB, angiotensin-II receptor blockers; CCR-2, chemokine receptor 2; FXR, farnesoid X receptor; GLP, glucagonlike peptide-1; GR-MD-02, galactoarabino-rhamnogalacturnate; LXRα, liver X receptor alpha; n-3 PUFAs, n-3 polyunsaturated fatty acids; NCAN, NCAN locus G-protein couple receptor; PNPLA3, patatin-like phospholipase domain-containing protein 3; PPAR, peroxisome proliferator–activated receptors; SREBR, sterol regulatory element-binding protein; TG, triglyceride; TNF, tumor necrosis factor.

measurable. Reversal of fibrosis is not rapid, and studies of longer duration are more likely to show differences between treated and untreated groups. However, this is not particularly appealing to drug companies engaged in new therapeutics for NASH, because lengthy studies increase cost and slow down the overall rate of therapeutic advancement. Thus, in balancing the desire to advance the field and keep drug development costs down while simultaneously using end points that are surrogates for disease severity and risk of progression, most experts recommend trials be at least of 1 to 2 years in duration.

NEW DRUGS UNDER STUDY FOR TREATMENT OF NONALCOHOLIC STEATOHEPATITIS
Farnesoid X Receptor Agonists

Farnesoid X is the nuclear receptor for bile acids that play a critical role in carbohydrate, lipid metabolism and regulation of insulin sensitivity[7] (see **Table 1**). Preclinical studies have shown that farnesoid X receptor (FXR) activation improves insulin sensitivity and reduces levels of plasma glucose, free fatty acids (FFA), triglycerides, and total cholesterol.[8,9] FXR has been proposed as a target for the treatment of NASH because of these metabolic effects.[10] Obeticholic acid (OCA) in animal models of NAFLD been shown to decrease hepatic fat and fibrosis.[11,12]

OCA, 6-ethylchenodeoxycholic acid, a synthetic variant of the natural bile acid chenodeoxycholic acid (CDCA), is a first-in-class selective FXR agonist and the most

Table 2
Clinical trials currently underway in persons with NASH

Agent	Phase of Study	Population	Target N	Treatment Arms	Duration	ClinicalTrials Identifier
Aramchol	2b	NASH with prediabetes/diabetes	240	400 mg vs 600 mg vs placebo	1 y	NCT02279524
Cenicriviroc	2b	NASH without cirrhosis	252	150 mg vs placebo	2 y	NCT02217475
Cysteamine	2b	NASH, ages 8–17 y	160	Weight based. 600 mg/d for ≤ 65 kg, 750 mg/d for >65–80 kg, 900 mg/d for >80 kg vs placebo	52 wk	NCT01529268
Emricasan (IDN-6556)	2b	NAFLD on imaging with increased ALT level	38	25 mg BID vs placebo	28 d	NCT02077374
GFT505	2b	NASH, noncirrhotics	270	80 mg vs 120 mg vs placebo	52 wk	NCT01694849
GR-MD-02	2b	Portal hypertension (HVPG >6 mm Hg) with NASH cirrhosis and advanced fibrosis (Ishak stage 5–6)	156	2 mg/kg lean body mass vs 8 mg/kg lean body mass vs placebo, intravenous	52 wk	NCT02462967
Liraglutide	2b	Overweight ± diabetics. Noncirrhotics	50	1.8 mg qd vs placebo	48 wk	NCT01237119
Losartan	3	NASH with fibrosis (1–3 Kleiner stage)	240	50 mg vs placebo	2 y	NCT01051219
Oltipraz	3	NAFLD with increased ALT level, noncirrhotics	276	90 mg tid vs 120 tid vs placebo	24 wk	NCT02068339
Simtuzumab (GS-6624)	2b	NASH with advance fibrosis (Ishak score 3–4) without cirrhosis	225	75 mg vs 120 mg vs placebo, subcutaneous	96 wk	NCT01672866
Simtuzumab (GS-6624)	2b	NASH cirrhosis (Ishak stage 5–6)	225	200 mg vs 700 mg vs placebo, intravenous	96 wk	NCT01672879

Abbreviations: ALT, alanine aminotransferase; BID, twice a day; HVPG, hepatic venous pressure gradient; qd, every day; tid, 3 times a day.

Table 3
Primary outcomes used in current randomized controlled trials in NASH

Agent	Target Population	Primary Outcome
Simtuzumab (GS-6624)	NASH cirrhosis (Ishak stage 5–6)	Mean change from baseline in HVPG; Event-free survival
Simtuzumab (GS-6624)	NASH with advanced fibrosis (Ishak score, 3–4) without cirrhosis	Change from baseline in morphometric quantitative collagen on liver biopsy; Event-free survival
GR-MD-02	Portal hypertension (HVPG >6 mm Hg) with NASH cirrhosis and advanced fibrosis (Ishak stage 5–6)	Reduction in HVPG
Liraglutide	Overweight ± diabetics. Noncirrhotics	Resolution of definite NASH and no worsening of fibrosis
Oltipraz	NAFLD with increased ALT level, noncirrhotics	Change in quantity of liver fat (percentage change) assessed by MRS
Cenicriviroc	NASH without cirrhosis	2-point improvement in NAS with at least a 1-point improvement in more than 1 category with no worsening of fibrosis
Aramchol	NASH with prediabetes/diabetes	Change in the average liver fat concentration measured by NMRS (13C nuclear magnetic resonance spectroscopy)
Losartan	NASH with fibrosis (stage 1–3)	Change in Kleiner fibrosis score based on histologic fibrosis stage
GFT505	NASH, noncirrhotics	Resolution of definite NASH and no worsening of fibrosis
Cysteamine	NASH, age 8–17 y	2-point improvement in NAS with at least a 1-point improvement in more than 1 category with no worsening of fibrosis
Emricasan	NAFLD on imaging with increased ALT level	Changes in alanine aminotransferase from baseline

Abbreviation: MRS, magnetic resonance spectroscopy.

extensively studied.[12,13] OCA has an approximately 100-fold greater FXR agonistic activity than CDCA.[9] In a small, randomized, placebo-controlled clinical trial in patients with NAFLD and type II diabetes, the effect of OCA on insulin sensitivity was investigated. Patients received 25 mg of OCA, 50 mg of OCA, or placebo, once daily for 6 weeks. Insulin sensitivity significantly improved by 28% and 20% from baseline in the 25-mg and 50-mg OCA groups, respectively, compared with only a 5.5% improvement in the placebo group. A significant reduction in both alanine aminotransferase (ALT) and gamma-glutamyltranspeptidase levels were seen in the treatment groups.[13]

The FLINT study (Farnesoid X nuclear receptor ligand obeticholic acid for noncirrhotic, non-alcoholic steatohepatitis) conducted by the NASH Clinical Research Network (NASH CRN) was a placebo-controlled, randomized clinical trial of 283 patients with histologically proven NASH randomized to receive OCA 25 mg/d (n = 141) or placebo (n = 142) for 72 weeks.[14] The primary outcome was improvement in liver histology, defined as a decrease in NAS by at least 2 points without worsening of fibrosis from baseline to the end of treatment. The final 64 patients did not undergo a liver biopsy because a preplanned interim analysis showed a highly significant difference in the primary end point. At 72 weeks, 45% of patients in the OCA group had improvement in liver histology compared with 21% in the placebo group (*P* = .0002). Treatment with OCA improved all features of NAS (steatosis, hepatocellular ballooning, and lobular inflammation). Importantly, there was a reduction in fibrosis score (1 stage) in 35% of OCA-treated patients versus 19% in the placebo arm. However, complete resolution of NASH was not achieved in a substantial proportion of patients. Pruritus, a known side effect of OCA, developed in 23% in the OCA arm versus 6% in the placebo arm (*P*<.0001). A decrease in the high-density lipoprotein level and an increase in the total cholesterol and low-density lipoprotein levels were observed in patients in the OCA arm compared with placebo.[14] Additional metabolic changes were a decrease in body weight by 2.3 kg at week 72 in the OCA group. The changes in liver biochemistry and metabolic profile mostly returned to pretreatment levels after stopping OCA from week 72 to week 96. A phase 3 clinical trial is planned (the Evaluate the Impact on NASH with Fibrosis of Obeticholic Acid Treatment study [REGENERATE]), with approximately 2500 patients anticipated to be enrolled.

FXR, in addition to being expressed in the liver, is also expressed in other tissues including kidney, stomach, small intestine, and large intestine.[15] In the intestine, expression of FXR regulates production of the endocrine hormone FGF19 (fibroblast growth factor 19) in humans, which in conjunction with hepatic FXR is thought to control bile acid synthesis, transport, and metabolism.[16,17] Fexaramine, a gut-restricted FXR agonist, does not activate FXR target genes in the liver and solely works in the intestine.[18] In animal studies, fexaramine was shown to slow diet-induced weight gain, inflammation, and hepatic glucose production.[19] Gut-restricted FXR agonists like fexaramine potentially offer improved safety profiles by achieving higher systemic efficacy without systemic toxicity.

Insulin Sensitizers

Insulin resistance is a key factor in the pathogenesis of NAFLD because it favors high rates of FFA flux to the liver from increased adipose tissue lipolysis.[20] The current understanding is that the insulin resistance originates at the level of adipose tissue, eventually involving the skeletal muscle, the pancreas, and the liver.[21] Peripheral insulin resistance (ie, adipose tissue) is likely more relevant to the pathogenesis of NASH than hepatic insulin resistance.[22,23] Given the central role of insulin resistance in NAFLD, drugs that improve insulin sensitivity have been a primary focus for drug development in the treatment of NASH. There are 2 classes of insulin sensitizers that are approved for the treatment of diabetes and have been evaluated as therapies for NASH with variable results: metformin and thiazolidinediones (TZDs).[24–27] Metformin is biguanide, the insulin-sensitizing effect of which is related to its ability to activate the adenosine monophosphate–activated protein kinase (AMPK) pathway, resulting in inhibition of gluconeogenesis and lipogenesis.[28] TZDs are agonists for peroxisome proliferator–activated receptor (PPAR) gamma, improving both hepatic and peripheral insulin sensitivity.[29]

Peroxisome proliferator–activated receptor agonists

The PPARs are members of the nuclear receptor superfamily that function as fatty acid–activated transcription factors.[30] The PPAR nuclear receptor subfamily is composed of 3 members: PPARα, PPARγ, and PPARδ, with different tissue distributions. PPARα is highly expressed in liver and controls genes involved in lipid and lipoprotein metabolism. PPARα ligands like fibrates are used for treatment of hyperlipidemia.[31] PPARγ is abundant in adipose tissues and is a key transcriptional factor for adipogenesis. PPARγ ligands, including TZDs, are used for treatment of type 2 diabetes. PPARδ is widely expressed and plays a critical role in mitochondrial function, fatty acid oxidation, and insulin sensitivity in mice.[32,33] PPARδ activation also improves hepatic inflammation and reduces hepatic glucose production.[34,35]

The limitations of TZDs and other PPARγ agonists in the treatment of NASH are the associated weight gain seen in up to 60% to 70% patients[36] and the concerns regarding safety with longer-term use, including risk of congestive heart failure, osteoporosis, and possibly bladder cancer.[37–39] Elafibranor (GFT505) is a dual PPARα/PPARδ agonist, liver-targeted insulin sensitizer that seems to be a promising candidate for the treatment of NAFLD. In an earlier study, GFT505 improved fasting plasma glucose and insulin resistance (HOMA-IR [homeostasis model assessment-estimated insulin resistance]), in abdominally obese patients.[40] In a recent study of 22 patients with abdominal obesity and insulin resistance, with or without diabetes, GFT505 improved hepatic and peripheral insulin sensitivity and dyslipidemia. GFT505 significantly reduced liver enzyme concentrations (gamma-glutamyltranspeptidase: -30.4%, $P = .003$. ALT: -20.5%, $P = .004$). A highly significant reduction of alkaline phosphatase levels also was observed after GFT505 treatment (effect size, -19.3%; $P<.0001$).[41] The safety profile of GFT505 is reassuring, with no specific adverse events with treatment up to 8 weeks. In contrast with what is observed with PPARγ agonists, there was neither body weight gain nor fluid retention. GFT505 also has hepatoprotective effects in animal models, with reduction in steatosis, hepatic inflammation, and antifibrotic properties.[42] Based on these results, a randomized, double-blind, placebo-controlled, 1-year phase 2b study is currently ongoing to assess the efficacy and safety of GFT505 in patients with histologically proven NASH. The primary end point is the reversal of NASH without worsening of fibrosis, based on liver biopsy assessments.

Sodium glucose-dependent renal transporter 2 inhibitors
Remogliflozin etabonate is an inhibitor of sodium glucose-dependent renal transporter 2 (SGLT2), which improves insulin sensitivity in type 2 diabetics.[43] In preclinical studies, remogliflozin etabonate reduced fat accumulation in the liver and caused a marked reduction in the levels of circulating markers of oxidative stress.[44] Unlike other drugs of its class (SGLT2 inhibitors), remogliflozin etabonate has intrinsic antioxidant activity that may reverse the steatohepatitis and oxidative stress.

In a clinical study of 336 treatment-naive patients with type 2 diabetes and hemoglobin A1c levels between 7.0% and 9.5%, 12 weeks of remogliflozin etabonate improved insulin sensitivity by 6% to 33% and beta-cell function by 23% to 43%. Patients receiving remogliflozin etabonate also had significant weight loss (1.4–3.6 kg vs placebo).[45] Recent post-hoc analysis of changes in ALT levels in this study indicated that remogliflozin etabonate–treated subjects with increased baseline ALT levels showed statistically significant ($P<.049$) mean reductions of 32% to 42% at week 12 compared with placebo.[46] Given its ability to reverse insulin resistance and lower ALT levels, remogliflozin etabonate may be a potential treatment of patients with NASH.[47]

Incretin analogues, including glucagonlike peptide-1 (liraglutide)
Glucagonlike peptide-1 (GLP-1) is an incretin hormone secreted from intestinal L cells in response to nutrient ingestion. This hormone has multiple activities, including enhancing insulin secretion, inhibiting glucagon secretion, slowing gastric emptying, and controlling food intake. GLP-1 agonists that improve diabetic control and facilitate

weight loss have been suggested as therapies in NASH. GLP-1–based therapies are beneficial for body-weight control, improving insulin sensitivity and dyslipidemia, and preventing oxidative stress in patients with type 2 diabetes.[48–50]

GLP-1 has a short half-life because of rapid degradation by dipeptidyl-peptidase IV (DPPIV). GLP-1 receptor agonists (exenatide, liraglutide) are long acting because they are DPPIV resistant and allow once-daily dosing. Liraglutide was developed for type 2 diabetes mellitus, for optimization of blood glucose levels. In animal models, glucose-induced GLP-1 secretion was dramatically decreased in patients with NAFLD or NASH compared with the controls, suggesting a deficiency of GLP-1 signaling in patients with NAFLD.[51] Recently, GLP-1 receptors have been found in human hepatocytes and liver tissue, suggesting that GLP-1 may exert a direct effect on hepatocytes. The number of GLP-1 receptors has been found to be decreased in liver biopsy specimens of patients with NASH compared with normal patients.[52,53]

Liraglutide improves liver enzyme levels in patients with type 2 diabetes. A recent meta-analysis assessed the safety and efficacy of 26 weeks of liraglutide on liver parameters using data from 6 phase 3 trials comprising the Liraglutide Effect and Action in Diabetes (LEAD) program. Of 4442 patients analyzed, 2241 (50.8%) patients had abnormal ALT levels at baseline. Liraglutide dose dependently reduced ALT levels in these patients. In a substudy of LEAD-2 in which hepatic steatosis was measured by computed tomography scan, liraglutide showed a trend toward improving hepatic steatosis compared with placebo. These effects were mainly mediated by weight loss and better glucose control.[54]

Liraglutide also has significant effect on weight loss. In a recent 56-week, double-blind trial study involving 3731 patients without diabetes and with a body mass index (BMI) of 30 kg/m^2 or a BMI of greater than or equal to 27 kg/m^2 with either dyslipidemia or hypertension, the liraglutide group lost a mean of 8.4 $\pm$ 7.3 kg of body weight, versus 2.8 $\pm$ 6.5 kg in the placebo group ($P<.001$). A total of 63.2% of the patients in the liraglutide group compared with 27.1% in the placebo group lost at least 5% of their body weight ($P<.001$).[46]

The results of the Liraglutide Efficacy and Action in NASH (LEAN) trial were recently presented. This multicenter trial studied the efficacy and safety of liraglutide in overweight patients with biopsy-proven NASH. Fifty-two patients were randomized 1:1 to receive a 48-week treatment with daily subcutaneous injections of either 1.8 mg of liraglutide or placebo. The primary end point was resolution of definite NASH and no worsening in fibrosis. The primary end point was achieved in 9 of 23 (39%) in the liraglutide group compared with 2 of 22 (9%) in the placebo arm. Liraglutide had greater weight loss (−5.3 vs 0.6 kg; $P = .001$), reduction in BMI ($P = .003$), and reduced fasting glucose levels ($P = .005$) compared with placebo. No serious adverse events were reported. Based on these encouraging results, the investigators concluded that a phase 3 clinical trial in NASH was warranted.[55]

Angiotensin-converting enzyme inhibitors and angiotensin-II receptor blockers

The renin-angiotensin system may promote insulin resistance and modulate cytokine and adipokine production.[56] The beneficial effects of angiotensin-II receptor blockers on insulin resistance may be related to the selective stimulation of PPAR-γ.[57] The renin-angiotensin system can also cause activation of stellate cells.[58,59] Thus, there are several pathways by which angiotensin-receptor inhibitors may be beneficial for NAFLD treatment.

In a pilot study of 7 hypertensive patients with NASH treated with losartan 50 mg daily for 48 weeks, improvements in the levels of aspartame aminotransferase (AST), ALT, and biomarkers of hepatic fibrosis were observed, in addition to improvement in systolic blood pressure. On liver biopsy, improvements in necroinflammation, ballooning, and fibrosis were seen in some patients but there was no change in steatosis.[60]

The angiotensin-II receptor blocker, telmisartan, has unique qualities of a PPAR-γ modulator.[61] In a blinded pilot study, 54 patients with biopsy-proven NASH and mild-moderate hypertension were randomly assigned to either telmisartan (20 mg/d) or valsartan (80 mg/d). Both medications improved transaminase levels and insulin resistance but this improvement was more profound in the telmisartan group, which also showed a significant decrease of NASH activity score and fibrosis. Valsartan did not improve liver histology except steatosis.[62] This finding is likely related to the modulation of PPAR-γ by telmisartan. Indirect evidence for the beneficial effects of telmisartan in hepatic steatosis was shown in a study in rats on a high-fat, high-carbohydrate diet, comparing the effects of telmisartan and valsartan. Telmisartan, but not valsartan, promoted increases in caloric expenditure and protected against diet-induced weight gain. Telmisartan reduced the accumulation of visceral fat, decreased adipocyte size, and reduced hepatic triglyceride levels to a much greater extent than valsartan.[63]

In contrast, a recent 12-month, randomized, open-label study in 137 patients with NASH showed no additional benefit on liver histology with combination therapy with rosiglitazone and losartan (50 mg/d) compared with rosiglitazone alone.[64] Thus, data from human studies are limited and contradictory. At present, there is a large, ongoing, phase III, randomized clinical trial in the United Kingdom underway to determine whether 24 months of treatment with losartan are effective in improving liver fibrosis in patients with NASH. It is hoped that this will provide a better insight into the potential beneficial effects of this class of drugs in NASH.

Modulators of Lipogenesis

N-3 polyunsaturated fatty acids

N-3 polyunsaturated fatty acids (n-3 PUFAs) are PPARα ligands, and are suggested to play a role in improving NAFLD by reducing insulin resistance and lipogenesis. In animal models of NASH, supplementation with n-3 PUFAs improved hepatic steatosis and liver injury.[65] Ethyl-eicosapentaenoic acid (EPA-E) is a synthetic polyunsaturated fatty acid that reduces hypertriglyceridemia. Administration of purified EPA (2700 mg/d) in a 12-month pilot study of 23 patients with biopsy-proven NASH (NAS score >5) showed a 26% decrease in serum ALT levels (79 ± 36 U/L vs 50 ± 20 U/L; $P = .002$) with improvement in steatosis, lobular inflammation, ballooning, and fibrosis in the 7 patients who had a follow-up biopsy.[66] In a larger phase 2 trial, these benefits were not confirmed. A total of 243 patients with biopsy-proven NASH were randomly assigned to placebo (n = 75), low-dosage EPA-E (1800 mg/d; n = 82), or high-dosage EPA-E (2700 mg/d; n = 86) for 1 year.[67] The primary efficacy end point was NASH activity score less than or equal to 3, without worsening of fibrosis; or a decrease in NASH activity score by greater than or equal to 2 with contribution from greater than 1 parameter, without worsening of fibrosis. Similar proportions of patients in each group met the primary end point (40%, 37%, and 35.9% for placebo, low-dosage, and high-dosage EPA-E, respectively). EPA-E had no significant effects on steatosis, inflammation, ballooning, or fibrosis scores. There were no significant effects on levels of liver enzymes, insulin resistance, adiponectin, and cytokeratin 18 (CK-18).[67] Thus, the fate of future studies with n-3 PUFAs is uncertain.

Aramchol

Aramchol (3b-arachidyl-amido, 7a-12a-dihydroxy, 5b-cholan-24-oic acid) is a novel synthetic lipid molecule obtained by conjugating 2 natural components, cholic acid (bile acid) and arachidic acid (saturated fatty acid), through a stable amide bond. Aramchol significantly reduces hepatic fat content in animals with a high-fat diet model.[68] In a recent phase II randomized, double-blind, placebo-controlled clinical trial, aramchol was safe and effective in reducing liver fat content, as measured by magnetic resonance spectroscopy (MRS), in patients with NAFLD after 12 weeks of daily administration of 300 mg.[69] There is an ongoing phase IIb study using 3 treatments arms: aramchol 400 and 600 mg daily and placebo tablets (2:2:1) for 1 year. The primary outcome measure is the change in the average liver fat concentration measured by MRS and not histology.

Inhibitors of liver X receptor alpha

Oltipraz is a synthetic dithiolethione, with an antisteatotic effect by inhibiting the activity of liver X receptor alpha (LXR-α), therefore disrupting LXR-α–dependent lipogenesis in hepatocytes. Dithiolethiones, a novel class of AMPK activators, prevents insulin resistance through AMPK-dependent p70 ribosomal S6 kinase-1 (S6K1) inhibition.[70] It also exerts antioxidative activity and enhances glutathione (GSH) biosynthesis. Oltipraz has been shown to protect against hepatotoxicity caused by carbon tetrachloride or acetaminophen.[71]

In a phase II study evaluating the efficacy and safety of oltipraz in adults with NAFLD, persons with imaging diagnosis of NAFLD with liver fat content of greater than 20% and increased aminotransferase levels were randomly allocated to 3 groups given either placebo (n = 22), 30 mg (n = 22), or 60 mg (n = 24) for 24 weeks. The change of liver fat amount from baseline to 24 weeks was quantified using MRS. Absolute reductions in liver fat content tended to occur in a dose-dependent manner ($-3.21 \pm 11.09\%$ in a placebo group, $-7.65 \pm 6.98\%$ in a low dose group, and $-13.91 \pm 10.65\%$ in a high dose group). Percentage reduction in liver fat content was significantly greater in the high-dose group than in the placebo group, but NAS, insulin resistance, and levels of liver enzymes, lipids, and cytokines were not significantly different among the groups.[72] There is an ongoing phase 3 study to evaluate the efficacy of oltipraz on change in quantity of liver fat (percentage change) assessed by MRS from baseline to 24 weeks in patients with NASH.

Antioxidants

One of the key factors in NAFLD progression is increased oxidative stress, either caused by excessive production of reactive oxygen species (ROS) or decreased production of antioxidants.[73] GSH is the most abundant intracellular antioxidant and its depletion is implicated in the development of hepatocellular injury and fibrosis.[74,75] Restoring GSH levels can have a protective effect through the reduction of ROS. Drugs such as N-acetylcysteine and cysteamine are able to restore GSH and can be effective in the treatment of conditions in which GSH depletion occurs (such as acetaminophen toxicity).

Cysteamine

Cysteamine, a precursor to GSH, is currently available for the treatment of cystinosis. In an open-label pilot trial of cysteamine bitartrate for biopsy-proven pediatric NAFLD with increased ALT levels to evaluate the safety and potential efficacy of enteric-coated cysteamine, 11 of 13 children enrolled completed therapy. In these 11 children, the mean ALT levels decreased between baseline and 24 weeks from 120.2 and 55 IU/L respectively ($P = .002$), and the AST levels decreased from 60 and 36 IU/L respectively ($P = .007$) after 6 months of treatment.[76] These encouraging preliminary results led to a multicenter, phase

2b, double-blind, placebo-controlled study conducted by the NASH CRN in children with histologically confirmed NAFLD (NCT01529268). Enrollment is complete and results are awaited. The primary outcome is histologic improvement, defined as a decrease in NAS of 2 or more and no worsening of fibrosis after 52 weeks of treatment.

Inhibitors of Inflammation and/or Apoptosis

C-C chemokine receptor 2 inhibitor

Liver inflammation in NASH activates Kupffer cells and other proinflammatory macrophages that ultimately activate hepatic stellate cells causing liver fibrosis. The signaling pathways of CC chemokine receptors, CCR2 and CCR5, play a central role in this process. Experimental fibrosis and inflammation models have shown that disruption of chemokine pathways such as CCL2 (chemokine (C-C motif) ligand 2) or its receptor CCR2, CCR5, and others may prevent collagen deposition.[77] Patients with simple steatosis and patients with NASH had increased serum levels of interleukin (IL)-6, CCL2/MCP-1 (monocyte chemotactic protein 1), and CCL19 compared with healthy controls.[78] Drugs designed to inhibit CCR2 and CCR5 may be effective in the treatment of NASH. A small-molecule inhibitor of CCR2, CCX872, in a mice model showed improved insulin sensitivity as well as significantly decreased ALT levels.[79]

Cenicriviroc, a novel, dual inhibitor of CCR2 and CCR5, is an immunomodulator that is being evaluated for the treatment of NASH. Cenicriviroc is primarily metabolized by the liver. In a phase 1 study of safety in patients with mild and moderate hepatic impairment (Child-Pugh A or B), patients received cenicriviroc 150 mg orally once daily for 14 days. Cenicriviroc concentrations were not affected by mild hepatic impairment but were increased by moderate impairment. Cenicriviroc was safe and well tolerated.[80] A phase II study is currently evaluating cenicriviroc in noncirrhotic patients with NASH and liver fibrosis.

Caspase inhibitors

Hepatocyte apoptosis is one of the hallmarks of NASH, which leads to liver injury and fibrosis. There are multiple apoptotic pathways involved in the pathogenesis of NASH, and the final common step of apoptosis is executed by a family of cysteine proteases termed caspases.

Emricasan (IDN-6556) is a first-in-class, orally active, irreversible pancaspase protease inhibitor designed to reduce the activity of enzymes that mediate inflammation and cell death, or apoptosis. In animal models, hepatic fibrosis and liver injury were reduced by emricasan by inhibiting hepatocyte apoptosis.[81] In a multicenter, double-blind, placebo-controlled, dose-ranging study of emricasan with a 14-day dosing period,[82] a total of 105 patients were enrolled in the study; 79 received active drug; 80 patients had chronic hepatitis C and 25 had other liver diseases including nonalcoholic steatohepatitis (NASH). In the patients with HCV, all doses of emricasan significantly reduced ALT and AST levels (P = .0041 to $P<$.0001 for various dosing groups). Declines in aminotransferase activity were also seen in patients with NASH. Emricasan was well tolerated and there were no differences in adverse events between emricasan and placebo. In a study of 204 patients with chronic hepatitis C treated with placebo or emricasan (5, 25, or 50 mg) orally twice daily for up to 12 weeks, significant reductions in serum AST and ALT levels were observed in all treatment groups ($P<$.0001) and the drug was well tolerated over 12 weeks.[83]

The results of a phase II study of emricasan in patients with NAFLD and increased transaminase levels were recently presented. Subjects were randomized 1:1 to emricasan 25 mg twice daily or placebo (19 per group) for 28 days.[84] The median absolute reduction in ALT levels from baseline was greater for emricasan than for placebo at day 7 (36.65 vs 8.65 U/L) and at day 28 (25.80 vs 9.40 U/L). Mean relative change from baseline in activated serum caspases and cleaved CK18 (cCK18 a caspase-cleaved substrate) were 28% reduction versus 5% increase at day 28 for emricasan versus placebo respectively. Emricasan was safe and well tolerated. Emricasan is also currently being studied in patients with liver cirrhosis and portal hypertension.

GS-9450 is a caspase inhibitor with selective activity against caspases 1, 8, and 9. In a small, randomized, proof-of-concept study, 124 subjects with biopsy-proven NASH were randomized to once-daily placebo or 1, 5, 10, or 40 mg of GS-9450 for 4 weeks. Treatment with GS-9450 resulted in significant decline in ALT levels and smaller non–statistically significant reductions in levels of AST and CK-18 fragments.[85] GS-9450 was safe and well tolerated in this trial; however, in a 6-month study in subjects with hepatitis C, episodes of drug-induced liver injury attributable to GS-9450 occurred, and the trial was terminated early.[86] There are no further studies planned with GS-9450 in patients with NASH at this time, likely because of concerns of drug-associated hepatotoxicity.

Antifibrotic Agents

Recognizing that fibrosis is a dynamic and reversible process, there is a great enthusiasm for developing effective antifibrotic drugs for NASH (**Fig. 3**).[87] Patients with NASH who have advanced fibrosis or cirrhosis are in greatest need of treatment to prevent progression of fibrosis or ideally reverse it with the ultimate goal of preventing hepatic decompensation and liver-related outcomes. Regression of fibrosis and even cirrhosis has been documented in patients with various chronic liver diseases, including NASH. Paired biopsy studies of patients with NAFLD who have undergone bariatric surgery showed significant improvement in fibrosis 1 year after the surgery. Among the 82 patients who underwent paired biopsies, NASH disappeared in 85% of cases with improvement of fibrosis (1.2 ± 1.1 to 0.9 ± 1.1; $P<.001$).[88] Controlling the underlying cause for liver injury remains the most effective antifibrotic treatment. However, this is less frequently achieved in patients with NAFLD than in patients with hepatitis B virus or HCV, for example. Thus, agents for NASH that achieve a decrease in hepatocyte injury, inflammation, and apoptosis would be predicted to achieve antifibrotic effects.[89] The FXR agonist OCA in a recent clinical trial (FLINT) showed clear improvement in the NAFLD activity and in fibrosis stage.[14] However, more direct targeting of fibrosis may be an alternative management strategy.

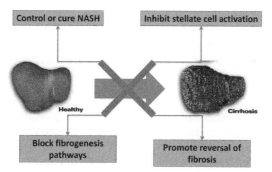

Fig. 3. Potential therapeutic approaches to stop worsening of fibrosis or promote its regression. (*Adapted from* Lee YA, Wallace MC, Friedman SL. Pathobiology of liver fibrosis: a translational success story. Gut 2015;64(5):830–41.)

The membrane and nuclear receptors expressed by stellate cells are potential targets of new antifibrotic therapies. Neurochemical receptors like cannabinoids, the renin-angiotensin system, and nuclear receptor stellate cells are some of the new and promising targets. Stellate cells express a diverse group of nuclear transcription factor receptors, including PPAR-γ and FXR. A combined PPAR-α/PPAR-δ agonist has shown promise in animal models and is currently in clinical trials.[42] In addition, agents that promote resolution of fibrosis by increasing matrix degradation or stimulating clearance of activated stellate cells are under development. A monoclonal antibody that inhibits the collagen cross-linking enzyme lysyl oxidase 2 has shown impressive results in animal models and is undergoing clinical trials.[90]

Simtuzumab

Lysyl oxidase–like-2 (LOXL2) is an extracellular matrix enzyme that causes cross-linkage of type 1 collagen and elastin, leading to remodeling of the extracellular matrix and promoting fibrosis.[91–93] Its serum level correlates with the stage of hepatic fibrosis.[94] An anti-LOXL2 murine monoclonal antibody (AB0023) inhibited fibrosis in mice and increased survival.[90] Simtuzumab is a humanized antifibrotic monoclonal antibody (immunoglobulin G4) against LOXL2. Simtuzumab was studied in a phase 1 study in patients with liver diseases of diverse cause.[95] Twenty patients, 18 to 65 years old, with Metavir fibrosis stage 1 to 3 were included in 2 cohorts treated with simtuzumab 10 mg/kg (cohort 1) or 3 mg/kg (cohort 2) infused every 2 weeks for a total of 3 infusions. Simtuzumab was well tolerated at doses up to 10 mg/kg.

Current multicenter clinical trials are examining the safety and efficacy of simtuzumab in patients with cirrhosis and advance fibrosis with NASH. In a phase 2b study currently underway, patients with NASH compensated cirrhosis are randomized to 2 doses of simtuzumab (75 mg vs 120 mg) intravenously versus placebo every 2 weeks for 96 weeks (double-blind phase) with an optional open-label phase (additional 240 weeks). The primary end point is mean change from baseline in HVPG at week 96 and event-free survival. In the other phase 2b study, simtuzumab is used in patients with NASH with advanced fibrosis (Ishak score, 3–4) without cirrhosis. Simtuzumab is administered subcutaneously weekly at doses of 200 mg versus 700 mg versus placebo. The study also has 2 phases: a randomized double-blind phase (96 weeks) and an optional open-label phase (240 weeks). The primary outcome is change from baseline in morphometric quantitative collagen on liver biopsy at week 96 and event-free survival.

Galactoarabino-rhamnogalacturnate

Galectin-3 protein (gal-3), a member of a family of proteins that have the property of binding to terminal galactose residues in glycoproteins,[96] has been implicated in the pathogenesis of liver fibrosis as well as in other organ fibrogenesis. Galactoarabino-rhamnogalacturnate (GR-MD-02), a complex carbohydrate drug that binds to and inhibits galectin proteins, with the greatest effect on gal-3, is associated with reduced fat accumulation, hepatocellular inflammation, and fibrosis in a mouse model of NASH. These effects are likely associated with a reduction in gal-3-expressing macrophages, reduction in inducible nitric oxide synthase expression, and reduction in activated stellate cells.[97]

GR-MD-02 was studied in a recent phase I study in patients with biopsy-proven NASH and stage 3 fibrosis. In the first cohort, 8 patients were randomized to receive 4 doses of either placebo (2 patients) or 2 mg/kg of GR-MD-02 (6 patients) by intravenous infusion on days 0, 28, 35, and 42. GR-MD-02 was safe and well tolerated following 4 doses of 2 mg/kg with no treatment-associated adverse events. In addition, patients on GR-MD-02 had significant reductions in the levels of inflammatory serum biomarkers compared with placebo, including IL-6 (-16% vs 6.5%; $P = .02$) and tumor necrosis factor alpha (-16% vs 20%; $P = .06$).[98]

A phase 2, multicenter, randomized, placebo-controlled, double-blind, 3-arm study of patients with compensated cirrhosis caused by NASH with portal hypertension (HVPG $\geq$6 mm Hg) is underway. GR-MD-02 is given in a dose of 2 mg/kg lean body mass, or in a dose of 8 mg/kg lean body mass administered via intravenous infusions every 2 weeks over a 52-week period and compared with placebo. The primary end point analysis is the reduction of portal pressure as a surrogate for a reduction in fibrosis.

SUMMARY

NAFLD is the most common liver disease in the Western world, with increasing prevalence worldwide. There is wealth of information accumulated in the past 10 years on the pathogenesis of NASH but, despite that, no approved therapy for NASH is available. OCA has shown promise in early studies in improving liver histology of NASH, including liver fibrosis, which was not seen with other treatments, including vitamin E or pioglitazone. Many other classes of drugs are in development and some promising phase 2 results have been seen. Future studies need to define primary outcomes, predictors of response, duration of studies, and whether combination therapy is more effective than monotherapy. In addition, longer-term studies are essential to establish safety and the effects of other metabolic comorbidities.

Overall, the future is looking bright for NASH therapeutics with several promising drug candidates but whether these will achieve the desired efficacy end points and be safe in these metabolically complex patients remains unknown. In the future, a more personalized treatment approach can be envisioned, based on a specific metabolic and liver disease profile. Combinations of drugs working in complimentary or synergistic ways are likely to be the future of effective NASH therapy.

REFERENCES

1. Williams CD, Stengel J, Asike MI, et al. Prevalence of nonalcoholic fatty liver disease and nonalcoholic steatohepatitis among a largely middle-aged population utilizing ultrasound and liver biopsy: a prospective study. Gastroenterology 2011;140(1):124–31.
2. Chalasani N, Younossi Z, Lavine JE, et al. American Gastroenterological Association; American Association for the Study of Liver Diseases; American College of Gastroenterology. The diagnosis and management of non-alcoholic fatty liver disease: practice guideline by the American Gastroenterological Association, American Association for the Study of Liver Diseases, and American College of Gastroenterology. Gastroenterology 2012;142(7):1592–609.
3. Vernon G, Baranova A, Younossi ZM. Systematic review: the epidemiology and natural history of non-alcoholic fatty liver disease and non-alcoholic steatohepatitis in adults. Aliment Pharmacol Ther 2011;34:274–85.
4. Ratziu V, Goodman Z, Sanyal A. Current efforts and trends in the treatment of NASH. J Hepatol 2015;62(1 Suppl):S65–75.
5. Kleiner DE, Brunt EM, Van Natta M, et al. Design and validation of a histological scoring system for nonalcoholic fatty liver disease. Hepatology 2005;41:1313–21.

6. Sanyal A, Brunt E, Kleiner D, et al. Endpoints and clinical trial design for nonalcoholic steatohepatitis. Hepatology 2011;54(1):344–53.
7. Lefebvre P, Cariou B, Lien F, et al. Role of bile acids and bile acid receptors in metabolic regulation. Physiol Rev 2009;89:147–91.
8. Zhang Y, Lee FY, Barrera G, et al. Activation of the nuclear receptor FXR improves hyperglycemia and hyperlipidemia in diabetic mice. Proc Natl Acad Sci U S A 2006;103:1006–11.
9. Cariou B, van Harmelen K, Duran-Sandoval D, et al. The farnesoid X receptor modulates adiposity and peripheral insulin sensitivity in mice. J Biol Chem 2006;281:11039–49.
10. Pellicciari R, Costantino G, Camaioni E, et al. Bile acid derivatives as ligands of the farnesoid X receptor. Synthesis, evaluation, and structure-activity relationship of a series of body and side chain modified analogues of chenodeoxycholic acid. J Med Chem 2004;47:4559–69.
11. Cipriani S, Mencarelli A, Palladino G, et al. FXR activation reverses insulin resistance and lipid abnormalities and protects against liver steatosis in Zucker (fa/fa) obese rats. J Lipid Res 2010;51:771–84.
12. Verbeke L, Farre R, Trebicka J, et al. Obeticholic acid, a farnesoid X receptor agonist, improves portal hypertension by two distinct pathways in cirrhotic rats. Hepatology 2014;59:2286–98.
13. Mudaliar S, Henry RR, Sanyal AJ, et al. Efficacy and safety of the farnesoid X receptor agonist obeticholic acid in patients with type 2 diabetes and nonalcoholic fatty liver disease. Gastroenterology 2013;145:574–82.
14. Neuschwander-Tetri BA, Loomba R, Sanyal AJ, et al, NASH Clinical Research Network. Farnesoid X nuclear receptor ligand obeticholic acid for non-cirrhotic, non-alcoholic steatohepatitis (FLINT): a multicentre, randomised, placebo-controlled trial. Lancet 2015;385:956–65.
15. Forman BM, Goode E, Chen J, et al. Identification of a nuclear receptor that is activated by farnesol metabolites. Cell 1995;81:687–93.
16. Kim I, Ahn SH, Inagaki T, et al. Differential regulation of bile acid homeostasis by the farnesoid X receptor in liver and intestine. J Lipid Res 2007;48:2664–72.
17. Song KH, Li T, Owsley E, et al. Bile acids activate fibroblast growth factor 19 signaling in human hepatocytes to inhibit cholesterol 7α-hydroxylase gene expression. Hepatology 2009;49:297–305.
18. Downes M, Verdecia MA, Roecker AJ, et al. A chemical, genetic, and structural analysis of the nuclear bile acid receptor FXR. Mol Cell 2003;11:1079–92.
19. Fang S, Suh JM, Reilly SM, et al. Intestinal FXR agonism promotes adipose tissue browning and reduces obesity and insulin resistance. Nat Med 2015;21:159–65.
20. Fabbrini E, Mohammed BS, Magkos F, et al. Alterations in adipose tissue and hepatic lipid kinetics in obese men and women with nonalcoholic fatty liver disease. Gastroenterology 2008;134(2):424–31.
21. Cusi K. Role of obesity and lipotoxicity in the development of nonalcoholic steatohepatitis: pathophysiology and clinical implications. Gastroenterology 2012; 142:711–25.
22. Lomonaco R, Ortiz-Lopez C, Orsak B, et al. Effect of adipose tissue insulin resistance on metabolic parameters and liver histology in obese patients with nonalcoholic fatty liver disease. Hepatology 2012;55:1389–97.
23. Gastaldelli A, Harrison SA, Belfort-Aguilar R, et al. Importance of changes in adipose tissue insulin resistance to histological response during thiazolidinedione treatment of patients with nonalcoholic steatohepatitis. Hepatology 2009;50: 1087–93.

24. Marchesini G, Brizi M, Bianchi G, et al. Metformin in non-alcoholic steatohepatitis. Lancet 2001;358:893–4.
25. Haukeland J, Konopski Z, Eggesbø H, et al. Metformin in patients with non-alcoholic fatty liver disease: a randomized, controlled trial. Scand J Gastroenterol 2009;44:853–60.
26. Belfort R, Harrison SA, Brown K, et al. A placebo-controlled trial of pioglitazone in subjects with nonalcoholic steatohepatitis. N Engl J Med 2006;355:2297–307.
27. Boettcher E, Csako G, Pucino F, et al. Metaanalysis: pioglitazone improves liver histology and fibrosis in patients with non-alcoholic steatohepatitis. Aliment Pharmacol Ther 2012;35:66–75.
28. Viollet B, Guigas B, Sanz Garcia N, et al. Cellular and molecular mechanisms of metformin: an overview. Clin Sci (Lond) 2012;122:253–70.
29. Juurinen L, Kotronen A, Granér M, et al. Rosiglitazone reduces liver fat and insulin requirements and improves hepatic insulin sensitivity and glycemic control in patients with type 2 diabetes requiring high insulin doses. J Clin Endocrinol Metab 2008;93:118–24.
30. Willson TM, Brown PJ, Sternbach DD, et al. The PPARs: from orphan receptors to drug discovery. Med Chem 2000;43:527–50.
31. Lefebvre P, Chinetti G, Fruchart JC, et al. Sorting out the roles of PPAR alpha in energy metabolism and vascular homeostasis. J Clin Invest 2006;116:571–80.
32. Tanaka T, Yamamoto J, Iwasaki S, et al. Activation of peroxisome proliferator-activated receptor delta induces fatty acid beta-oxidation in skeletal muscle and attenuates metabolic syndrome. Proc Natl Acad Sci U S A 2003;100:15924–9.
33. Lee CH, Olson P, Hevener A, et al. PPARdelta regulates glucose metabolism and insulin sensitivity. Proc Natl Acad Sci U S A 2006;103:3444–9.
34. Barish GD, Narkar VA, Evans RM. PPAR delta: a dagger in the heart of the metabolic syndrome. J Clin Invest 2006;116:590–7.
35. Bojic LA, Huff MW. Peroxisome proliferator-activated receptor delta: a multifaceted metabolic player. Curr Opin Lipidol 2013;24:171–7.
36. Musso G, Gambino R, Cassader M, et al. A meta-analysis of randomized trials for the treatment of nonalcoholic fatty liver disease. Hepatology 2010;52(1):79–104.
37. Cariou B, Charbonnel B, Staels B. Thiazolidinediones and PPARγ agonists: time for a reassessment. Trends Endocrinol Metab 2012;23:205–15.
38. Aubert RE, Herrera V, Chen W, et al. Rosiglitazone and pioglitazone increase fracture risk in women and men with type 2 diabetes. Diabetes Obes Metab 2010;12(8):716–21.
39. Lewis JD, Ferrara A, Peng T, et al. Risk of bladder cancer among diabetic patients treated with pioglitazone: interim report of a longitudinal cohort study. Diabetes Care 2011;34(4):916–22.
40. Cariou B, Zaïr Y, Staels B, et al. Effects of the new dual PPAR α/δ agonist GFT505 on lipid and glucose homeostasis in abdominally obese patients with combined dyslipidemia or impaired glucose metabolism. Diabetes Care 2011;34:2008–14.
41. Cariou B, Hanf R, Lambert-Porcheron S, et al. Dual peroxisome proliferator-activated receptor alpha/delta agonist GFT505 improves hepatic and peripheral insulin sensitivity in abdominally obese subjects. Diabetes Care 2013;36:2923–30.
42. Staels B, Rubenstrunk A, Noel B, et al. Hepatoprotective effects of the dual peroxisome proliferator-activated receptor alpha/delta agonist, GFT505, in rodent models of nonalcoholic fatty liver disease/nonalcoholic steatohepatitis. Hepatology 2013;58:1941–52.

43. Dobbins RL, O'Connor-Semmes R, Kapur A, et al. Remogliflozin etabonate, a selective inhibitor of the sodium-dependent transporter 2 reduces serum glucose in type 2 diabetes patients. Diabetes Obes Metab 2012;14:15–22.

44. Nakano S, Katsuno K, Isaji M, et al. Remogliflozin etabonate improves fatty liver disease in diet-induced obese male mice. J Clin Exp Hepatol 2015. http://dx.doi.org/10.1016/j.jceh.2015.02.005.

45. Sykes AP, O'Connor-Semmes R, Dobbins R, et al. Randomized trial showing efficacy and safety of twice-daily remogliflozin etabonate for the treatment of type 2 diabetes. Diabetes Obes Metab 2015;17(1):94–7.

46. Pi-Sunyer X, Astrup A, Fujioka K, et al. A randomized, controlled trial of 3.0 mg of liraglutide in weight management. N Engl J Med 2015;373(1):11–22.

47. Wilkison W, Cheatham B, Walker S. Remogliflozin etabonate reduces insulin resistance and liver function enzymes: role for treatment of NASH. J Hepatol 2015;62:S211–2.

48. Drucker DJ, Sherman SI, Gorelick FS, et al. Incretin-based therapies for the treatment of type 2 diabetes: evaluation of the risks and benefits. Diabetes Care 2010;33:428–33.

49. Kolterman OG, Buse JB, Fineman MS, et al. Synthetic exendin-4 (exenatide) significantly reduces postprandial and fasting plasma glucose in subjects with type 2 diabetes. J Clin Endocrinol Metab 2003;88:3082–9.

50. Ratner RE, Maggs D, Nielsen LL, et al. Long-term effects of exenatide therapy over 82 weeks on glycaemic control and weight in over-weight metformin-treated patients with type 2 diabetes mellitus. Diabetes Obes Metab 2006;8:419–28.

51. Bernsmeier C, Meyer-Gerspach AC, Blaser LS. Glucose-induced glucagon-like peptide 1 secretion is deficient in patients with non-alcoholic fatty liver disease. PLoS One 2014;9:e87488.

52. Gupta NA, Mells J, Dunham RM, et al. Glucagon-like peptide-1 receptor is present on human hepatocytes and has a direct role in decreasing hepatic steatosis in vitro by modulating elements of the insulin signaling pathway. Hepatology 2010;51:1584–92.

53. Svegliati-Baroni G, Saccomanno S, Rychlicki C, et al. Glucagon-like peptide-1 receptor activation stimulates hepatic lipid oxidation and restores hepatic signalling alteration induced by a high-fat diet in nonalcoholic steatohepatitis. Liver Int 2011;31:1285–97.

54. Armstrong MJ, Houlihan DD, Rowe IA, et al. Safety and efficacy of liraglutide in patients with type 2 diabetes and elevated liver enzymes: individual patient data metaanalysis of the LEAD program. Aliment Pharmacol Ther 2013;37:234–42.

55. Armstrong MJ, Gaunt P, Aithal GP, et al. Liraglutide is effective in the histological clearance of non-alcoholic steatohepatitis in a multicentre, double blinded, randomised, placebo-controlled phase II trial. J Hepatol 2015;62:S271 [LB-Abstract G01].

56. Georgescu EF. Angiotensin receptor blockers in the treatment of NASH/NAFLD: could they be a first-class option? Adv Ther 2008;25:1141–74.

57. Rong X, Li Y, Ebihara K, et al. Angiotensin II type 1 receptor-independent beneficial effects of telmisartan on dietary-induced obesity, insulin resistance and fatty liver in mice. Diabetologia 2010;53(8):1727–31.

58. Hirose A, Ono M, Saibara T, et al. Angiotensin II type 1 receptor blocker inhibits fibrosis in rat nonalcoholic steatohepatitis. Hepatology 2007;45:1375–81.

59. Yokohama S, Tokusashi Y, Nakamura K, et al. Inhibitory effect of angiotensin II receptor antagonist on hepatic stellate cell activation in non-alcoholic steatohepatitis. World J Gastroenterol 2006;12:322–6.

60. Yokohama S, Yoneda M, Haneda M, et al. Therapeutic efficacy of an angiotensin II receptor antagonist in patients with nonalcoholic steatohepatitis. Hepatology 2004;40:1222–5.
61. Kobayashi N, Ohno T, Yoshida K, et al. Cardioprotective mechanism of telmisartan via PPAR-gamma-eNOS pathway in Dahl salt-sensitive hypertensive rats. Am J Hypertens 2008;21:576–81.
62. Georgescu EF, Ionescu R, Niculescu M, et al. Angiotensin-receptor blockers as therapy for mild-to-moderate hypertension-associated non-alcoholic steatohepatitis. World J Gastroenterol 2009;15:942–54.
63. Sugimoto K, Qi NR, Kazdova L, et al. Telmisartan but not valsartan increases caloric expenditure and protects against weight gain and hepatic steatosis. Hypertension 2006;47:822–3.
64. Torres DM, Jones FJ, Shaw JC, et al. Rosiglitazone versus rosiglitazone and metformin versus rosiglitazone and losartan in the treatment of nonalcoholic steatohepatitis in humans: a 12-month randomized, prospective, open- label trial. Hepatology 2011;54:1631–9.
65. Svegliati-Baroni G, Candelaresi C, Saccomanno S, et al. A model of insulin resistance and nonalcoholic steatohepatitis in rats: role of peroxisome proliferator-activated receptor-alpha and n-3 polyunsaturated fatty acid treatment on liver injury. Am J Pathol 2006;169:846–60.
66. Tanaka N, Sano K, Horiuchi A, et al. Highly purified eicosapentaenoic acid treatment improves nonalcoholic steatohepatitis. J Clin Gastroenterol 2008;42:413–8.
67. Sanyal AJ, Abdelmalek MF, Suzuki A, et al, EPE-A Study Group. No significant effects of ethyl-eicosapentanoic acid on histologic features of nonalcoholic steatohepatitis in a phase 2 trial. Gastroenterology 2014;147(2):377–84.
68. Konikoff FM, Gilat T. Effects of fatty acid bile acid conjugates (FABACs) on biliary lithogenesis: potential consequences for non-surgical treatment of gallstones. Curr Drug Targets Immune Endocr Metabol Disord 2005;5:171–5.
69. Safadi R, Konikoff FM, Mahamid M, et al, FLORA Group. The fatty acid–bile acid conjugate aramchol reduces liver fat content in patients with nonalcoholic fatty liver disease. Clin Gastroenterol Hepatol 2014;12:2085–91.
70. Hwahng SH, Ki SH, Bae EJ, et al. Role of adenosine monophosphate-activated protein kinase-p70 ribosomal S6 kinase-1 pathway in repression of liver X receptor-alpha-dependent lipogenic gene induction and hepatic steatosis by a novel class of dithiolethiones. Hepatology 2009;49(6):1913–25.
71. Ansher SS, Dolan P, Bueding E. Chemoprotective effects of two dithiolthiones and of butylhydroxyanisole against carbon tetrachloride and acetaminophen toxicity. Hepatology 1983;3(6):932–5.
72. Kim W, Sung Lee J, Kyon Lee C, et al. Antisteatotic efficacy and safety of the liver X receptor alpha inhibitor, dithiolethione in patients with nonalcoholic fatty liver disease. Hepatology 2014;60(Suppl 1):224A–7A [abstract: 55].
73. Sanyal AJ, Campbell-Sargent C, Mirshahi F, et al. Nonalcoholic steatohepatitis: association of insulin resistance and mitochondrial abnormalities. Gastroenterology 2001;120:1183–92.
74. Wu G, Fang YZ, Yang S, et al. Glutathione metabolism and its implications for health. J Nutr 2004;134:489–92.
75. Liu RM, Gaston Pravia KA. Oxidative stress and glutathione in TGF-beta-mediated fibrogenesis. Free Radic Biol Med 2010;48:1–15.
76. Dohil R, Schmeltzer S, Cabrera BL, et al. Enteric-coated cysteamine for the treatment of paediatric non-alcoholic fatty liver disease. Aliment Pharmacol Ther 2011; 33:1036–44.

77. Zimmermann HW, Tacke F. Modification of Chemokine pathways and immune cell infiltration as a novel therapeutic approach in liver inflammation and fibrosis. Inflamm Allergy Drug Targets 2011;10(6):509–36.
78. Haukeland JW, Damås JK, Konopski Z, et al. Systemic inflammation in nonalcoholic fatty liver disease is characterized by elevated levels of CCL2. J Hepatol 2006;44(6):1167–74.
79. Parker R, Walters M, Ertl L, et al. Therapeutic use of a clinical stage CCR2 inhibitor, CCX872, in obesity-associated steatohepatitis. Lancet 2014;383:S78.
80. Lefebvre E, Smith P, Willett MS, et al. Pharmacokinetics and safety of multiple-dose cenicriviroc, a novel, oral, once-daily CCR2 and CCR5 antagonist, in adults with mild or moderate hepatic impairment. Hepatology 2013;58: 219A–22A.
81. Barreyro FJ, Holod S, Finocchietto PV, et al. The pan-caspase inhibitor Emricasan (IDN-6556) decreases liver injury and fibrosis in a murine model of non-alcoholic steatohepatitis. Liver Int 2015;35(3):953–66.
82. Pockros PJ, Schiff ER, Shiffman ML, et al. Oral IDN-6556, an antiapoptotic caspase inhibitor, may lower aminotransferase activity in patients with chronic hepatitis C. Hepatology 2007;46:324–9.
83. Shiffman ML, Pockros P, McHutchison J, et al. Clinical trial: the efficacy and safety of oral PF-03491390, a pancaspase inhibitor - a randomized placebo-controlled study in patients with chronic hepatitis C. Aliment Pharmacol Ther 2010;31: 969–78.
84. Shiffman M, Freillich B, Vuppalanchi R, et al. A placebo-controlled, multicenter, double-blind, randomized trial of emricasan (IDN-6556) in subjects with non-alcoholic fatty liver disease (NAFLD) and raised transaminases. J Hepatol 2015;62:S271 [abstract: LP37].
85. Ratziu V, Sheikh MY, Sanyal AJ, et al. A phase 2, randomized, double-blind, placebo-controlled study of GS-9450 in subjects with nonalcoholic steatohepatitis. Hepatology 2012;55(2):419–28.
86. Manns M, Lawitz E, Hoepelman AIM, et al. Short term safety, tolerability, pharmacokinetics and preliminary activity of GS-9450, a selective caspase inhibitor, in patients with chronic HCV infection. J Hepatol 2010;52(Suppl 1):S133.
87. Schuppan D, Kim YO. Evolving therapies for liver fibrosis. J Clin Invest 2013;123: 1887–901.
88. Lassailly G, Caiazzo R, Buob D, et al. Effects of bariatric surgery on severe liver injury in morbid obese patients with proven NASH: a prospective study. Hepatology 2014;60 [abstract: 213].
89. Lee YA, Wallace MC, Friedman SL. Pathobiology of liver fibrosis: a translational success story. Gut 2015;64(5):830–41.
90. Barry-Hamilton V, Spangler R, Marshall D, et al. Allosteric inhibition of lysyl oxidase-like-2 impedes the development of a pathologic microenvironment. Nat Med 2010;16:1009–17.
91. Mehal WZ, Iredale J, Friedman SL. Scraping fibrosis: expressway to the core of fibrosis. Nat Med 2011;17:552–3.
92. Kagan HM, Li W. Lysyl oxidase: properties, specificity, and biological roles inside and outside of the cell. J Cell Biochem 2003;88(4):660–72.
93. Vadasz Z, Kessler O, Akiri G, et al. Abnormal deposition of collagen around hepatocytes in Wilson's disease is associated with hepatocyte specific expression of lysyl oxidase and lysyl oxidase like protein-2. J Hepatol 2005;43(3): 499–507.

94. Murawaki Y, Kusakabe Y, Hirayama C. Serum lysyl oxidase activity in chronic liver disease in comparison with serum levels of prolyl hydroxylase and laminin. Hepatology 1991;14:1167–73.
95. Talal AH, Feron-Rigodon M, Madere J, et al. 1319 Simtuzumab, an antifibrotic monoclonal antibody against lysyl oxidase-like 2 (LOXL2) enzyme, appears safe and well tolerated in patients with liver disease of diverse etiology [abstract]. J Hepatol 2013;58(Suppl 1):S532.
96. Di Lella S, Sundblad V, Cerliani JP, et al. When galectins recognize glycans: from biochemistry to physiology and back again. Biochemistry 2011;50:7842–57.
97. Traber PG, Zomer E. Therapy of experimental NASH and fibrosis with galectin inhibitors. PLoS One 2013;8(12):e83481.
98. Harrison SA, Chalasani NP, Lawitz E, et al. Early phase 1 clinical trial results of GR-MD-02, a galectin-3 inhibitor, in patients having non-alcoholic steatohepatitis (NASH) with advanced fibrosis. Hepatology 2014;60(Suppl 1):224A–7A.

Extrahepatic Complications of Nonalcoholic Fatty Liver Disease

Kristina R. Chacko, MD, John Reinus, MD*

KEYWORDS

- Nonalcoholic fatty liver disease (NAFLD) • Extrahepatic complications
- Metabolic syndrome • Cardiovascular disease

KEY POINTS

- Non-alcoholic fatty liver disease is the hepatic manifestation of the metabolic syndrome.
- Individuals with NAFLD have increased mortality due to cardiovascular disease and malignancy and have lower rates of hepatic decompensation and liver-related death compared to other types of chronic liver disease.
- Visceral adiposity and hepatic fat result in a systemic inflammatory state which appears to predispose individuals with NAFLD to extra-hepatic disease.
- Strong associations between NAFLD and the development of cardiovascular disease, DM, CKD, CRC and endocrinopathies have been found independent of the metabolic syndrome.

Nonalcoholic fatty liver disease (NAFLD) is an important cause of liver injury, with a worldwide prevalence that varies in proportion to those of obesity and diabetes mellitus (DM). Originally thought of as the hepatic manifestation of the metabolic syndrome, which is a cluster of traits that includes disproportionately large waist circumference, high serum triglyceride and fasting glucose levels, low high-density lipoprotein (HDL) cholesterol levels, and hypertension,[1] there is now a growing awareness that NAFLD is associated with the development of cardiovascular disease, DM, chronic kidney disease (CKD), and malignancies. Compared with patients with cirrhosis from hepatitis C, those with cirrhosis secondary to NAFLD have lower rates of clinical decompensation and hepatocellular carcinoma, but similar overall mortality.[2] In more than 11,000 individuals with NAFLD included in the National Health and Nutrition Examination Survey (NHANES) followed for a median of 14.5 years,[3] the leading causes of mortality were cardiovascular disease (9.3%) and malignancy (5%), whereas complications of liver disease accounted for only 0.4% of deaths. The presence of advanced fibrosis

Disclosure: The authors have nothing to disclose.
Department of Medicine, Albert Einstein College of Medicine, 111 East 210th Street, Rosenthal 2C, Bronx, NY 10467, USA
* Corresponding author.
E-mail address: JREINUS@montefiore.org

Clin Liver Dis 20 (2016) 387–401
http://dx.doi.org/10.1016/j.cld.2015.10.004
1089-3261/16/$ – see front matter © 2016 Elsevier Inc. All rights reserved.

liver.theclinics.com

(diagnosed using noninvasive fibrosis scores) compared with only hepatic steatosis (diagnosed by ultrasonography) was associated with an increase in mortality. Mortalities during long-term follow-up (median 24 years) of patients with biopsy-proven NAFLD were 69% greater than those in the general population, with 30% of deaths caused by cardiovascular disease, 28% caused by extrahepatic malignancy, and 19% caused by complications of liver disease.[4] Patients with nonalcoholic steatohepatitis (NASH) have better survival than patients with viral hepatitis or alcoholic liver disease and are less likely to die of liver-related complications; however, their survival is poorer than that of individuals with simple hepatic steatosis, autoimmune hepatitis, or liver disease secondary to alpha1-antitrypsin deficiency.[4]

CARDIOVASCULAR DISEASE

There is a growing recognition of the strong association between NAFLD and cardiovascular disease. Numerous studies have been undertaken to identify individuals who may develop cardiovascular disease and to discover the mechanisms by which liver disease influences this process. Because cardiovascular disease is the most common cause of death in patients with NAFLD, the ability to identify and modify cardiovascular risk is important in the management of patients with NAFLD.

Several prospective trials have been conducted to study the connection between cardiovascular disease and NAFLD using a variety of diagnostic techniques, including ultrasonography, liver biopsy, and increased serum alanine aminotransferase (ALT) and serum gamma-glutamyltransferase (GGT) levels. Increased ALT levels are caused by hepatocyte injury or death, whereas an increased GGT level is thought to be an indicator of oxidative stress.[5] Use of ALT and GGT as markers of NAFLD has yielded mixed results. Haring and colleagues[6] found abnormal GGT levels to be associated with a greater than 2-fold increase in the risk of cardiovascular mortality, and superior to hepatic ultrasonography in predicting mortality risk. In a large study from South Korea, increased ALT levels (>40 U/L) were associated with a significant decrease in cardiovascular and diabetes-related survival, whereas no association of ALT level with cardiovascular disease or all-cause mortality was identified at 20-year follow-up of patients in the Framingham Offspring Study cohort.[7,8]

Ultrasonography is a sensitive and specific method for detecting liver fat; however, it is limited by its inability to differentiate between steatohepatitis and simple steatosis.[9] In a large prospective study, patients diagnosed with NAFLD based on ultrasonography had a significantly higher incidence of serious cardiovascular events during follow-up, independent of other known risk factors, including smoking, hypertension, low-density lipoprotein (LDL) cholesterol level, metabolic syndrome, age, and gender.[10] Retrospective review of NHANES data showed an increased risk of cardiovascular disease in patients with NAFLD diagnosed by ultrasonography independent of liver enzyme levels but without an increase in mortality.[11]

Liver biopsies can determine the degree of steatohepatitis and liver fibrosis, and allow clinicians to examine their effect on cardiovascular risk. In a longitudinal study assessing the mortality of patients with NAFLD compared with that in the general population and individuals with other types of liver disease, patients with NASH with or without advanced fibrosis on biopsy had a significantly increased mortality caused by cardiovascular disease.[4,12]

EVALUATION OF SUBCLINICAL CARDIOVASCULAR RISK

Various noninvasive tests have been used in patients with NAFLD to diagnose subclinical cardiovascular disease. These tests include measurements of carotid intima-media thickness, arterial stiffness, flow-mediated vasodilatation, coronary-artery calcification (CAC), and epicardial fat. Use of these and similar tests may allow clinicians to stratify the atherosclerotic risk in patients with NAFLD and prevent disease progression.

A systematic review of 7 studies that included 1427 patients with NAFLD and 2070 age-matched and sex-matched controls showed a significant association between NAFLD and increased carotid intima-media thickness, a marker of carotid atherosclerosis, as well as the presence of carotid plaques.[13] Increased serum ALT and GGT levels strongly correlated with the degree of carotid intima-media thickness, suggesting a relationship between the severity of liver disease and the risk of atherosclerotic disease. Another study found no significant increase in carotid intima-media thickness in patients with ultrasonography-diagnosed NAFLD, after correcting for the presence of the metabolic syndrome.[14] Based on the results of these studies, there is a clear increase in carotid atherosclerosis in patients with NAFLD, although the degree of risk associated with abnormal serum liver enzyme levels, advanced fibrosis, and presence of the metabolic syndrome remains less certain.

In a study of young men aged 20 to 40 years with NAFLD, both NASH and hepatic steatosis were significantly associated with subclinical atherosclerosis using vascular assessments, including carotid intima-media thickness, flow-mediated vasodilatation (a marker of endothelial dysfunction), and arterial stiffness.[15] CAC is another surrogate marker of subclinical cardiovascular disease that has been linked to an increased risk of cardiac events.[16] The substantial increased prevalence of CAC in patients with NAFLD seems to equal that in patients with well-established cardiac risk factors, such as smoking and diabetes.[17] Patients with NAFLD but without independent cardiac risk factors had a higher incidence of CAC, although the strength of this association may be attenuated after adjusting for visceral adiposity.[18,19]

Visceral fat has been shown to be a key factor in the pathophysiology of the metabolic syndrome and the pathogenesis of NAFLD. In a cohort study of patients with and without NAFLD, increased hepatic fat, as defined by an advanced MRI-based biomarker, correlated with increased prevalence of the metabolic syndrome. This finding was independent of the presence of NASH, suggesting that increased hepatic fat may directly contribute to the development of the metabolic syndrome and its associated cardiovascular risk.[20] Epicardial fat has recently been evaluated as a potential cardiometabolic risk factor, and was noted to be associated with advanced hepatic fibrosis in patients with NAFLD.[21] Those subjects with NAFLD and stage 3 to 4 fibrosis had impaired cardiac morphology and function, even after correcting for other metabolic risk factors.

CLINICAL MANIFESTATIONS AND EFFECT ON CARDIOVASCULAR DISEASE

Longitudinal studies have found an increased risk of cardiac events in patients with NAFLD. In a large cohort study of individuals with type 2 DM, the presence of NAFLD was found to be an independent risk factor for cardiovascular disease after controlling for other known risk factors, such as dyslipidemia, smoking, body mass index (BMI), and metabolic syndrome.[22] NAFLD has been associated with an increased prevalence of coronary, cerebrovascular, and peripheral vascular diseases. A substantial number of retrospective and prospective studies have found NAFLD to be an independent risk factor for cardiovascular disease; the presence of advanced fibrosis or NASH may further increase the risk of cardiovascular mortality.[23]

Given its importance to long-term survival, evaluation and management of cardiovascular disease in patients with NAFLD is essential. Traditional cardiac risk calculators and current guidelines do not account for the effect of NAFLD on cardiovascular risk and for this reason may underestimate patient survival. Suggested screening includes annual assessments of blood pressure, waist circumference, fasting lipid profile, smoking history, and family history of cardiovascular disease.[23]

PATHOPHYSIOLOGY

The relationship between NAFLD and cardiovascular disease does not seem to be purely related to overlapping risk factors, but to an atherosclerotic effect of hepatic steatosis and steatohepatitis (**Fig. 1**). Putative mechanisms for accelerated atherosclerotic disease in patients with NAFLD include a systemic proinflammatory state and disordered lipid metabolism.

Insulin resistance, a key component of the metabolic syndrome, is closely linked to the development and progression of NAFLD.[24] Obesity, specifically visceral adiposity, results in increased hepatic free fatty acid accumulation as well as decreased free fatty acid oxidation and impaired glucose metabolism, contributing to hepatic insulin resistance.[25] Visceral obesity is associated with the production of proinflammatory cytokines (eg, tumor necrosis factor alpha [TNFα], interleukin-6) and adipokines by adipocytes and infiltrating macrophages, resulting in chronic systemic inflammation, as shown in **Fig. 2**.[26,27] Activation of 2 transcription-factor pathways, nuclear factor kappa-B (NF-κB) and JNK (jun-n-terminal kinase pathway), by proinflammatory cytokines and free fatty acids results in insulin resistance.[26] Intrahepatic inflammation may lead to hepatic production of proatherogenic molecules, such as C-reactive protein, procoagulant plasminogen-activator inhibitor-1 (PAI-1), and fibrinogen.[28] Increased levels of PAI-1 and soluble intercellular adhesion molecule (sICAM-1), known biomarkers of endothelial dysfunction and atherosclerosis, have been found in patients with NAFLD.[29] The increase in cardiovascular risk in patients with NASH compared with simple steatosis seems to support a proatherogenic role for these proinflammatory and procoagulant biomarkers.[5]

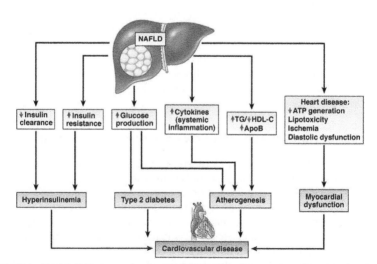

Fig. 1. NAFLD directly influences the development of cardiovascular risk through a variety of pathologic mechanisms. ApoB, apolipoprotein B; HDL-C, high density lipoprotein cholesterol; TG, triglyceride. (*From* Cusi K. Role of obesity and lipotoxicity in the development of nonalcoholic steatohepatitis: pathophysiology and clinical implications. Gastroenterology 2012;142(4):711–25; with permission.)

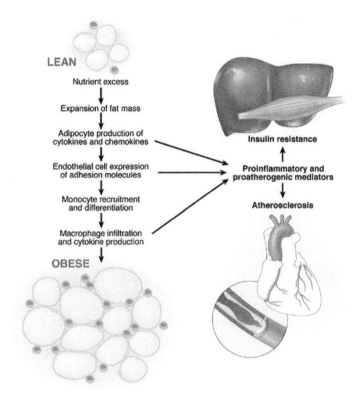

Fig. 2. Obesity and NAFLD are considered proinflammatory states. Through the production of a variety of adipokines and proinflammatory cytokines, individuals with NAFLD develop insulin resistance within skeletal and liver tissues. The production of certain proatherogenic cytokines results in an increase in atherosclerotic disease. (*From* Shoelson SE, Herrero L, Naaz A. Obesity, inflammation, and insulin resistance. Gastroenterology 2007;132:2169–80; with permission.)

DIABETES MELLITUS

The worldwide prevalence of type 2 DM has grown rapidly as a result of an increasing incidence of obesity. As components of the metabolic syndrome, DM and insulin resistance are strongly related to the prevalence of NAFLD and, furthermore, NAFLD has been shown to be an independent risk factor for development of DM. The cluster of insulin resistance, obesity, and fatty liver further increases this risk.[30] Overweight and obese individuals with NAFLD who underwent screening for diabetes with an oral glucose tolerance test were found to have significantly higher rates of prediabetes compared with an overweight and obese control group without NAFLD (75% vs 25%).[31]

Fatty liver and diabetes are significantly associated with the presence of hepatic insulin resistance, suggesting that increased hepatic fat plays a role in the development of DM. In a meta-analysis of 18 prospective studies that investigated the risk of DM in persons with abnormal serum ALT and GGT levels, or ultrasonography findings of steatosis, all three were found to be predictors of incident DM.[32] Limitations of many published studies include a lack of baseline data on the presence of insulin resistance and DM; however, NAFLD is estimated to carry a 2-fold to 5-fold increase in risk of DM.[23] A 4-year longitudinal study found that the combination of an abnormal serum ALT level and the appearance of steatosis on ultrasonography correlated with development of DM (hazard ratio, 1.64).[33] Given the significant risk of developing diabetes in patients with NAFLD, screening for DM with annual hemoglobin A1C or oral glucose challenge test is recommended.[23]

PATHOGENESIS

There is a mutual association of adipose tissue dysfunction, NAFLD, and the development of impaired glucose tolerance and type 2 DM. The association of NASH and advanced fibrosis with DM seems to be independent of obesity and is linked to the presence of insulin resistance.[24] Individuals with DM and NAFLD are significantly more likely to have severe fatty liver disease than persons with DM or NAFLD alone, something that may be caused by the inflammatory mediators TNFα and adiponectin.[34] Lipotoxicity results from the accumulation of toxic metabolites of triglycerides in muscle, liver, and pancreatic beta cells with activation of inflammatory pathways resulting in insulin resistance.[35,36] The excess of free fatty acids in NAFLD leads to skeletal muscle insulin resistance that is proportional to the degree of adipose tissue insulin resistance; in contrast, individuals with insulin-sensitive adipose tissue seem to not have the metabolic syndrome and hepatic steatosis.[36] As the result of adipose tissue dysfunction, metabolic abnormalities develop, including dyslipidemia, hepatic and muscle insulin resistance, hepatic steatosis, and NASH. In addition, increased plasma free fatty acid concentration induces pancreatic beta-cell dysfunction, affecting insulin secretion.[35]

CHRONIC KIDNEY DISEASE

CKD often affects persons with known metabolic risk factors, including hypertension and DM. New studies reveal that NAFLD is independently associated with an increased prevalence of CKD. CKD, defined either as a reduced estimated glomerular filtration rate (eGFR), or microalbuminuria or proteinuria, seems to occur at higher rates in patients with NAFLD (20%–55%) compared with those without NAFLD.[37] However, marked differences in the relationship between CKD and NAFLD have been found in retrospective, cross-sectional studies. An NHANES study of 11,469 US adults showed no increased risk of CKD in patients with ultrasonography-diagnosed NAFLD, after correcting for the presence of the metabolic syndrome.[38] In contrast, a large prospective cohort study of 8329 Korean men without DM, hypertension, or CKD at baseline followed for 4 years showed that those patients with NAFLD had a significantly higher risk of developing CKD, after correcting for the presence of the metabolic syndrome, obesity, incident DM, and hypertension.[39]

Although most studies have used imaging or liver enzyme levels to diagnose NAFLD, several biopsy studies found that the presence of NASH and the degree of fibrosis were associated with a higher prevalence of CKD.[40–42] A meta-analysis of 63,902 participants in 20 cross-sectional studies and 13 longitudinal studies revealed NAFLD to be an independent risk factor for CKD (odds ratio [OR], 2.12). NASH (OR, 2.53) and advanced fibrosis (OR, 5.20) further increased the risk.[43] Only 2 studies have included the clinical outcomes of end-stage renal disease and nephrotic syndrome in patients with NAFLD.[44,45] Screening for CKD with annual assessment of eGFR and microalbuminuria is recommended in patients with NAFLD, based on their propensity to develop CKD.[23]

PATHOGENESIS

Although the reasons why individuals with NAFLD develop CKD have not been fully elucidated, currently available data suggest that NAFLD is a mediator, rather than a marker, of CKD. The underlying lipotoxicity, oxidative stress, and chronic inflammation in NAFLD are considered important contributors to CKD pathogenesis through activation of inflammatory pathways, promotion of endothelial dysfunction, abnormal fetuin-A and adiponectin levels, and upregulated adhesion molecules.[46,47]

Adiponectin and fetuin-A, both mediators of insulin resistance, are key links between obesity and liver and kidney disease. Fetuin-A, a promoter of insulin resistance, is secreted by the liver and regulates adiponectin production by adipose tissue. Production of adiponectin, an adipokine acting as an insulin sensitizer that seems to orchestrate crosstalk between adipose tissue, the kidney, and the liver, is often reduced in NAFLD.[48] Low levels of adiponectin correlate with microalbuminuria and proteinuria.[49] The mechanism seems to be a decrease in 5′-AMP–activated protein kinase in podocytes, resulting in foot process effacement and albuminuria.[50]

EXTRAHEPATIC MALIGNANCY

Obesity is thought to increase the risk of mortality from all types of cancer.[51] Although advanced fibrosis and cirrhosis are clearly related to the development of hepatocellular carcinoma, patients with NAFLD seem to have higher rates of extrahepatic malignancy.[52] In particular, colorectal neoplasm has been found to have a strong association with NAFLD.

COLORECTAL CANCER

Colorectal cancer, the third most common cancer worldwide, has known modifiable risk factors, including obesity, physical inactivity, and a diet rich in animal fat and low in fiber.[53] Several large, retrospective studies have examined the risk of colorectal neoplasm in patients with NAFLD. Wong and colleagues[54] found that individuals with biopsy-proven NASH had a significantly higher prevalence of colorectal adenomas (51% vs 25.6%) and neoplasms (34.7% vs 14%) compared with those with hepatic steatosis, a finding that persisted after correcting for other identifiable risk factors, including age, gender, smoking, diabetes, obesity, and family history. Although a smaller US study of 94 patients with biopsy-proven NAFLD did not find an increased prevalence of colorectal adenomas compared with controls, several large retrospective studies from Asia and Austria found ultrasonography-diagnosed NAFLD to be an independent risk factor for colorectal adenomas and adenocarcinoma.[55–58] In a study of patients with the metabolic syndrome and colorectal neoplasm, the presence of obesity and hepatic steatosis were independently associated with colorectal cancer.[59]

Despite a growing body of evidence suggesting a significant increase in risk of colorectal neoplasm in patients with NAFLD, a lack of prospective, long-term studies prevents establishment of a causal relationship. Current colorectal screening guidelines do not recommend adjustments made for patients with NAFLD or NASH; however, given this clear association, adherence to these guidelines should be strongly recommended.[60]

ENDOCRINOPATHIES

NAFLD is seen in association with a variety of endocrinopathies, including polycystic ovarian syndrome (PCOS), hypothyroidism, growth hormone deficiency, hypogonadism, hypopituitarism, and hypercortisolemia.[61] The relationship between these hormonal abnormalities and NAFLD is incompletely understood, and although these disorders may exist in patients with NAFLD, their role in the pathogenesis of NAFLD has not yet been established.

Androgen deficiency and excess both play a role in the development of hypogonadism in men and PCOS in women. A retrospective study of Korean men found an inverse relationship between testosterone level and the presence of NAFLD that persisted after adjusting for visceral obesity and insulin resistance.[17] One study of 122 patients with hypogonadism showed improvement in metabolic parameters and aminotransferase levels after supplementation with testosterone.[62]

POLYCYSTIC OVARIAN SYNDROME

In contrast, PCOS is a reproductive disease characterized by androgen excess and is associated with obesity and insulin resistance. Several cohort studies have shown that women with PCOS have a higher prevalence of NAFLD diagnosed by biochemical or ultrasonography abnormalities.[63,64] A case-control study from Greece did not find a difference in ALT and GGT levels between patients with PCOS and controls until subgroup analysis revealed a significant difference in the obese group that was absent in the lean group.[65] Importantly, most studies suggest that the association between NAFLD and PCOS is mediated by insulin resistance rather than androgen excess.[61] In contrast, 1 small case-control study did find an increase in liver fat in patients with androgen excess after controlling for obesity and insulin resistance.[66] At this time, there is limited evidence to suggest a direct effect of androgen excess on the pathogenesis of NAFLD but, given their shared risk factors, there should be a lower threshold for evaluation of PCOS in women with infertility and irregular menstruation.[23,64]

HYPOTHYROIDISM

Thyroid dysfunction, previously linked to obesity and the metabolic syndrome, seems to also have close associations with the development of NAFLD.[67,68] Subclinical hypothyroidism, defined as an increased thyroid-stimulating hormone (TSH) level with normal free T4 (FT4) level, and clinical hypothyroidism, with increased TSH and low FT4 levels, may be an independent risk factor for the development of NAFLD and NASH. The prevalence of hypothyroidism in patients with NAFLD is reported to range from 15.2% to 36.3% according to a recently published systematic review, compared with an estimated national prevalence of 3.7%.[69,70] One large cross-sectional study revealed a significant link between NAFLD and subclinical and clinical hypothyroidism.[71] A prospective case-control study found patients with subclinical hypothyroidism had a higher incidence of ultrasonography-diagnosed NAFLD when followed for a median of 4.92 years; a significant difference even after correcting for metabolic factors such as central obesity, dyslipidemia, or hypertension.[71] Both studies found that the TSH level correlated in a dose-dependent manner with the risk of NAFLD. A retrospective, case-control study found that biopsy-proven NAFLD, with a significant increase in the NASH subset, was associated with a higher prevalence of hypothyroidism (21% vs 9.5%) compared with matched controls.[72] Screening of patients with NAFLD with annual TSH should be considered.

OSTEOPOROSIS

Osteoporosis occurs frequently in patients with chronic liver disease, with reported prevalence rates of up to 55%, linked to known risk factors such as cholestatic liver disease, alcohol abuse, poor nutrition, and hypogonadism.[73] Both male and female patients with NAFLD have been shown to have an increased risk of osteoporosis and osteoporotic fracture.[74,75] Current guidelines recommend screening patients for low bone mineral density if symptomatic or undergoing liver transplant evaluation.[76]

OBSTRUCTIVE SLEEP APNEA

Obstructive sleep apnea (OSA) is strongly associated with NAFLD and seems to be a significant risk factor for the presence of NASH and advanced fibrosis.[77] A meta-analysis of 18 cross-sectional studies of 2183 participants found an increased risk of ultrasonography-diagnosed NAFLD (OR, 2.99), biopsy-proven NASH (OR, 2.37), and advanced fibrosis (OR, 2.30) in individuals with OSA.[78] There is emerging evidence that OSA may play a role in the pathogenesis of NASH and the development of advanced fibrosis. The chronic intermittent hypoxia of OSA results in increased proinflammatory cytokine production, oxidative stress, and insulin resistance, and directly affects fibrogenesis through hypoxia-inducible factors, a family of transcription factors targeting hepatocytes, hepatic stellate cells, and Kupffer cells to modulate gene transcription.[79,80] A recent study linked OSA severity to the degree of hepatic fibrosis independent of obesity and the metabolic syndrome.[81] At present, there are no prospective data regarding incident OSA in patients with NAFLD or showing that appropriate management of OSA could affect the progression of fatty liver disease.

CHOLESTERYL ESTER STORAGE DISEASE

Cholesteryl ester storage disease (CESD), an autosomal recessive deficiency of lysosomal acid lipase (LAL), is an underdiagnosed cause of liver disease and dyslipidemia. LAL deficiency is caused by various mutations in the LIPA gene (lipase A, lysosomal acid, cholesterol esterase) and has a heterogeneous presentation, including a fulminant presentation in infancy (Wolman disease) and liver dysfunction with accelerated atherosclerosis in childhood and adulthood, referred to as CESD.[82] Characterized by dyslipidemia, cardiovascular disease, and hepatomegaly with steatosis, CESD shares many similarities with NAFLD.

LAL is responsible for hydrolysis of cholesteryl esters and triglycerides in lysosomes. An absence or deficiency of LAL results in accumulation of cholesteryl esters and triglycerides within lysosomes as well as upregulation of endogenous cholesterol production, synthesis of apolipoprotein B, and increased production of very-low-density lipoprotein.[83] Individuals with LAL deficiency develop dyslipidemia with increased serum LDL, low HDL, and increased total cholesterol levels. The most common clinical manifestations of CESD include hepatomegaly, increased aminotransferase levels (ALT, aspartate aminotransferase), and dyslipidemia. Over time, affected individuals may develop cirrhosis and significant cardiovascular disease. Given the clinical overlap between patients with CESD and those with NAFLD, diagnosis is challenging; screening for LAL deficiency should be considered in individuals with NAFLD in the absence of obesity or the metabolic syndrome.

Diagnosis may be made by histology and confirmed with measurement of LAL activity or genetic testing for LIPA mutations. Liver biopsy specimens from individuals with CESD may have a striking yellow-orange color; microscopically, the disorder is characterized by microvesicular steatosis. Foamy Kupffer cells stain with the periodic acid–Schiff and cathepsin D stains, which identify lysosomal lipid accumulation.[84] Management of patients with CESD has primarily focused on treatment of dyslipidemia with limited affect on disease progression. A novel therapeutic agent, sebelipase alfa, is a recombinant LAL that has been shown to rapidly reduce serum transaminase and cholesterol levels with an acceptable safety profile.[85,86] It is

Table 1	
Potential screening model for extrahepatic complications in patients with NAFLD	
Extrahepatic Disease	**Screening/Evaluation**
Type 2 DM	Hemoglobin A1C (annual)
CKD	Urinalysis with microalbumin, eGFR (annual)
CVD	Assess CV risk factors (annual) • Blood pressure • Lipid panel • Smoking history • Family history • Central obesity
CRC	Assess CRC risk factors • Family history • Smoking and diet history • BMI Adhere to current CRC screening guidelines
Endocrinopathies	TSH (annual) Evaluate for PCOS in symptomatic women of childbearing age DEXA scan in patients with cirrhosis or with pathologic fracture
OSA	Clinical awareness of symptoms • Epstein Sleep Scale • Refer for sleep study

Because of increased risk, all patients with NAFLD should be screened for diabetes, CKD, and CVD annually. Recognizing the increased prevalence of colorectal cancer, OSA, and certain endocrinopathies such as hypothyroidism, PCOS, and osteoporosis in this population should lead to earlier recognition of these conditions in patients showing clinical signs of disease.

Abbreviations: CRC, colorectal cancer; CV, cardiovascular; CVD, cardiovascular disease; DEXA, dual-energy x-ray absorptiometry; eGFR, estimated glomerular filtration rate.

Adapted from Armstrong M, Adams L, Canbay A, et al. Extrahepatic complications of nonalcoholic fatty liver disease. Hepatology 2014;59:1174–97.

currently in phase-3 clinical trials and undergoing review by the US Food and Drug Administration.

SUMMARY

As the hepatic manifestation of the metabolic syndrome, NAFLD has shown clear associations with cardiovascular disease, DM, and CKD. Further study has shown clearly that NAFLD, independent of known risk factors, is significantly associated with the pathogenesis and development of incident cardiovascular disease, DM, CKD, colorectal neoplasm, and endocrinopathies such as hypothyroidism and PCOS. Individuals with NAFLD have higher cardiovascular mortality and lower rates of liver-related complications compared with those with other types of chronic liver disease. By acknowledging these clinical implications, the evaluation and monitoring of extrahepatic complications becomes a vital part of the care of patients with NAFLD. **Table 1** outlines a screening model for long-term management of individuals with NAFLD. Modification of cardiac risk factors as well as screening for the development of incident extrahepatic complications optimizes the care of individuals with NAFLD.[87]

REFERENCES

1. Chalasani N, Younossi Z, Lavine JE, et al. The diagnosis and management of non-alcoholic fatty liver disease: practice guideline by the American Association

for the Study of Liver Diseases, American College of Gastroenterology, and the American Gastroenterological Association. Hepatology 2012;55(6):2005–23.

2. Bhala N, Angulo P, van der Poorten D, et al. The natural history of nonalcoholic fatty liver disease with advanced fibrosis or cirrhosis: an international collaborative study. Hepatology 2011;54(4):1208–16.

3. Kim D, Kim WR, Kim HJ, et al. Association between noninvasive fibrosis markers and mortality among adults with nonalcoholic fatty liver disease in the United States. Hepatology 2013;57:1357–65.

4. Soderberg C, Stål P, Askling J, et al. Decreased survival of subjects with elevated liver function tests during a 28-year follow-up. Hepatology 2010;51:595–602.

5. Targher G, Day C, Bonora E. Risk of cardiovascular disease in patients with nonalcoholic fatty liver disease. N Engl J Med 2010;363:1341–50.

6. Haring R, Wallaschofski H, Nauck M, et al. Ultrasonographic hepatic steatosis increases prediction of mortality risk from elevated serum gamma-glutamyl transpeptidase levels. Hepatology 2009;50:1403–11.

7. Yun KE, Shin CY, Yoon YS, et al. Elevated alanine aminotransferase levels predict mortality from cardiovascular. Atherosclerosis 2009;205:533–7.

8. Goessling W, Massaro JM, Vasan RS, et al. Aminotransferase levels and 20-year risk of metabolic syndrome. Gastroenterology 2008;135:1935–44.

9. Saadeh S, Younossi Z, Remer E, et al. The utility of radiological imaging in nonalcoholic fatty liver disease. Gastroenterology 2002;123(3):745–50.

10. Hamaguchi M, Kojima T, Takeda N, et al. Nonalcoholic fatty liver disease is a novel predictor of cardiovascular disease. World J Gastroenterol 2007;13: 1579–84.

11. Stepanova M, Younossi Z. Independent association between nonalcoholic fatty liver disease and cardiovascular disease in the US population. Clin Gastroenterol Hepatol 2012;10:646–50.

12. Ekstedt M, Franzén LE, Mathiesen UL. Long-term follow-up of patients with NAFLD and elevated liver enzymes. Hepatology 2006;44:865–73.

13. Sookoian S, Pirola CJ. Non-alcoholic fatty liver disease is strongly associated with carotid atherosclerosis: a systematic review. J Hepatol 2008;49:600–7.

14. Kim H, Kim D, Huh K. Association between nonalcoholic fatty liver disease and carotid intima-media thickness according to the presence of metabolic syndrome. Atherosclerosis 2009;204:521–5.

15. Ozturk K, Uygun A, Guler AK, et al. Nonalcoholic fatty liver disease is an independent risk factor for atherosclerosis in young adult men. Atherosclerosis 2015;240: 380–6.

16. Yeboah J, McClelland R, Polonsky T, et al. Comparison of novel risk markers for improvement in cardiovascular risk assessment in intermediate-risk individuals. JAMA 2012;308:788–95.

17. Kim D, Choi SY, Park EH, et al. Nonalcoholic fatty liver disease is associated with coronary artery calcification. Hepatology 2012;56:605–13.

18. VanWagner L, Ning H, Lewis C, et al. Associations between nonalcoholic fatty liver disease and subclinical atherosclerosis in middle-aged adults: the Coronary Artery Risk Development in Young Adults Study. Atherosclerosis 2014;235: 599–605.

19. Mellinger J, Pencina K, Massaro J, et al. Hepatic steatosis and cardiovascular disease outcomes: an analysis of the Framingham Heart Study. J Hepatol 2015;63(2):470–6.

20. Arulanandan A, Ang B, Bettencourt R, et al. Association between quantity of liver fat and cardiovascular risk in patients with nonalcoholic fatty liver disease

independent of nonalcoholic steatohepatitis. Clin Gastroenterol Hepatol 2015; 13(8):1513–20.e1.

21. Petta S, Argano C, Colomba D, et al. Epicardial fat, cardiac geometry and cardiac function in patients with non-alcoholic fatty liver disease: association with the severity of liver disease. J Hepatol 2015;62:928–33.

22. Targher G, Bertolini L, Padovani R, et al. Prevalence of nonalcoholic fatty liver disease and its association with cardiovascular disease among type 2 diabetic patients. Diabetes Care 2007;30:1212–8.

23. Armstrong M, Adams L, Canbay A, et al. Extrahepatic complications of nonalcoholic fatty liver disease. Hepatology 2014;59:1174–97.

24. Chitturi S, Abeygunasekera S, Farrell GC, et al. NASH and insulin resistance: insulin hypersecretion and specific association with the insulin resistance syndrome. Hepatology 2002;35:373–9.

25. Gastaldelli A, Cusi K, Pettiti M, et al. Relationship between hepatic/visceral fat and hepatic insulin resistance in nondiabetic and type 2 diabetic subjects. Gastroenterology 2007;133(2):496–506.

26. Shoelson SE, Herrero L, Naaz A. Obesity, inflammation, and insulin resistance. Gastroenterology 2007;132(6):2169–80.

27. Tilg H, Moschen AR. Insulin resistance, inflammation, and non-alcoholic fatty liver disease. Trends Endocrinol Metab 2008;19(10):371–9.

28. Yoo HJ, Choi KM. Hepatokines as a link between obesity and cardiovascular diseases. Diabetes Metab J 2015;39:10–5.

29. Sookoian S, Castaño GO, Burgueño AL, et al. Circulating levels and hepatic expression of molecular mediators of atherosclerosis in nonalcoholic fatty liver disease. Atherosclerosis 2010;209:585–91.

30. Sung KC, Jeong WS, Wild SH, et al. Combined influence of insulin resistance, overweight/obesity, and fatty liver as risk factors for type 2 diabetes. Diabetes Care 2012;35(4):717–22.

31. Ortiz-Lopez C, Lomonaco R, Orsak B, et al. Prevalence of prediabetes and diabetes and metabolic profile of patients with nonalcoholic fatty liver disease (NAFLD). Diabetes Care 2012;35(4):873–8.

32. Fraser A, Harris R, Sattar N, et al. Alanine aminotransferase, gamma-glutamyltransferase, and incident diabetes: the British Women's Heart and Health Study and meta-analysis. Diabetes Care 2009;32(4):741–50.

33. Choi JH, Rhee EJ, Bae JC, et al. Increased risk of type 2 diabetes in subjects with both elevated liver enzymes and ultrasonographically diagnosed nonalcoholic fatty liver disease: a 4-year longitudinal study. Arch Med Res 2013;44(2):115–20.

34. Lin X, Zhang Z, Chen JM, et al. Role of APN and TNF-α in type 2 diabetes mellitus complicated by nonalcoholic fatty liver disease. Genet Mol Res 2015;14(2):2940–6.

35. Cusi K. Role of obesity and lipotoxicity in the development of nonalcoholic steatohepatitis: pathophysiology and clinical implications. Gastroenterology 2012;142(4):711–25.e6.

36. Lomonaco R, Ortiz-Lopez C, Orsak B, et al. Effect of adipose tissue insulin resistance on metabolic parameters and liver histology in obese patients with nonalcoholic fatty liver disease. Hepatology 2012;55(5):1389–97.

37. Targher G, Chonchol MB, Byrne CD. CKD and nonalcoholic fatty liver disease. Am J Kidney Dis 2014;64(4):638–52.

38. Sirota JC, McFann K, Targher G, et al. Association between non-alcoholic liver disease and chronic kidney disease: an ultrasound analysis from NHANES 1988–1994. Am J Nephrol 2012;36(5):466–71.

39. Chang Y, Ryu S, Sung E, et al. Nonalcoholic fatty liver disease predicts chronic kidney disease in nonhypertensive and nondiabetic Korean men. Metabolism 2008;57(4):569–76.
40. Machado MV, Gonçalves S, Carepa F, et al. Impaired renal function in morbid obese patients. Liver Int 2012;32(2):241–8.
41. Yilmaz Y, Alahdab YO, Yonal O, et al. Microalbuminuria in nondiabetic patients with nonalcoholic fatty liver disease: association with liver fibrosis. Metab Clin Exp 2010;59(9):1327–30.
42. Targher G, Bertolini L, Rodella S, et al. Relationship between kidney function and liver histology in subjects with nonalcoholic steatohepatitis. Clin J Am Soc Nephrol 2010;5(12):2166–71.
43. Musso G, Gambino R, Tabibian JH, et al. Association of non-alcoholic fatty liver disease with chronic kidney disease: a systematic review and meta-analysis. PLoS Med 2014;11(7):1–26.
44. Targher G, Mantovani A, Pichiri I, et al. Nonalcoholic fatty liver disease is independently associated with an increased incidence of chronic kidney disease in patients with type 1 diabetes. Diabetes Care 2014;37(6):1729–36.
45. Targher G, Chonchol M, Bertolini L, et al. Increased risk of CKD among type 2 diabetics with nonalcoholic fatty liver disease. J Am Soc Nephrol 2008;19(8):1564–70.
46. Ix JH, Sharma K. Mechanisms linking obesity, chronic kidney disease, and fatty liver disease: the roles of fetuin-A, adiponectin, and AMPK. J Am Soc Nephrol 2010;21(3):406–12.
47. Moschen AR, Wieser V, Tilg H. Adiponectin: key player in the adipose tissue-liver crosstalk. Curr Med Chem 2012;19(32):5467–73.
48. Tsioufis C, Dimitriadis K, Chatzis D, et al. Relation of microalbuminuria to adiponectin and augmented C-reactive protein levels in men with essential hypertension. Am J Cardiol 2005;96(7):946–51.
49. Hui JM, Hodge A, Farrell GC, et al. Beyond insulin resistance in NASH: TNF-alpha or adiponectin? Hepatology 2004;40(1):46–54.
50. Sharma K, Ramachandrarao S, Qiu G, et al. Adiponectin regulates albuminuria and podocyte function in mice. J Clin Invest 2008;118(5):1645–56.
51. Taghizadeh N, Boezen HM, Schouten JP, et al. BMI and lifetime changes in BMI and cancer mortality risk. PLoS One 2015;10(4):e0125261.
52. Seko Y, Sumida Y, Tanaka S, et al. Predictors of malignancies and overall mortality in Japanese patients with biopsy-proven non-alcoholic fatty liver disease. Hepatol Res 2014;45(7):728–38.
53. Haggar FA. 2009.
54. Wong VW, Wong GL, Tsang SW, et al. High prevalence of colorectal neoplasm in patients with non-alcoholic steatohepatitis. Gut 2011;60(6):829–36.
55. Lin XF, Shi KQ, You J, et al. Increased risk of colorectal malignant neoplasm in patients with nonalcoholic fatty liver disease: a large study. Mol Biol Rep 2014; 41(5):2989–97.
56. Touzin NT, Bush KN, Williams CD, et al. Prevalence of colonic adenomas in patients with nonalcoholic fatty liver disease. Therap Adv Gastroenterol 2011;4(3): 169–76.
57. Huang KW, Leu HB, Wang YJ, et al. Patients with nonalcoholic fatty liver disease have higher risk of colorectal adenoma after negative baseline colonoscopy. Colorectal Dis 2013;15(7):830–5.
58. Lee YI, Lim YS, Park HS. Colorectal neoplasms in relation to non-alcoholic fatty liver disease in Korean women: a retrospective cohort study. J Gastroenterol Hepatol 2012;27(1):91–5.

59. Fiori E, Lamazza A, De Masi E, et al. Association of liver steatosis with colorectal cancer and adenoma in patients with metabolic syndrome. Anticancer Res 2015; 35(4):2211–4.

60. Lieberman DA, Rex DK, Winawer SJ, et al. United States Multi-Society Task Force on Colorectal Cancer. Guidelines for colonoscopy surveillance after screening and polypectomy: a consensus update by the US Multi-Society Task Force on Colorectal Cancer. Gastroenterology 2012;143(3):844–57.

61. Hazlehurst JM, Tomlinson JW. Non-alcoholic fatty liver disease in common endocrine disorders. Eur J Endocrinol 2013;169(2):R27–37.

62. Haider A, Gooren LJ, Padungtod P, et al. Improvement of the metabolic syndrome and of non-alcoholic liver steatosis upon treatment of hypogonadal elderly men with parenteral testosterone undecanoate. Exp Clin Endocrinol Diabetes 2010; 118(3):167–71.

63. Zueff LF, Martins WP, Vieira CS, et al. Ultrasonographic and laboratory markers of metabolic and cardiovascular disease risk in obese women with polycystic ovary syndrome. Ultrasound Obstet Gynecol 2012;39(3):341–7.

64. Vassilatou E. Nonalcoholic fatty liver disease and polycystic ovary syndrome. World J Gastroenterol 2014;20(26):8351–63.

65. Economou F, Xyrafis X, Livadas S, et al. In overweight/obese but not in normal-weight women, polycystic ovary syndrome is associated with elevated liver enzymes compared to controls. Hormones 2009;8(3):199–206.

66. Jones H, Sprung VS, Pugh CJ, et al. Polycystic ovary syndrome with hyperandrogenism is characterized by an increased risk of hepatic steatosis compared to nonhyperandrogenic PCOS phenotypes and healthy controls, independent of obesity and insulin resistance. J Clin Endocrinol Metab 2012;97(10):3709–16.

67. Erdogan M, Canataroglu A, Ganidagli S, et al. Metabolic syndrome prevalence in subclinic and overt hypothyroid patients and the relation among metabolic syndrome parameters. J Endocrinol Invest 2011;34(7):488–92.

68. Chung GE, Kim D, Kim W, et al. Non-alcoholic fatty liver disease across the spectrum of hypothyroidism. J Hepatol 2012;57(1):150–6.

69. Eshraghian A, Hamidian JA. Non-alcoholic fatty liver disease and thyroid dysfunction: a systematic review. World J Gastroenterol 2014;20(25):8102–9.

70. Aoki Y, Belin RM, Clickner R, et al. Serum TSH and total T4 in the United States population and their association with participant characteristics: National Health and Nutrition Examination Survey (NHANES 1999-2002). Thyroid 2007;17(12): 1211–23.

71. Xu L, Xu C, Yu C, et al. Association between serum growth hormone levels and nonalcoholic fatty liver disease: a cross-sectional study. PLoS One 2012;7(8).

72. Pagadala MR, Zein CO, Dasarathy S, et al. Prevalence of hypothyroidism in nonalcoholic fatty liver disease. Dig Dis Sci 2012;57(2):528–34.

73. Collier J. Bone disorders in chronic liver disease. Hepatology 2007;46(4): 1271–8.

74. Moon SS, Lee YS, Kim SW. Association of nonalcoholic fatty liver disease with low bone mass in postmenopausal women. Endocrine 2012;42(2):423–9.

75. Li M, Xu Y, Xu M, et al. Association between nonalcoholic fatty liver disease (NAFLD) and osteoporotic fracture in middle-aged and elderly Chinese. J Clin Endocrinol Metab 2012;97(6):2033–8.

76. Martin P, DiMartini A, Feng S, et al. Evaluation for liver transplantation in adults: 2013 practice guideline by the American Association for the Study of Liver Diseases and the American Society of Transplantation. Hepatology 2014;59(3): 1144–65.

77. Corey KE, Misdraji J, Gelrud L, et al. Obstructive Sleep Apnea Is Associated with Nonalcoholic Steatohepatitis and Advanced Liver Histology. Dig Dis Sci 2015; 60(8):2523–8.
78. Musso G, Cassader M, Olivetti C, et al. Association of obstructive sleep apnoea with the presence and severity of non-alcoholic fatty liver disease. A systematic review and meta-analysis. Obes Rev 2013;14(5):417–31.
79. Musso G, Olivetti C, Cassader M, et al. Obstructive sleep apnea-hypopnea syndrome and nonalcoholic fatty liver disease: emerging evidence and mechanisms. Semin Liver Dis 2012;32(1):49–64.
80. Paschetta E, Belci P, Alisi A, et al. OSAS-related inflammatory mechanisms of liver injury in nonalcoholic fatty liver disease. Mediators Inflamm 2015. [Epub ahead of print].
81. Agrawal S, Duseja A, Aggarwal A, et al. Obstructive sleep apnea is an important predictor of hepatic fibrosis in patients with nonalcoholic fatty liver disease in a tertiary care center. Hepatol Int 2015;9(2):283–91.
82. Reynolds T. Cholesteryl ester storage disease: a rare and possibly treatable cause of premature vascular disease and cirrhosis. J Clin Pathol 2013;66(11): 918–23.
83. Reiner Ž, Guardamagna O, Nair D, et al. Lysosomal acid lipase deficiency–an under-recognized cause of dyslipidaemia and liver dysfunction. Atherosclerosis 2014;235(1):21–30.
84. Bernstein DL, Hülkova H, Bialer MG, et al. Cholesteryl ester storage disease: review of the findings in 135 reported patients with an underdiagnosed disease. J Hepatol 2013;58(6):1230–43.
85. Valayannopoulos V, Malinova V, Honzík T, et al. Sebelipase alfa over 52 weeks reduces serum transaminases, liver volume and improves serum lipids in patients with lysosomal acid lipase deficiency. J Hepatol 2014;61(5):1135–42.
86. Balwani M, Breen C, Enns GM, et al. Clinical effect and safety profile of recombinant human lysosomal acid lipase in patients with cholesteryl ester storage disease. Hepatology 2013;58(3):950–7.
87. Armstrong M, Adams L, Canbay A, et al. Extrahepatic complications of nonalcoholic fatty liver disease. Hepatology 2014;59:1174–97.

Nonalcoholic Fatty Liver Disease and Liver Transplantation

Tuan Pham, MD[a], Travis B. Dick, PharmD, MBA, BCPS[b],
Michael R. Charlton, MD, FRCP[c],*

KEYWORDS

- Nonalcoholic fatty liver disease • Liver transplantation • The metabolic syndrome
- Nonalcoholic steatohepatitis

KEY POINTS

- Nonalcoholic fatty liver disease (NAFLD) is on a trajectory to become the most common indication for liver transplantation.
- Although features of NAFLD are common after liver transplantation for nonalcoholic steatohepatitis (NASH), recurrence of NASH with progressive fibrosis is unusual.
- Management of obesity and components of the metabolic syndrome are essential in achieving optimal posttransplant outcomes.
- Minimization of immunosuppression is a cornerstone of posttransplant management of patients undergoing liver transplantation for NAFLD.

INTRODUCTION

Nonalcoholic fatty liver disease (NAFLD) is a complication of obesity[1,2] and is widely considered to be the hepatic manifestation of the metabolic syndrome. It is a frequent cause of chronic liver disease in the United States with a changing prevalence mirroring the rising obesity trend.[3–5] NAFLD has a variable natural history, but in some patients can progress to nonalcoholic steatohepatitis (NASH) with progressive fibrosis and eventual complications of cirrhosis, including liver failure and hepatocellular carcinoma.[6–8] NASH is also thought to be the underlying etiology for cryptogenic cirrhosis in patients with features of the metabolic syndrome.[6] Compared with the general population, patients with NASH have an increased risk for cardiovascular-related death,

Disclosures: Drs T.B. Dick and T. Pham have nothing to disclose. Dr M.R. Charlton has received research support from Gilead Sciences, Merck, and Janssen.
a Division of Gastroenterology and Hepatology, University of Utah, 30 N 1900 E, Salt Lake City, UT 84132, USA; b Department of Pharmacy, Intermountain Medical Center, 5121 South Cottonwood Street, Murray, UT 84107-5701, USA; c Hepatology and Liver Transplantation, Intermountain Transplant Center, Intermountain Medical Center, 5121 South Cottonwood Street, Murray, UT 84107-5701, USA
* Corresponding author.
E-mail address: michael.charlton@imail.org

liver-related death,[9] overall mortality, and death in association with hepatocellular carcinoma.[10] The significant impact on mortality, magnified by the growing prevalence of the disease, has led to NASH being the third most common indication for liver transplantation, with a trajectory to become the most common (**Fig. 1**).[11]

Aside from its role in causing primary liver disease, concomitant NAFLD has been linked with a greater severity of liver disease in patients with chronic hepatitis C infection,[12] as well as treatment failure in patients with chronic hepatitis B infection.[13] Furthermore, the increasing prevalence of NAFLD in the population at large may lead to a reduced pool of suitable donor organs, because moderate to severe steatosis in the donor organ can significantly impact allograft viability.[14] Taken in sum, the ever-growing burden and far-reaching impact of NAFLD underscores the need for evolving new considerations in liver transplant management. This article reviews these considerations as well as our current understanding of the physiology and management of patients with NASH before and after liver transplantation.

NONALCOHOLIC FATTY LIVER DISEASE AND PRE LIVER TRANSPLANT CONSIDERATIONS

The median wait-list time has increased over recent years along with the number of candidates removed from the list for being too sick to undergo liver transplantation.[15] The increased frequency of medical comorbidities in patients with NAFLD make them especially susceptible to being delisted or dying while awaiting surgery.[16] Recognition of these comorbidities and their respective impact is essential for improving pretransplant survivorship, in addition to minimizing posttransplant complications.

Impact of Weight and Body Composition

An increased body mass index (BMI) in cirrhosis can lead to an increased rate of clinical decompensation and risk of dying or being delisted while awaiting

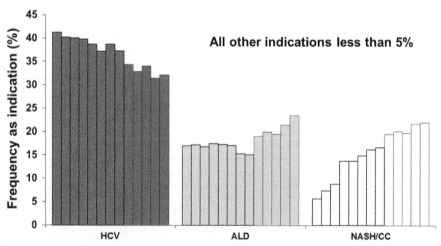

Fig. 1. Longitudinal trends in the frequency of indications for liver transplantation in the United States are shown for 2002 through 2014. Nonalcoholic steatohepatitis (NASH) and cryptogenic cirrhosis (CC) have been combined to account for the high frequency of NASH as a cause of cryptogenic cirrhosis. Alcoholic liver disease (ALD) has also had a surge as an indication for liver transplantation. HCV, hepatitis C virus. (*Data from* Scientific Registry of Transplant Recipients.)

liver transplantation.[16,17] Conversely, weight reduction can lead to an improvement in the histologic features of NASH.[18] In the posttransplant setting, Nair and colleagues[19] demonstrated through a large scale analysis of the United Network for Organ Sharing database that patients with class III obesity (BMI $\geq$40 kg/m^2) at the time of transplant have significantly higher rates of posttransplant primary graft nonfunction and mortality at 1 and 2 years. This same study also noted increased mortality at 5 years posttransplant in recipients with class II obesity (BMI >35 kg/m^2). These observations may have been confounded by the presence of ascites. After correcting for ascites, a large, prospective, multicenter study found BMI does not confer any independent risk of mortality or allograft failure.[20] Hakeem and colleagues[21] also confirmed a lack of correlation between BMI corrected for ascites and posttransplant graft and patient survival, although the authors did note a significant increase in postoperative complications and greater duration of hospital stay in overweight and obese patients compared with those with normal weight (BMI 18–25 kg/m^2). By extension, weight reduction should have important implications for pretransplant survivorship as well as reducing postoperative morbidity and mortality.

Overnutrition and obesity, the primary effectors of NAFLD, are also strongly associated with sarcopenia through shared mechanisms such as insulin resistance, physical inactivity, chronic inflammation, vitamin D deficiency, and oxidative stress.[22,23] Tandon and colleagues[24] found sarcopenia to be highly prevalent (41%) and predictive of mortality (hazard ratio, 2.36; 95% CI, 1.23–4.53) in patients awaiting liver transplantation. In situations of refractory ascites and hyponatremia where a conventional Model for End-stage Liver Disease (MELD) score underestimates death,[25] the addition of a sarcopenic index to MELD significantly improves pretransplant prognostication.[26] Furthermore, patients with sarcopenia have a higher risk of posttransplant infection, longer postoperative hospitalizations, and unclear risk for posttransplant death.[27–29] Several tools have been described for evaluating sarcopenia and malnutrition, including skeletal muscle mass on imaging, strength testing on functional assessments, and anthropomorphic measurements. Of these, abdominal imaging with computed tomography has been the most studied with regards to relevant clinical outcomes in the pretransplant and posttransplant populations, and is considered the gold standard despite concerns for operationalization beyond clinical research.[24,26,29,30] The reproducibility of measurements and high likelihood of use within a liver transplant program make abdominal computed tomography a good candidate tool for concomitant sarcopenia management. Other promising modalities include dual energy x-ray absorptiometry,[22] bioelectrical impedance analysis,[31] hand-grip strength,[32] and triceps skinfold thickness.[33] Regardless of the diagnostic test, recognition and reversing sarcopenia has been associated with a survival benefit.[34] Because sarcopenia has been linked to protein malnutrition and physical inactivity in patients with advanced liver disease, the mainstays of treatment to date have focused on caloric/amino acid supplementation and increased physical activity. A moderate exercise regimen, such as walking 5000 steps per day in combination with respective energy and protein intakes of 35 to 40 kcal/kg of body weight per day and 1.2 to 1.5 g/kg of body weight per day, can increase musculoskeletal mass in patients with compensated cirrhosis.[31] In those patients with compensated cirrhosis and concomitant obesity, exercise for weight loss in combination with total caloric restriction and branched chain amino acid supplementation has been advocated. Owing to the inherent exercise intolerance associated with decompensated liver disease, a primary nutritional strategy of branched chain amino acid and caloric supplementation may be the best option for treating sarcopenia.[35]

Chronic Kidney Disease

A recent metaanalysis by Musso and colleagues[36] demonstrated an increased prevalence (odds ratio [OR], 2.12; 95% CI, 1.69–2.66) and incidence (HR, 1.79; 95% CI, 1.65–1.95) of chronic kidney disease (CKD) in patients with NAFLD. Worsening NAFLD severity was associated with a higher prevalence and incidence of CKD, with the highest prevalence (OR, 5.20; 95% CI, 3.14–8.61) and incidence (HR, 3.29; 95% CI, 2.30–4.71) seen in cases of more advanced fibrosis. The effect of this seems to be an increase in NASH-related cirrhosis as an indication for simultaneous liver–kidney transplantation based on an analysis of the United Network for Organ Sharing database during the years 2002 to 2011.[37] This study also observed a lesser 5-year liver graft (HR, 2.50; 95% CI, 1.10–5.80), kidney graft (HR, 2.30; 95% CI, 1.10–5.10), and patient (HR, 2.20; 95% CI, 1.02–5.79) survival for NASH patients in comparison with transplantation for other causes of cirrhosis. This observation is supported by several studies demonstrating a direct impact on allograft and patient survival by the presence of renal insufficiency at the time of transplant[38,39] and by NASH itself.[40]

The relationship between CKD and posttransplant outcomes highlight the need for improved recognition. Direct measurement of the glomerular filtration rate (GFR) with exogenous markers of clearance such as inulin, iothalamate, or iohexol is considered the gold standard for assessing renal function. However, the cost and complexity of these techniques typically preclude their routine use at many transplant centers. Owing to ease of testing and availability, serum creatinine is widely used for estimating GFR. Current consensus recommendations for simultaneous liver–kidney transplant evaluation endorse the use of serum creatinine in the Modified Diet in Renal Disease equation to estimate renal function.[41] However, concern for conventional serum creatinine levels underestimating GFR in patients with cirrhosis and sarcopenia has driven efforts to evaluate other markers in this population. Cystatin C is a low-molecular-weight protein filtered by the kidneys that has been shown to improve estimated GFR over serum creatinine.[42] In 1 study by Mindikoglu and colleagues,[43] a new equation developed by the Chronic Kidney Epidemiology Collaboration (CKD-EPI) using both serum creatinine and cystatin C (CKD-EPI creatinine-cystatin C equation) was found to be more accurate for estimating GFR compared with conventional creatinine-based equations such as creatinine clearance, the Cockcroft-Gault equation, and the Modified Diet in Renal Disease equation. Cystatin C has also been demonstrated to outperform MELD regardless of the severity of ascites and in the presence of significant renal dysfunction (GFR <60 mL/min/1.73 m^2).[44] Future efforts should further validate the use of cystatin C–containing equations for better predicting pretransplant mortality, posttransplant renal disease, and need for simultaneous liver–kidney transplants.

Cardiovascular Disease

The shared association with the metabolic syndrome leads to a high concurrence of atherosclerotic disease in patients with NAFLD. In a NAFLD cohort of 129 patients, Ekstedt and colleagues[45] found a 15.5% rate of cardiovascular-related mortality during a mean follow-up of 13.7 years. Another cross-sectional study of 250 patients after at an outpatient diabetes clinic found a higher prevalence of overt coronary, cerebrovascular, and peripheral vascular disease in patients with NAFLD compared with those without (10.8% vs 1.1%; 37.3% vs 5.5%, 24.5% vs 2.5% respectively; P<.001).[46] NAFLD, independent of the metabolic syndrome, has been highly associated with subclinical atherosclerotic disease as well.[47]

Current recommendations from the American Association for the Study of Liver Diseases advocate noninvasive testing with dobutamine stress echocardiography in patients with traditional cardiac risk factors (chronic smokers, age >50 years, and a clinical or family history of heart disease or diabetes), followed by coronary angiography if preliminary screening is abnormal or inconclusive. However, noninvasive testing modalities such as dobutamine stress echocardiography and single photon emission computed tomography–technetium-99m–sestamibi imaging have poor sensitivity in detecting coronary artery disease in cirrhotic patients.[48,49] They are even less likely to detect subclinical atherosclerosis, although the presence of such may still carry implications for postoperative cardiovascular events.[50] Based on the poor sensitivity of noninvasive testing, Raval and colleagues[51] advocated for proceeding directly to coronary angiography in patients with known coronary artery disease, diabetes mellitus, or 2 or more other cardiovascular risk factors. However, although cardiac catheterization can be performed in patients with end-stage liver disease despite coagulopathy, there remains an increased risk for major bleeding complications and pseudoaneurysms. As such, current consensus recommendations from the American Heart Association and American College of Cardiology do not recommend routine angiography in the absence of symptoms; noninvasive testing can be considered in the presence of 3 or more relevant risk factors (diabetes mellitus, prior cardiovascular disease, left ventricular hypertrophy, age >60 years, tobacco use, hypertension, and dyslipidemia).[52] Given these constraints, serum biomarkers may have a role in supplementing a risk stratification scheme for predicting postoperative cardiovascular complications. Data from Cross et al[53] found that, among other cardiovascular risk factors (age, diabetes, history of cardiovascular disease), a serum troponin I level of greater than 0.07 was also predictive of post liver transplant cardiac events (HR, 2.00; $P = .023$). Although this lends credence to the usefulness of serum biomarkers in predicting relevant cardiovascular events, more evidence is needed before use of biomarkers can be routinely incorporated into decision-making schemes for tempering coronary artery evaluation or transplant eligibility.

NONALCOHOLIC FATTY LIVER DISEASE AND POST LIVER TRANSPLANT CONSIDERATIONS
Transplant Outcomes

Published center outcomes for NAFLD-related liver disease have varied widely. Heuer and colleagues[54] analyzed data from 432 consecutive patients transplanted between 2007 and 2011, of which 40 patients had underlying NASH. They found that 25% of their NASH patients died within the first month from cardiogenic shock and infectious complications, and had a 1-year survival rate of 42%. A large number of these patients (22%) had a BMI of greater than 35 kg/m² at the time of surgery. Barritt and colleagues[55] demonstrated that patients transplanted for NAFLD had an increased risk for death with adjusted hazard ratios of 8.96, 1.49, and 1.05, respectively, at 30 days, 1 year, and 3 years posttransplant. However, in a larger cohort followed for 10 years, Bhagat and colleagues[56] found no difference in survival ($P = .17$) or graft failure ($P = .40$) compared with those transplanted for alcoholic liver disease. Vanwagner and colleagues[57] also found no difference in patient, graft, or cardiovascular mortality between patients transplanted for NASH and alcohol related cirrhosis during a 12-month or longer follow-up, but the authors did note that NASH patients were more likely to have the metabolic syndrome at the time of transplantation and to experience a cardiovascular event within the first postoperative year (OR, 4.12; 95% CI, 1.91–8.90).

Results from large registry studies portray more comparable posttransplant outcomes. Quillin and colleagues[58] queried the Ohio Solid Organ Transplantation

Consortium and examined a total of 2356 patients transplanted for NASH, hepatitis C virus, and alcoholic liver disease. They found no difference in survival among the 3 groups at 30 days and 1 year posttransplantation; patients with NASH had improved survival at 3 and 5 years posttransplantation, as well as graft survival compared with those with hepatitis C virus liver disease. An analysis of 35,781 adult patients from the Scientific Registry of Transplant Recipients who underwent primary liver transplant from 2001 to 2009, showed similar 1- and 3-year survival rates between those transplanted for NASH (84% and 78%, respectively) compared with non-NASH indications (87% and 78%, respectively; $P = .67$).[11] The most common causes of long-term mortality are malignancy, cardiovascular disease, infections, and renal insufficiency (**Fig. 2**). Data encompassing 53,738 patients demonstrated 1-, 3-, and 5-year survival rates of 87.6%, 82.2%, and 76.7% respectively for NASH, which was in turn found to be superior to the survival of patients transplanted for hepatocellular carcinoma, hepatitis C infection, and alcoholic liver disease among others.[59] On balance, based on the results of analyses of large, prospective registries, short- and medium-term morbidity notwithstanding, posttransplant mortality and graft loss seems to be comparable for patients undergoing liver transplantation for other indications.

Recurrence of Nonalcoholic Fatty Liver Disease and Nonalcoholic Steatohepatitis

Although features of NAFLD are common after liver transplantation for NASH, recurrence of NASH with progressive fibrosis is unusual. In contrast, simple steatosis (grade $\geq$2) is very common, occurring in two-thirds of recipients in the first postoperative year, a frequency that is significantly more frequent than observed in other indications.[60] The prevalence of steatohepatitis is also high, occurring in about one-half of transplant recipients with NASH by the second postoperative year. NASH with a

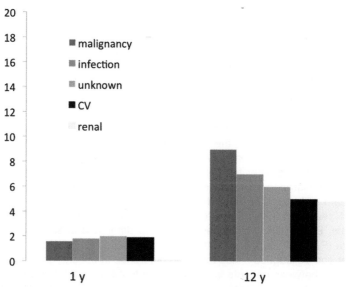

Fig. 2. The frequency of nonhepatic causes of mortality among liver transplant recipients, including those with nonalcoholic steatohepatitis (NASH) or cryptogenic cirrhosis are shown. Malignancy, infections, cardiovascular disease, and renal insufficiency, all exacerbated by the metabolic syndrome and immunosuppression, are common causes of mortality at 1 and 12 years posttransplantation. Recurrence of NASH is an unusual cause of mortality. CV, cardiovascular.

fibrosis stage of 2 or greater occurs in only 5% of recipients by postoperative year 5,[60] with cirrhosis occurring in only 2% to 3% of NASH recipients in the medium term.[61] Recurrence of NASH is thus much less aggressive than recurrence of hepatitis C virus.

An important exception to the low frequency of progressive fibrosing NASH in liver transplant recipients are patients with hypopituitarism, who frequently experience rapid recurrence of NASH and advanced fibrosis and graft loss, commonly associated with hepatopulmonary syndrome. Recurrence of NASH and hepatopulmonary syndrome has been reported to be responsive to growth hormone supplementation in patients with hypopituitarism.[62]

Posttransplant Imaging and Liver Biopsies

The low frequency of clinically important recurrence of NASH reduces the yield of routine or protocol based liver biopsies to screen for recurrence of disease. A combination of normal alanine aminotransferase (<40 IU/L) and an ultrasound examination that is negative for hepatic steatosis has been reported to have a 100% negative predictive value for recurrence of NASH.[62] Liver biopsies should only be considered in patients with steatosis on ultrasound and/or persistently elevated transaminases. In the nontransplant setting, MR elastography has emerged as a dynamic, sensitive, and specific tool for screening for and determining the amount of fibrosis secondary to NASH.[63,64]

APPROACH TO RECURRENCE OF NONALCOHOLIC FATTY LIVER DISEASE AND NONALCOHOLIC STEATOHEPATITIS AFTER LIVER TRANSPLANTATION

An algorithm for an overall approach to the posttransplant management of patients undergoing liver transplantation for NASH is presented in **Fig. 3**. There are, as of yet, no Food and Drug Administration–approved therapies for NASH. Although weight loss has been shown to attenuate the histologic features of NASH in the nontransplant setting,[65] the impact of chronic fatigue and the metabolic effects of immunosuppression make sustained reduction of weight difficult for the majority of liver transplant recipients, who more typically develop progressively increasing BMIs after liver transplantation. Difficulties with weight reduction aside, optimized weight and nutrition are cornerstones of the approach to posttransplant NASH because even modest reductions in BMI, for example, a reduction of 20% to 40%, can produce improvement in transaminases and histologic features of NASH.[66–69]

Pharmacologic Considerations

Glycemic control is an important consideration in patients with NASH who have type 2 diabetes mellitus; even in the absence of weight loss, metformin has been reported to improve the histologic features of NASH.[70] Alternatively, vitamin E (800 IU/d α-tocopherol) was superior to both pioglitazone and placebo in improving histologic features of NASH in patients with type 2 diabetes mellitus in a large, multicenter study.[71] Longer term vitamin E use is associated with an increased risk of tumors (eg, prostate cancer) and cardiovascular disease and should therefore not be used in the long periods, for example, for longer than 1 year. Pioglitazone use is associated with weight gain[71] and has a signal for potential hepatotoxicity.[72] The weight gain associated with thiazolidinediones may, in the medium and long term, negate their modest reported histologic benefits. For these reasons, we suggest that vitamin E (800 IU/d of α-tocopherol) be considered in all patients with histologically proven recurrence of NASH. Pioglitazone should only be considered in patients with recurrence of NASH and who have type 2 diabetes mellitus. Growth hormone therapy should be considered for patients with NASH secondary to hypopituitarism after liver transplantation.[62]

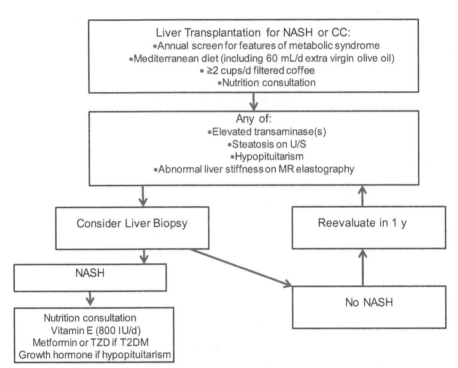

Fig. 3. An algorithm for the general management of patients who undergo liver transplantation for nonalcoholic steatohepatitis (NASH) or cryptogenic cirrhosis (CC) is shown. Features of the metabolic syndrome are common and are a common source of morbidity and mortality. The low frequency of progressive recurrence of NASH mandates a selective approach to obtaining liver biopsies. T2DM, type 2 diabetes mellitus; TZD, thiazolidinedione; U/S, ultrasonography.

Key considerations in prescribing immunosuppression and pharmacotherapy of the metabolic syndrome are presented in **Table 1**. For further information see, Hameed B, Terrault N: Emerging Therapies for Nonalcoholic Fatty Liver Disease, in this issue.

Dietary Considerations

Cholesterol

There is overwhelming evidence that cholesterol is a key lipotoxic trigger for NASH. Mechanisms of cholesterol lipotoxicity include sensitization of hepatocytes to tumor necrosis factor-α and Fas,[73] depletion of mitochondrial glutathione with subsequent loss of mitochondrial membrane function, ultimately leading to cytochrome C translocation to the cytosol.[74,75] The importance of cholesterol-induced glutathione depletion is further implied by the observation that supplementation of mitochondrial glutathione restores mitochondrial function and attenuates the histologic features of NASH.[74] Increases in hepatic and hepatocyte mitochondrial cholesterol have been a highly reproducible finding in animal models of NASH.[73,76–78] In the absence of an approved pharmacotherapy and based on the substantial evidence implicating dietary cholesterol as a lipotoxic trigger for NASH, dietary cholesterol intake should be minimized routinely in patients with fatty liver disease, including liver transplant recipients.

Table 1
Immunosuppression and pharmacotherapy of the metabolic syndrome

Drug	HMG-CoA Reductase Inhibitors (Statins)	Metformin	Thiazolidinediones	ACEi	ARB	CCB	PPI
CNI Tacrolimus Cyclosporine	Increase in HMG-CoA reductase inhibitor concentrations	No drug–drug interactions	No drug–drug interactions	Increased risk of elevated serum creatinine and serum potassium	Increased risk of elevated serum creatinine and serum potassium	Increase in CNI concentrations	CNI exposure can increase
Antiproliferative Mycophenolate	No drug–drug interaction		Case report of increased anemia with rosiglitazone	No drug–drug interactions	No drug–drug interactions	No drug–drug interactions	Decreased mycophenolate concentrations
mTORi Everolimus Sirolimus	No clinically significant interactions	No drug–drug interactions	No drug–drug interactions	Increased risk of angioedema		Increase in mTORi concentrations	No drug–drug interactions

CNI can inhibit the metabolism of most statins. The safest combination with CNI is pravastatin owing to its metabolism being less dependent upon CYP3A4. Reduction of other statin doses may be necessary and monitoring of myotoxicity is important. mTORi can cause angioedema and risk is increased with concomitant administration of ACEi. There is no metabolic drug–drug interaction described in the literature. CNI vasoconstrict the afferent arteriole and both ACEi and ARBs vasodilate the efferent renal arteriole. Concomitant administration may result in decreased renal perfusion causing an elevated serum creatinine. Both agents can lead to hyperkalemia owing to this mechanism and the CNI's ability to induce distal renal tubular acidosis. Combination therapy has been used safely, but judicious monitoring of renal function is imperative. Both dihydropyridine and nondihydropyridine CCB inhibit CYP3A metabolism of CNI and increase CNI whole blood concentrations. Dihydropyridine CCB in combination with CNI are not routinely clinically significant. Nondihydropyridine CCB, both verapamil and diltiazem, are potent inhibitors and usually require dose adjustments of CNI when initiating, titrating, or discontinuing these agents. Nondihydropyridine CCB, both verapamil and diltiazem, potently inhibit the metabolism of both mTORi. Empiric dose adjustments of the mTORi are warranted when initiating, titrating, or discontinuing these agents. Dihydropyridine CCB can inhibit metabolism of mTORi but are generally not clinically significant. PPI, particularly omeprazole and lansoprazole, can increase concentrations of CNI by potentially inhibiting CYP3A4 metabolism of tacrolimus, particularly in those that are poor or intermediate metabolizers at CYP2C19. Coadministration of mycophenolate mofetil with PPI, particularly lansoprazole and pantoprazole, can reduce exposure of mycophenolate. Increased gastric pH may contribute to decreased mycophenolate solubility. Pantoprazole administered with mycophenolic acid in healthy volunteers did not alter pharmacokinetics of a single dose of mycophenolic acid.

Abbreviations: ACEi, angiotensin-converting enzyme inhibitors; ARB, angiotensin receptor antagonists; CCB, calcium channel blockers; CNI, calcineurin inhibitor; HMG-CoA, 3-hydroxy-3-methyl-glutaryl-coenzyme A; mTORi, mammalian target of rapamycin inhibitors; PPI, proton pump inhibitors.

Coffee

Empiric pharmacotherapy of NAFLD with insulin-sensitizing agents or vitamin E is of marginal benefit (at best) and confers substantial risk (eg, weight gain). Several nonpharmacologic interventions have, however, emerged as beneficial for obesity and for reducing histologic severity and impact in NAFLD. The most compelling evidence is for coffee consumption; 2 to 4 cups of coffee consumed daily has been associated with improved histologic features of NAFLD and a reduction in the severity of components of the metabolic syndrome. Regardless of mechanism, coffee consumption is associated independently with a 12% decrease in mortality when compared with no coffee consumption.[79] The benefit seems to be greatest with filtered coffee rather than consumption of espresso or tea.[80] Consumption of 2 or more cups of coffee per day is also associated with decreased rates of hepatic fibrosis for patients with chronic liver diseases,[81] including NASH.[82] Although cause and effect is not established, a systematic review reported improved serum transaminases, decreased frequency of progression to cirrhosis and HCC, and lowered overall mortality in association with regular coffee consumption.[83] Although multiple components of coffee may contribute to the beneficial effects, coffee polyphenols and caffeine have been demonstrated to have antioxidant effects,[84] downregulate transforming growth factor-beta1 and SMAD2/3, increase peroxisome proliferator activated receptor-gamma receptor expression,[85] and to decrease activation of hepatic stellate cells.[86,87] Based on the substantial sum of these observations, recipients with obesity and/or NAFLD should be encouraged to consume 2 or more cups of coffee per day.

Mediterranean diet and olive oil

A Mediterranean diet is defined by a diet composed of primarily fruits, vegetables, whole grains, legumes, and nuts and replacement of butter with extra virgin olive oil. Herbs and spices replace salt to flavor foods. Red meat is largely replaced by fish and poultry, which are eaten at least twice a week. A large (n = 7447), prospective study in which diets were supplemented with extra virgin olive oil ($\sim$60 mL/d) versus no supplementation of olive oil, observed that olive oil supplementation reduced the incidence of major cardiovascular events by 30%.[80] The hazard ratio for all-cause mortality was 0.70 (95% CI, 0.54–0.92) for the group assigned to a Mediterranean diet with extra virgin olive oil when compared with the control group in multivariate analysis. Olive oil also has specific benefits in patients with NAFLD, reducing hepatic steatosis and improving inflammatory markers.[88–90] On the basis of these observations and in the absence of any risk associated with consumption of extra virgin olive oil, we recommend a Mediterranean diet, including approximately 60 mL/d of olive oil for liver transplant recipients.

REFERENCES

1. Wanless IR, Lentz JS. Fatty liver hepatitis (steatohepatitis) and obesity: an autopsy study with analysis of risk factors. Hepatology 1990;12:1106–10.
2. Williams CD, Stengel J, Asike MI, et al. Prevalence of nonalcoholic fatty liver disease and nonalcoholic steatohepatitis among a largely middle-aged population utilizing ultrasound and liver biopsy: a prospective study. Gastroenterology 2011;140:124–31.
3. Byron D, Minuk GY. Clinical hepatology: a profile of an urban, hospital-based practice. Hepatology 1996;24:813–5.
4. Bell BP, Manos MM, Zaman A, et al. The epidemiology of newly diagnosed chronic liver disease in gastroenterology practices in the United States: results from population-based surveillance. Am J Gastroenterol 2008;103:2727–36.

5. Younossi ZM, Stepanova M, Afendy M, et al. Changes in the prevalence of the most common causes of chronic liver disease in the United States from 1988 to 2008. Clin Gastroenterol Hepatol 2011;9:524–30.

6. Powell EE, Cooksley WG, Hanson R, et al. The natural history of nonalcoholic steatohepatitis: a follow-up study of forty-two patients for up to 21 years. Hepatology 1990;11:74–80.

7. Fassio E, Alvarez E, Domínguez N, et al. Natural history of nonalcoholic steatohepatitis: a longitudinal study of repeat liver biopsies. Hepatology 2004;40:820–6.

8. Bugianesi E, Leone N, Vanni E, et al. Expanding the natural history of nonalcoholic steatohepatitis: from cryptogenic cirrhosis to hepatocellular carcinoma. Gastroenterology 2002;123:134–40.

9. Haflidadottir S, Jonasson JG, Norland H, et al. Long-term follow-up and liver-related death rate in patients with non-alcoholic and alcoholic related fatty liver disease. BMC Gastroenterol 2014;14:166.

10. Onnerhag K, Nilsson PM, Lindgren S. Increased risk of cirrhosis and hepatocellular cancer during long-term follow-up of patients with biopsy-proven NAFLD. Scand J Gastroenterol 2014;49:1111–8.

11. Charlton MR, Burns JM, Pedersen RA, et al. Frequency and outcomes of liver transplantation for nonalcoholic steatohepatitis in the United States. Gastroenterology 2011;141:1249–53.

12. Sanyal AJ, Contos MJ, Sterling RK, et al. Nonalcoholic fatty liver disease in patients with hepatitis C is associated with features of the metabolic syndrome. Am J Gastroenterol 2003;98:2064–71.

13. Jin X, Chen YP, Yang YD, et al. Association between hepatic steatosis and entecavir treatment failure in Chinese patients with chronic hepatitis B. PLoS One 2012;7:e34198.

14. Strasberg SM, Howard TK, Molmenti EP, et al. Selecting the donor liver: risk factors for poor function after orthotopic liver transplantation. Hepatology 1994;20:829–38.

15. Kim WR, Smith JM, Skeans MA, et al. OPTN/SRTR 2012 Annual data report: liver. Am J Transplant 2014;14(Suppl 1):69–96.

16. O'Leary JG, Landaverge C, Jennings L, et al. Patients with NASH and cryptogenic cirrhosis are less likely than those with hepatitis C to receive liver transplants. Clin Gastroenterol Hepatol 2011;9:700–4.

17. Berzigotti A, Garcia-Tsao G, Bosch J, et al. Obesity is an independent risk factor for clinical decompensation in patients with cirrhosis. Hepatology 2011;54:555–61.

18. Promrat K, Kleiner DE, Niemeier HM, et al. Randomized controlled trial testing the effects of weight loss on nonalcoholic steatohepatitis. Hepatology 2010;51:121–9.

19. Nair S, Verma S, Thuluvath PJ. Obesity and its effect on survival in patients undergoing orthotopic liver transplantation in the United States. Hepatology 2002;35:105–9.

20. Leonard J, Heimbach JK, Malinchoc M, et al. The impact of obesity on long-term outcomes in liver transplant recipients-results of the NIDDK liver transplant database. Am J Transplant 2008;8:667–72.

21. Hakeem AR, Cockbain AJ, Raza SS, et al. Increased morbidity in overweight and obese liver transplant recipients: a single-center experience of 1325 patients from the United Kingdom. Liver Transpl 2013;19:551–62.

22. Hong HC, Hwang SY, Choi HY, et al. Relationship between sarcopenia and nonalcoholic fatty liver disease: the Korean Sarcopenic Obesity Study. Hepatology 2014;59:1772–8.

23. Kim TN, Park MS, Lim KI, et al. Relationships between sarcopenic obesity and insulin resistance, Inflammation, and vitamin D status: the Korean Sarcopenic Obesity Study. Clin Endocrinol (Oxf) 2013;78:525–32.
24. Tandon P, Ney M, Irwin I, et al. Severe muscle depletion in patients on the liver transplant wait list: its prevalence and independent prognostic value. Liver Transpl 2012;18:1209–16.
25. Heuman DM, Abou-Assi SG, Habib A, et al. Persistent ascites and low serum sodium identify patients with cirrhosis and low MELD scores who are at high risk for early death. Hepatology 2004;40:802–10.
26. Durand F, Buyse S, Francoz C, et al. Prognostic value of muscle atrophy in cirrhosis using psoas muscle thickness on computed tomography. J Hepatol 2014;60:1151–7.
27. Englesebe MJ, Patel SP, He K, et al. Sarcopenia and mortality after liver transplantation. J Am Coll Surg 2010;211:271–8.
28. Krell RW, Kaul DR, Martin AR, et al. Association between sarcopenia and the risk of serious infection among adults undergoing liver transplantation. Liver Transpl 2013;19:1396–402.
29. Montano-Loza AJ, Meza-Junco J, Baracos VE, et al. Severe muscle depletion predicts postoperative length of stay but is not associated with survival after liver transplantation. Liver Transpl 2014;20:640–8.
30. Abellan van Kan G, Houles M, Vellas B. Identifying sarcopenia. Curr Opin Clin Nutr Metab Care 2012;15:436–41.
31. Hayahi F, Matsumoto Y, Momoki C, et al. Physical inactivity and insufficient dietary intake are associated with the frequency of sarcopenia in patients with compensated viral liver cirrhosis. Hepatol Res 2013;43:1264–75.
32. Alvares-da-Silva MR, Reverbel da Silveira T. Comparison between handgrip strength, subjective global assessment, and prognostic nutritional index in assessing malnutrition and predicting clinical outcome in cirrhotic outpatients. Nutrition 2005;21:113–7.
33. Figueiredo F, Dickson ER, Pasha TM, et al. Utility of standard nutritional parameters in detecting body cell mass depletion in patients with end-stage liver disease. Liver Transpl 2000;6:575–81.
34. Tsien C, Shah SN, McCullough AJ, et al. Reversal of sarcopenia predicts survival after a transjugular intrahepatic portosystemic stent. Eur J Gastroenterol Hepatol 2013;25:85–93.
35. Toshikuni N, Arisawa T, Tsutsumi M. Nutrition and exercise in the management of liver cirrhosis. World J Gastroenterol 2014;20:7286–97.
36. Musso G, Gambino R, Tabibian JH, et al. Association of non-alcoholic fatty liver disease chronic kidney disease: a systematic review and meta-analysis. PLoS Med 2014;11:e1001680.
37. Singal AK, Salameh H, Kuo YF, et al. Evolving frequency and outcomes of simultaneous liver kidney transplants based on liver disease etiology. Transplantation 2014;98:216–21.
38. Nair S, Verma S, Thuluvath PJ. Pretransplant renal function predicts survival in patients undergoing orthotopic liver transplantation. Hepatology 2002;35:1179–85.
39. Giusto M, Berenquer M, Merkel C, et al. Chronic kidney disease after liver transplantation: pretransplantation risk factors and predictors during follow-up. Transplantation 2013;95:1148–53.
40. Houlihan DD, Armstrong MJ, Davidov Y, et al. Renal function in patients undergoing transplantation for nonalcoholic steatohepatitis cirrhosis: time to reconsider immunosuppression regimens? Liver Transpl 2011;17:1292–8.

41. Nadim MK, Sung RS, Davis CL, et al. Simultaneous liver-kidney transplantation summit: current state and future directions. Am J Transplant 2012;12:2901–8.
42. Inker LA, Schmid CH, Tighiouart H, et al. Estimating glomerular filtration rate from serum creatinine and cystatin C. N Engl J Med 2012;367:20–9.
43. Mindikoglu AL, Dowling TC, Weir MR, et al. Performance of chronic kidney disease epidemiology collaboration creatinine-cystatin C equation for estimating kidney function in cirrhosis. Hepatology 2014;59:1532–42.
44. De Souza V, Hadj-Aissa A, Dolomanova O, et al. Creatinine- versus cystatin C-based equations in assessing the renal function of candidates for liver transplantation with cirrhosis. Hepatology 2014;59:1522–31.
45. Ekstedt M, Franzen LE, Mathiesen UL, et al. Long-term follow-up of patients with NAFLD and elevated liver enzymes. Hepatology 2006;44:865–73.
46. Targher G, Bertolini L, Padovani R, et al. Prevalence of non-alcoholic fatty liver disease and its association with cardiovascular disease in patients with type 1 diabetes. J Hepatol 2010;53:713–8.
47. Oni ET, Agatston AS, Blaha MJ, et al. A systematic review: burden and severity of subclinical cardiovascular disease among those with nonalcoholic fatty liver; should we care? Atherosclerosis 2013;230:258–67.
48. Harrinstein ME, Flaherty JD, Ansari AH, et al. Predictive value of dobutamine stress echocardiography for coronary artery disease detection in liver transplant candidates. Am J Transplant 2008;8:1523–8.
49. Davidson CJ, Gheorghiade MI, Flaherty JD, et al. Predictive value of stress myocardial perfusion imaging in liver transplant candidates. Am J Cardiol 2002;89:359–60.
50. Rubin DA, Schulman DS, Edwards TD, et al. Myocardial ischemia after orthotopic liver transplantation. Am J Cardiol 1994;74:53–6.
51. Raval Z, Harrinstein ME, Skaro AI, et al. Cardiovascular risk assessment of the liver transplant candidate. Cardiology 2011;58:223–31.
52. Lentine KL, Costa SP, Weir MR, et al. Cardiac disease evaluation and management among kidney and liver transplantation candidates. J Am Coll Cardiol 2012;60:434–80.
53. Cross E, Watt KD, Pedersen R, et al. Predictors of cardiovascular events after liver transplantation: a role for pretransplant serum troponin levels. Liver Transpl 2011;17:23–31.
54. Heuer M, Kaiser GM, Kahraman A, et al. Liver transplantation in nonalcoholic steatohepatitis is associated with mortality and post-transplant complications: a single-center experience. Digestion 2012;86:107–13.
55. Barritt AS, Dellon ES, Kozlowski T, et al. The influence of nonalcoholic fatty liver disease and its associated comorbidities on liver transplant outcomes. J Clin Gastroenterol 2011;45:372–8.
56. Bhagat V, Mindikoglu AL, Nudo CG, et al. Outcomes of liver transplantation in patients with cirrhosis due to nonalcoholic steatohepatitis versus patients with cirrhosis due to alcoholic liver disease. Liver Transpl 2009;15:1814–20.
57. VanWagner LB, Bhave M, Te HS, et al. Patients transplanted for nonalcoholic steatohepatitis are at increased risk for postoperative cardiovascular events. Hepatology 2012;56:1741–50.
58. Quillin RC, Wilson GC, Sutton JM, et al. Increasing prevalence of nonalcoholic steatohepatitis as an indication for liver transplantation. Surgery 2014;156:1049–56.
59. Afzali A, Berry K, Ioannou GN. Excellent posttransplant survival for patients with nonalcoholic steatohepatitis in the United States. Liver Transpl 2012;18:29–37.

60. Maor-Kendler Y, Batts KP, Burgart LJ, et al. Comparative allograft histology after liver transplantation for cryptogenic cirrhosis, alcohol, hepatitis C, and cholestatic liver diseases. Transplantation 2000;70:292–7.
61. Dumortier J, Giostra E, Belbouab S, et al. Non-alcoholic fatty liver disease in liver transplant recipients: another story of "seed and soil". Am J Gastroenterol 2010; 105:613–20.
62. Singal AW, Watt KD, Heimbach JH, et al. Recurrence of metabolic syndrome and non-alcoholic steatohepatitis after liver transplantation – a comparative analysis. Hepatology 2012;53(Suppl):636.
63. Loomba R, Wolfson T, Ang B, et al. Magnetic resonance elastography predicts advanced fibrosis in patients with nonalcoholic fatty liver disease: a prospective study. Hepatology 2014;60:1920–8.
64. Loomba R, Sirlin CB, Ang B, et al. Ezetimibe for the treatment of nonalcoholic steatohepatitis: assessment by novel magnetic resonance imaging and magnetic resonance elastography in a randomized trial (MOZART trial). Hepatology 2015; 61:1239–50.
65. Ueno T, Sugawara H, Sujaku K, et al. Therapeutic effects of restricted diet and exercise in obese patients with fatty liver. J Hepatol 1997;27:103–7.
66. Vajro P, Fontanella A, Perna C, et al. Persistent hyperaminotransferasemia resolving after weight reduction in obese children. J Pediatr 1994;125:239–41.
67. Drenick EJ, Simmons F, Murphy JF. Effect on hepatic morphology of treatment of obesity by fasting, reducing diets and small-bowel bypass. N Engl J Med 1970; 282:829–34.
68. Hickman IJ, Jonsson JR, Prins JB, et al. Modest weight loss and physical activity in overweight patients with chronic liver disease results in sustained improvements in alanine aminotransferase, fasting insulin, and quality of life. Gut 2004;53:413–9.
69. Mummadi RR, Kasturi KS, Chennareddygari S, et al. Effect of bariatric surgery on nonalcoholic fatty liver disease: systematic review and meta-analysis. Clin Gastroenterol Hepatol 2008;6:1396–402.
70. Lin HZ, Yang SQ, Chuckaree C, et al. Metformin reverses fatty liver disease in obese, leptin-deficient mice. Nat Med 2000;6:998–1003.
71. Sanyal AJ, Chalasani N, Kowdley KV, et al. Pioglitazone, vitamin E, or placebo for nonalcoholic steatohepatitis. N Engl J Med 2010;362:1675–85.
72. Promrat K, Lutchman G, Uwaifo GI, et al. A pilot study of pioglitazone treatment for nonalcoholic steatohepatitis. Hepatology 2004;39:188–96.
73. Mari M, Caballero F, Colell A, et al. Mitochondrial free cholesterol loading sensitizes to TNF- and Fas-mediated steatohepatitis. Cell Metab 2006;4:185–98.
74. Caballero F, Fernandez A, Matías N, et al. Specific contribution of methionine and choline in nutritional nonalcoholic steatohepatitis: impact on mitochondrial S-adenosyl-L-methionine and glutathione. J Biol Chem 2010;285:18528–36.
75. Mari M, Morales A, Colell A, et al. Mitochondrial glutathione, a key survival antioxidant. Antioxid Redox Signal 2009;11:2685–700.
76. Mari M, Colell A, Morales A, et al. Mechanism of mitochondrial glutathione-dependent hepatocellular susceptibility to TNF despite NF-kappaB activation. Gastroenterology 2008;134:1507–20.
77. Charlton M, Krishnan A, Viker K, et al. Fast food diet mouse: novel small animal model of NASH with ballooning, progressive fibrosis, and high physiological fidelity to the human condition. Am J Physiol Gastrointest Liver Physiol 2011;301:G825–34.
78. Wouters K, van Gorp PJ, Bieghs V, et al. Dietary cholesterol, rather than liver steatosis, leads to hepatic inflammation in hyperlipidemic mouse models of nonalcoholic steatohepatitis. Hepatology 2008;48:474–86.

79. Freedman ND, Park Y, Abnet CC, et al. Association of coffee drinking with total and cause-specific mortality. N Engl J Med 2012;366:1891–904.
80. Anty R, Marjoux S, Iannelli A, et al. Regular coffee but not espresso drinking is protective against fibrosis in a cohort mainly composed of morbidly obese European women with NAFLD undergoing bariatric surgery. J Hepatol 2012;57: 1090–6.
81. Modi AA, Feld JJ, Park Y, et al. Increased caffeine consumption is associated with reduced hepatic fibrosis. Hepatology 2010;51:201–9.
82. Molloy JW, Calcagno CJ, Williams CD, et al. Association of coffee and caffeine consumption with fatty liver disease, nonalcoholic steatohepatitis, and degree of hepatic fibrosis. Hepatology 2012;55:429–36.
83. Saab S, Mallam D, Cox GA 2nd, et al. Impact of coffee on liver diseases: a systematic review. Liver Int 2014;34:495–504.
84. Kalthoff S, Ehmer U, Freiberg N, et al. Coffee induces expression of glucuronosyltransferases by the aryl hydrocarbon receptor and Nrf2 in liver and stomach. Gastroenterology 2010;139:1699–710.
85. Gressner OA, Lahme B, Rehbein K, et al. Pharmacological application of caffeine inhibits TGF-beta-stimulated connective tissue growth factor expression in hepatocytes via PPARgamma and SMAD2/3-dependent pathways. J Hepatol 2008;49: 758–67.
86. Shim SG, Jun DW, Kim EK, et al. Caffeine attenuates liver fibrosis via defective adhesion of hepatic stellate cells in cirrhotic model. J Gastroenterol Hepatol 2013;28:1877–84.
87. Estruch R, Ros E, Salas-Salvadó J, et al. Primary prevention of cardiovascular disease with a Mediterranean diet. N Engl J Med 2013;368:1279–90.
88. Buettner R, Ascher M, Gäbele E, et al. Olive oil attenuates the cholesterol-induced development of nonalcoholic steatohepatitis despite increased insulin resistance in a rodent model. Horm Metab Res 2013;45:795–801.
89. Kruse M, von Loeffelholz C, Hoffmann D, et al. Dietary rapeseed/canola-oil supplementation reduces serum lipids and liver enzymes and alters postprandial inflammatory responses in adipose tissue compared to olive-oil supplementation in obese men. Mol Nutr Food Res 2015;59:507–19.
90. Hernandez R, Martinez-Lara E, Cañuelo A, et al. Steatosis recovery after treatment with a balanced sunflower or olive oil-based diet: involvement of perisinusoidal stellate cells. World J Gastroenterol 2005;11:7480–5.

Moving?

Make sure your subscription moves with you!

To notify us of your new address, find your **Clinics Account Number** (located on your mailing label above your name), and contact customer service at:

Email: journalscustomerservice-usa@elsevier.com

800-654-2452 (subscribers in the U.S. & Canada)
314-447-8871 (subscribers outside of the U.S. & Canada)

Fax number: 314-447-8029

Elsevier Health Sciences Division
Subscription Customer Service
3251 Riverport Lane
Maryland Heights, MO 63043

*To ensure uninterrupted delivery of your subscription,
please notify us at least 4 weeks in advance of move.

ELSEVIER